D1234785

The Humanization Processes: *A Social, Behavioral Analysis of Children's Problems*

WILEY SERIES ON PSYCHOLOGICAL DISORDERS

IRVING B. WEINER, *Editor*
The University of Rochester Medical Center

Interaction in Families
by Elliot G. Mishler and Nancy E. Waxler

Social Status and Psychological Disorder: *A Causal Inquiry*
by Bruce P. Dohrenwend and Barbara Dohrenwend

Psychological Disturbance in Adolescence
by Irving B. Weiner

Assessment of Brain Damage: *A Neuropsychological Key Approach*
by Elbert W. Russell, Charles Neuringer, and Gerald Goldstein

Black and White Identity Formation
by Stuart Hauser

The Humanization Processes: *A Social, Behavioral Analysis of Children's Problems*
by Robert L. Hamblin, David Buckholdt, Daniel Ferritor, Martin Kozloff, and Lois Blackwell

Adolescent Suicide
by Jerry Jacobs

Toward the Integration of Psychotherapy
by John M. Reisman

Minimal Brain Dysfunction in Children
by Paul Wender

The Humanization Processes:

A Social, Behavioral Analysis of Children's Problems

Robert L. Hamblin
David Buckholdt
Daniel Ferritor
Martin Kozloff
Lois Blackwell

WILEY-INTERSCIENCE A Division of John Wiley & Sons, Inc.
New York · London · Sydney · Toronto

Library of Congress Catalogue Card Number: 74-149772
ISBN 0-471-34630-6

Printed in the United States of America.

10 9 8 7 6 5 4 3 2 1

to

George Caspar Homans
who gave us our first insights into
the way reinforcement functions
in every day social life.

Series Preface

This series of books is addressed to behavioral scientists concerned with understanding and ameliorating psychological disorders. Its scope should prove pertinent to clinicians and their students in psychology, psychiatry, social work, and other disciplines that deal with problems of human behavior as well as to theoreticians and researchers studying these problems. Although many facets of behavioral science have relevance to psychological disorder, the series concentrates on the three core clinical areas of psychopathology, personality assessment, and psychotherapy.

Each of these clinical areas can be discussed in terms of theoretical foundations that identify directions for further development, empirical data that summarize current knowledge, and practical applications that guide the clinician in his work with patients. The books in this series present scholarly integrations of such theoretical, empirical, and practical approaches to clinical concerns. Some pursue the implications of research findings for the validity of alternative theoretical frameworks or for the utility of various modes of clinical practice; others consider the implications of certain conceptual models for lines of research or for the elaboration of clinical methods; and others encompass a wide range of theoretical, research, and practical issues as they pertain to a specific psychological disturbance, assessment technique, or treatment modality.

University of Rochester
Rochester, New York

IRVING B. WEINER

Preface by the First Author

Many assume that an infant at birth is human in the full sense of the word. He is potentially human, but those most human qualities which differentiate man from other animals all have to be acquired or developed over a score or so years in a human society with an extant culture. This book is about the acculturation processes through which children develop the essential human characteristics—spoken and written language, logic as exemplified by mathematics, and intellect reflected in a great capacity to learn and to adapt. However, our definition of human includes that which is humane or truly civilized and we focus on the humane processes of humanization. It is our feeling that children can learn to be humane only in a social environment which is itself humane.

Style. We tried to write this book so that any interested person would find it understandable enough to read. In this respect we are following the tradition of Galileo, the father of modern science who was able to write in a fascinating style about his investigations in astronomy and his precedent-setting experiments in physics. While his dialogues sound a little stilted to the modern ear, they have inherent drama and movement which catch the interest of a reader, a witty sarcasm which adds a humanistic flavor, and a clarity of exposition which elucidates even his most complicated arguments. If anything, he suffered because he wrote too well for educated laymen. The churchmen of his day understood the revolutionary implications of his work, and after his humiliating Inquisition trial, he spent the last years of his life under house arrest.

In contrast, Newton wrote his *Principia* in a style so complex, so obscure, that only the very brightest of his fellow scientists could understand. Unfortunately, with few notable exceptions such as Pasteur who did public experiments most subsequent generations of natural scientists wrote in Newton's tradition rather than in Galileo's!

Social scientists who have done experiments or surveys, who have used statistics or mathematics, have generally adopted the difficult style of the natural scientists. Such a difficult style has been somewhat functional in the past because social scientists, and particularly, the experimentalists, have had little to say that has been genuinely relevant or useful to educated laymen. However, we feel the experiments reported herein are relevant, so following Pasteur's example, we want our experiments to be public.

Being less gifted in writing than Galileo, we have decided, except for the Appendix, to exclude statistics and mathematics from the presentation. Even so, for those with a more scientific bent we have included in footnotes, the essential information about inter-observer reliability and other methodological details.

Psychology? Sociology? Emile Durkheim in his classic book, *Suicide,* took what had generally been considered a psychological phenomenon, self-murder, and did what he argued was an essentially sociological or social systems analysis. In doing this he flattered a fledgling discipline with a sense of identity. Our work is no longer as pristine as Durkheim's. It is neither pure sociology nor pure psychology, but a blend of both.

Those readers who are familiar with modern psychology will recognize that our experimental work is somewhat in the Skinnerian tradition. We have been influenced most by Teodoro Ayllon, Nathan Azrin, Donald Baer, Sidney Bijou, Ivar Lovaas, Todd Risley, Arthur Staats, and Montrose Wolf, psychologists who made what we consider to be particularly exciting early applications of learning and conditioning theory to human problems.

Our work, while it follows the learning psychologists in many respects, differs in that we tend to think in exchange theoretical terms. Thus, we are always talking about structuring and restructuring social exchanges so as to condition or recondition a child in a certain way. Most of the members of our group feel that implicit in the Skinnerian version of learning theory is a more general version of exchange theory. It is no accident that many operant conditioners have turned their attention to social systems design because theirs is a very sophisticated systems theory. Their experiments always involve a repetitive or structured exchange between the subject and the experimenter. The subject initiates the exchange and the experimenter reciprocates; and the subject's behavior, which is always the focus of interest, turns out to be a function of the way in which the experimenter reciprocates. Thus, our group has often been led to observe that B. F. Skinner is as much an animal sociologist as an animal psychologist.

More specifically, our experiments while they involve learning demonstrate the intimate relationship between the structure of social exchange systems and acculturation. They show that to change man's behavior it is usually necessary to change the structure of the social exchange systems which man works. This is true even if those people who are involved have substantial biological deficits. Such deficits can be compensated for, in part at least, by structured social exchange systems which are scientifically, artfully designed.

In addition, we have suggested a new theory of deviant behavior, one that is supported strongly by experimental data for autistic and hyper-aggressive children and which seems to apply to inner-city and suburban children as well. This theory, which we will call the "inadvertent exchange theory of deviancy," suggests that the deviant pattern occurs in childhood in this culture because what the parent and teacher assume to be a punishment usually turns out to be a reward for the deviant child. So the more a parent or teacher "punishes" the child to inhibit a deviant behavior pattern, the more, in fact, he is rewarded and thus reinforced. This whole process is usually inadvertent, in that the parents and the teachers, as far as we can tell, seldom become aware of the reinforcing consequences of their actions. Even so, the consequences are real. As the child comes to work the pathogenic exchange at a rather high rate, the conditioning processes begin to have their effect. He gradually develops deviant abilities and tastes, and he is labeled a deviant, sometimes for the rest of his life.

His behavior is perceived and labeled deviant, apparently in part because it is so exploitive of the parents and others in his environment. The exchanges which people consider normal usually involve cost sharing and benefit sharing. For a number of understandable reasons, the deviant behavior is aversive or costly to the parent; but, as we have noted, the parents' reciprocation which is intended to be aversive or costly is, in fact, rewarding to the child.

The long-term result is tragedy for both the parents and the child if he is kept in the traditional social structure where normal behavior is "expected" and hence rewarded very little or quite haphazardly, and where deviant behavior is "punished." However, our experimental results show that the tragedy may be avoided if the child is placed in an alternative social structure where he is rewarded systematically and meaningfully for behaving normally and where he earns nothing for behaving deviantly.

Conditioning. While the operant conditioners are not explicit in their theories about the structured exchanges which are built into their experiments, they are explicit about the conditioning which always occurs as a person repeatedly works what we call a structured exchange. As a result of conditioning processes, his abilities change and so do his tastes and his feelings—the latter according to the laws of respondent or classical conditioning.

When the word conditioning is used, the educated layman often thinks nervously of Pavlov and his dogs, of Watson and his rather bizarre experiments with children or his extreme advice to parents on child-rearing, of Huxley's *Brave New World,* of Orwell's *1984,* of Packard's *Hidden Persuaders,* etc. There is no doubt that conditioning theory has had a bad press. The educated layman has, in effect, been negatively conditioned to conditioning theory. This bad press has been possible, in part, because in contrast to the word learning which implies a voluntary process, conditioning implies an involuntary process, something which happens to a person without his will or usually even without his knowledge. We have purposely chosen to continue with the word conditioning to refer to the processes of respondent or classical conditioning, in part to highlight the involuntary nature of the processes. However, we also wanted to educate people so that they might better understand how conditioning occurs, so they might have the option of voluntarily selecting social situations for their conditioning effects.

Conditioning theory is important because it is the key to understanding man's feelings, particularly how feelings change with changes in the social and physical environment. It is a key to man's developing likes and dislikes, his fluctuating loyalties and alienations, his waxing and waning loves and hates, his changing obsessions and phobias. While an understanding of conditioning may be put to malevolent use, the exciting applications are those which benefit mankind. For an example of the latter, respondent conditioning theory is now being used in treating certain of the more severe adult psychoses. The therapy is relatively inexpensive (typically it involves only five to thirty hours with the therapist) and relatively effective. These and other benefits have and will accrue because psychologists via basic experiments with human and lower animals have learned how to erase the effects of the negative conditioning that occur in traumatic and other situations.

However, the big problems of the world, the social problems which in effect threaten to destroy our very existence, are likely due to ineptly structured exchange systems which either fail to condition humankind to live together productively, creatively, or happily, or in fact, have conditioned them to live together exploitively, aggressively, destructively. The big job for the social scientist, as we see it, is to learn (1) about structured social exchange systems, particularly the ways in which such systems condition the people who live in them, and (2) how to structure social systems in a way that will benefit everyone concerned. There are those who may be frightened by such a prospect. However, a scientist always starts small, with protosystems which are tested and retested, much as we have done here. It would be foolish for us to advocate the legislation of any huge social structure without first trying and evaluating some prototypes.

Universals vs. Alternatives. Cultural universals are the minimal conventions required of *all* in a given culture, that is, all who wish to be considered minimally competent persons. For example, the ability to use the oral and written forms of the conventional language are cultural universals in most modern societies. Cultural alternatives, on the other hand, involve a true choice. For example, most persons in modern societies have the opportunity to select from among several occupations that which suits them most.

It is interesting to note that early education is ordinarily designed to help children acquire the cultural universals and that secondary and higher education helps them, as blossoming adults, to sample, to choose and to acquire alternative patterns which are suitable to themselves and to society. Hence the objective of early childhood education is to structure educational environments which are so attractive that the child will choose to work them and hence acquire the cultural universals. The parent, the teacher who fails to provide an environment which will allow the child to learn to talk, to read, to write, to do arithmetic and basic mathematics relegates him to pariah status and thereby *fails the child and society*. In contrast, at the secondary and higher levels of education, the teacher has a more complex responsibility to help students choose from suitable alternatives, and once choices are made, to structure attractive learning environments to enable students to develop the appropriate competencies. Thus our design objectives, which have been limited to early childhood education are not inclusive enough to be suitable for secondary and higher education. Even so, what we have learned about the operating characteristics of the biological learning mechanisms, about the dynamics of social learning environments, may be helpful to those who face these more complex design problems.

Scientific Proof. This book is written on the assumption that our experiments prove nothing, but that they are a vehicle of discovery and illustration. Proof, to the extent there is such a thing in science, must come in replications by other competent investigators. Galileo described his famous inclined plane experiment on one page. An elegant piece of writing, it contained enough detail of the method and results to illustrate the conditions under which he obtained his equation. What turned his equation into a scientific law was the work of hundreds of other competent scientists who subsequently replicated his experiment and invariably obtained the same results. This process is well understood in the physical sciences; for example, Robert Millikan invited competent physicists from all over the world to come to the California Institute of Technology to use his equipment to replicate his famous cloud chamber experiment which isolated the electron. Replicability establishes the lawfulness of an effect. Even so, the necessity of replication does not relieve original experimenters of the problems of exercising great care or achieving great accuracy in their work. On the contrary, only those experiments that are done with care and accuracy have a chance of being replicated. We have strived to maintain the highest possible standards in our work; it is just that no matter how much care and accuracy one exercises, no matter how clear one's results are, one can never prove one's own hypotheses.

About Us. We are human beings as well as scientists and we empathize with children and parents who have grave problems. We have not hesitated to allow our human feelings to show because to hide them would be dishonest and unwise. Certainly in science one is trained to be cold and dispassionate about facts, but one is not required to be cold and dispassionate about mankind. Scientists, as well as other people, are at their worst when they are unfeeling for others.

St. Louis, Missouri
January, 1971

ROBERT L. HAMBLIN

Acknowledgments

The research and development work reported in this book was done by the authors as employees of the Central Midwestern Regional Educational Laboratory, a private, nonprofit corporation supported in part as a Regional Educational Laboratory by funds from the U.S. Office of Education, Department of Health, Education, and Welfare. The opinions expressed here do not necessarily reflect the position or policy of the Office of Education, and no official endorsement by the Office of Education should be inferred.

In addition the first author wishes to acknowledge with appreciation the following support for the writing: a nine month sabbatical at full salary from Washington University, a Visiting Professorship with released time for writing at Southern Illinois University, Edwardsville, and some released time for writing during the summer as an investigator on an NIH grant (MH15561-01) with Lee Rainwater and others. Gratitude is also extended to those at Washington University who were instrumental in helping the first author to be relieved of administrative duties there. They also made this book possible.

We want to acknowledge the support, the encouragement, the personal help, and the wise advice of Wade Robinson, the Executive Director of CEMREL. Also, at CEMREL, the help of Thomas Johnson, Verna Smith, Jerry Thomas, and Harriet Doss. Harriet Doss joined the staff of our Program and in that capacity worked on an experiment reported in Chapter 3.

The following as graduate students have also benefited our research effort by doing excellent experiments with us, most for their Ph.D. dissertations: Janet Dehn, Desmond Ellis, June A. Hamblin, Gary Merritt, Carol Pfeiffer, Dennis Shea, Denis Stoddard, and Francis Shands. Also, the following former colleagues and graduate students contributed substantially to the tradition at Washington University which eventuated in our using learning and social exchange theory to study acculturation: Donald Bushell, Keith Miller, James A. Wiggins, Robert L. Burgess, David Schmidt, Bruce Chadwick and Harry Gyman. Donald Bushell was also a member of our staff at one point, and in that capacity worked on two experiments in Chapter 2.

The following professors at Washington University have been particularly encouraging and supportive of our work: in Sociology—Lee Rainwater, Irving Horowitz, and the late Jules Henry; in Anthropology—John Bennett; in Psychology—Lawrence Brock; in Social Work—Aaron Rosen; in Education—Bryce Hudgins, Joan Beaning, Hazel Sprandel, and Judd Shaplin. Also, Dean Wiley, Dean of the Education Division at Southern Illinois University at Edwardsville, has been very supportive.

We want to acknowledge the helpful suggestions, criticisms by Wells Hively, Chairman of our Program's National Advisory Committee, and of Steele Gow, Bernard Friedman, Ernst Rothkopf, and Robert Marker of the Board of Visitors of the U.S. Office of Education. Their reviews of our program have been most helpful.

The following, as teachers, have made substantial contributions to our experimental programs at Washington University: Joanne Walters, June A. Hamblin, Ellen Accurso, Annie Hubbard, and Martha Tucker. In our inner-city classrooms, the imaginative teaching and help of Marion Allen, Mary Jane Phillips, and a number of other dedicated teachers, who will remain nameless, have made great contributions to the success of this effort. We also thank them for putting up with us. Also, we deeply appreciate the support of Samuel Shepard, Gerald Moeller and Lamar Smith, the school administrators who helped us establish our research and development program in their school system.

Finally, the work which eventuated in this book could never have been done without the hundreds of wonderful little children who were the subjects of our experiments. We thank them for being themselves, and we thank their parents for their cooperation. In a very real sense, they share with us the responsibility for any contributions which may eventuate from this effort.

Contents

CHAPTER 1

Introduction

In the pool of potential school children in every American community there is a shadowy group of untouchables.[1] Educators soften the word: they are "unteachables." They are too "culturally deprived" to be taught, too aggressive or violent to be managed in the classroom or perhaps they are "disturbed" having a psychosis such as autism. They are the impossible children. The teachers give up on them and in many cases so do the counselors, the social workers, even the psychiatrists. They are, therefore, typically relegated to failure in school and to failure in life, exiled to a twilight, fringe existence. Some, perhaps most, are eventually put away, buried prematurely to vegetate in our mental hospitals or our prisons.

The problem is real enough from the teacher's point of view: such children simply do not respond to traditional educational programs. When faced with such a situation, however, one can rid oneself of the children, actually or figuratively, or one can try to devise new educational programs which do work. We have chosen to do the latter in the several experimental classrooms associated with the Central Midwestern Regional Educational Laboratory (CEMREL).

Since we started our program in March 1966, we have seen the following results. Preschoolers too shy, too withdrawn to talk in non-family situations were given language training which within a few months enabled them to acquire average speech patterns.

Disadvantaged children in several inner-city kindergarten classes were given training designed to help them acquire the kind of language that is useful as a medium of instruction and learning as well as for reasoning. The data suggest that over the seven month period of the experiment the acquisition rate of the general intellectual abilities measured as mental age (MA) increased markedly. Finally teachers in a number of inner-city classes were enabled via our training to accelerate substantially the rate at which their

[1] Hamblin took the major responsibility for writing this chapter.

children progressed. At the outset the average level of academic achievement in these classes was as much as a full year behind the national average. After seven to eight months in the program the classes of two thirds of the teachers were approximately at the national norm.

Our three classes of extraordinarily hyperaggressive boys, who had not previously responded to therapy, were tamed; they settled down and in the process turned into better than average students. Prior to entering our experimental classes these boys improved on the average .4 academic levels per year on standardized achievement tests. During the one year in our classes they improved, on the average, 1.2 levels.

Several autistic children, who in the beginning were either mute or could at best randomly parrot sounds, have developed functional speech, have lost their bizarre, disruptive behavior patterns, and their relationships with others have become relatively normal. This was accomplished by using our structured exchange procedures in the laboratory and by training their mothers to use the exchange procedures at home, to supplement the learning experiences which the child was undergoing in the laboratory.

The procedures we have developed using exchanges seem simple, but deceptively so. In fact, they may not even seem new in some ways. However, the teaching procedures and the theory upon which they are based are currently making rapid advances, in part because they are continually being subjected to experimental evaluation. Even so, the goals are simple. The teacher tries to structure an instructional exchange so that as the child moves forward step by step in the learning process (which progress the teacher values), she repeatedly reinforces his progress, that is, she gives him something which he enjoys each time he earns it. As a natural consequence of repetitive reinforcement, the child will pay attention to the teacher in a way that allows her to teach him something, and he works substantially harder at his studies thereby increasing his learning rate.

However, children's problems are not limited to deficits; sometimes they develop bizarre, disruptive patterns which ultimately will be troublesome both for them and for those who live with them. With such behavior the goal is also simple, to put an end to whatever has been reinforcing it. Study after study has shown that whenever a child persists in behaving badly some adult has, usually unintentionally, been repeatedly reinforcing him for it. Thus the evidence suggests that children behave badly primarily because they are inadvertently acculturated to behave badly.

Acculturation is a term used by social scientists to refer to the accumulative learning effects which occur as a result of a person's socio-cultural environment. It involves the acquisition of the behavior and the thought patterns of a particular culture or sub-culture. This would include the ability to perform such cultural roles as father or mother, worker, homemaker, citizen and consumer, and the facility for language which allows a person to communicate more or less accurately with others of his culture. More basically, however, acculturation refers to the process of transforming a newborn baby whose behavior is limited to such rudimentary reflexes as crying, eating, and sleeping into a functional adult with the ability to relate to other adults, to solve problems, and to exercise a measure of control over self and others.

The acculturation processes are subtle. They go on quite naturally, often without people even being aware of what is happening. Apparently these processes vary in some details from culture to culture, even from family to family, but by and large the result is at least moderately successful. It is only when the "normal" acculturation processes go awry that the disorders appear: the nonverbal children, the hyperaggressive children, the autistic children, and later on, delinquents, criminals, adult psychotics, etc. Thus in their normal form the acculturation processes are, in fact, synonymous with the humanization processes.

Historically, acculturation and humanization has been the implicit if not the explicit subject of the psychoanalytic theory of Sigmund Freud (1964; also see Erikson, 1950, 1968), the symbolic interaction theory of George Herbert Mead (1934, 1964; and for work in that tradition see Goffman, 1959, 1961), the differential association theory of E. H. Sutherland (cf. Sutherland and Cressey, 1960. Also Burgess and Akers, 1966), and the developmental theories of Gesell (1945, 1952, and Gesell and Thompson, 1938) and Piaget (cf. 1926, 1928, 1930, 1948, and 1952). While these theories have been both provocative and interesting, they have seldom led to powerful therapeutic or educational programs where the improvement rate of those in the program was significantly better than the improvement rate of those who received no specialized treatment at all (cf. Eysenck, 1965, and 1967; Levitt, 1963; and Lewis, 1965).

The reasons for this have become increasingly clear. First, the above theories have focused primarily on what is learned in typical or atypical acculturation while ignoring the operating characteristics of the biological learning mechanisms involved in acculturation. This may seem like a small point, but understanding the operation of these mechanisms seems to be crucial to an adequate understanding of behavior modification and maintenance, the key issues in acculturation. Second, while all of the above traditions were the result of brilliant observational studies, some of them involving contrived situations as in the case of Piaget, none have used rigorous experimentation, the essential method of the successful applied sciences.

LEARNING THEORY

When most people think of learning, they recall their own participation in formal educational systems which involved the acquisition of knowledge or understanding by listening to teachers, having discussions, reading books, working problems, taking notes, outlining, reviewing, taking tests, etc. While this symbolic or verbal learning is essential in later stages of an individual's development, it is not the only kind of learning. Man has biological mechanisms which allow him to learn directly via his own experience with his environment. It is through learning mediated by such mechanisms that human organisms develop habitual ways of working their environment for reinforcement—to obtain sustenance or pleasure and to avoid destruction or pain.

The reinforcement version of learning theory has developed rapidly in the last twenty years as the result of the brilliant animal experiments of B. F. Skinner and his colleagues (cf. Holland and Skinner, 1961 and Ferster and Skinner, 1957). More recently a number of people have been extending that tradition in experiments with human subjects. (For summary descriptions of this work see Bijou and Baer, 1961, Ullmann and Krasner, 1965 and Reese, 1966. Also for a summary of exchange theory, the social variant of reinforcement theory, which we tend to emphasize, see Homans, 1961.)

Although most of our thinking has been in reinforcement terms, there are many occasions to be encountered later in the book where the discoveries and the variables escape that language community. These theoretical developments, as well as the details of reinforcement theory, will be presented in later chapters in the context of our experimentation. However, a very brief overview of reinforcement theory is appropriate for our introductory purposes here.

An Overview

All learning environments, be they natural, mechanical or social, while differing in some ways are essentially similar in several ways. All such environments may be worked for reinforcers. Reinforcers may be defined as stimuli which induce changes in a person's feeling state. They are positive reinforcers if they induce a pleasant feeling state, negative reinforcers if they induce an aversive or painful feeling state. In general, people learn to work their environments to acquire positive reinforcers and to avoid or escape negative reinforcers. The learning occurs via discovering the behavior which will or will not produce the reinforcers, and then by repetitively working the environment. In general, the strength of a reinforcer is gauged by the size of the change it produces in the person's feeling state, and the stronger the reinforcers involved in the environmental response, the more quickly, the more easily the person will learn.

The repetitive production and nonproduction of reinforcers, as mentioned, provides a person with a kind of feedback which allows him to learn how to work his environment. However, in addition to reinforcement, learning environments generally provide other feedback, process cues which are predictive of reinforcement which may be somewhat delayed. Be that as it may, the immediacy of feedback, whether it is reinforcement per se or process cues predictive of later reinforcement, is an important determinant of the rate of learning. In general, learning will occur more easily and more rapidly, the more immediate the feedback.[2]

Learning environments also may vary in the consistency of their feedback; that is, the degree to which the environmental response pattern is invariant. In general, the more consistent the feedback, the more quickly, the more easily the person will learn. Learning environments may also vary in the degree to which a person is allowed to set his own pace in working for reinforcers. In other words, some environments allow a person more freedom than others in that the response pattern neither rushes nor delays his work pattern. In general, a person will learn more easily, more quickly the more freedom he has to set his own pace in working the environment for reinforcers.

On Optimal Social Learning Environments

As noted, the rate of learning increases as the strength of the reinforcer increases. Hence, in designing optimal social learning environments, one must devise a way of increasing the strength of reinforcers without sacrificing immediacy, consistency, and self-pacing. How might this be done?

Surprisingly, in the usual preschool or kindergarten classroom there is less a dearth of strong reinforcers than one might suspect. By the time they become students, most children are turned on by playing with other children, by doing certain types of art work, by cutting and pasting, by playing with Playdoh, by playing with climbing and swinging equipment, by playing with educational toys, and so on. Furthermore, some classes of young children are served a morning snack of juice and cookies, and some have television and movies. Thus the problem of structuring an optimal learning environment in the usual classroom is not so much the availability of strong reinforcers as the ability to make them part of an effective learning environment.

One simple, effective way to incorporate these potential reinforcers into

[2] Those familiar with O. K. Moore's work on human learning theory will notice the influence here of his formulations. (Cf. Moore and Anderson, 1966).

such an environment is to trade them for tokens, plastic disks about one and a quarter inches in diameter, which the child earns by doing his numbers, reading, or other academic work. Thus the day is split up into alternating earning and buying periods. During the buying periods, the child can trade his tokens for established reinforcers, which in this context we call backups.

An example of a backup is seeing a movie. The price for a movie varies in our experimental classes. For four tokens a student may watch sitting on the floor; for eight, sitting on a chair; for twelve, sitting on a table. Possibly because the view is better, the children almost always buy the table if they have earned enough. If they have dawdled through the earning period and thus have not earned four tokens, they now sit in an area of the room where they can hear but not see the movie while it is being shown. Thus, the children, particularly in preschool and in kindergarten, earn then spend throughout their school day.

However, when children are first introduced to tokens, they are meaningless. To establish their value as a conditioned reinforcer, we sometimes start by pairing them with M&M candies. As the child does his academic work, the teacher reciprocates with a "thank you," which signals a token and an M&M. At this juncture the children generally work for the M&M and, perhaps, the thank you. The token is just a curiosity. One indication of this: the children have to be urged, at first, to put them into the pockets of their smocks. However, when the teacher later sells admission to the movie, playdoh or whatever, she tells them the price in tokens and asks them to count out the appropriate number. As this process is repeated, the teacher "forgets" more and more to give the M&M's, until within a day or two the children are never given candy, just tokens. By then the children will have learned that if they want the movie, the treat, etc., they must pay for them with tokens which they have earned. Thus, the tokens eventually take on a value of their own; they become conditioned reinforcers, and their strength as reinforcers is proportional to the strength of the backups.

The tokens then are strong reinforcers which, because they can be passed out through time for academic work, allow the teacher to structure the situation for immediacy of feedback, self pacing, etc. Hence, a moderately well run token exchange should theoretically promote direct learning, whatever the content. The experiments in subsequent chapters are illustrative of how token exchanges may be operated, and of how, in fact, they do promote several rather basic types of direct learning.

Even so, some people are uneasy about the material reinforcers which are used as backups in a token exchange. Yet the reasons for using such backups are straightforward. First, as mentioned, material reinforcers are usually strong. Second, they are effective for all children, not just those who have been previously conditioned to value approval or getting the right answers. Third, a token exchange with powerful material backups is designed specifically to condition all of the children to respond to the same reinforcers which are used in the traditional classroom. Hence, the token exchange, as outlined here, is a starter mechanism designed to engage *all,* not just the advantaged children.

Reducing the Frequency of Offensive Behavior

The laboratories' teachers try to avoid the use of punishment. They are asked not to structure aversive exchanges—not to use mean, ego-bruising words, not to pinch, not to shake, not to slap, spank or whip, or otherwise apply pain-inducing stimuli to the child—in their efforts to get him to stop behaving badly. While complex, the procedures we recommend in place of punishment are humane and, usually, very effective.

In general, offensive behavior has an exchange function, that is, it earns the person something he wants from others. Thus, the first step in reducing the frequency of an offensive pattern is to try to identify the exact nature of that which reinforces it, e.g. teacher attention, a hurt look. The general finding has been that offensive behavior in children is really a pattern of malicious teasing.

The second step in reducing the frequency of offensive behavior is to structure what we call a counter exchange: that is, an exchange which if worked, will reinforce culturally prescribed behavior which is the opposite of and incompatible with the offensive behavior in question. Thus, to reduce the frequency of offensive teasing the teachers will structure an exchange which reinforces social but nonteasing patterns, e.g. cooperation or help. Thus, the counter exchange is a functional alternative to the exchange which maintains the offensive behavior—i.e. it allows the individual to earn something equivalent to that earned by the offensive behavior and it strengthens or reinforces the non offensive behavior.

The third step is to terminate the offensive interchange identified in the first step via one or more non exchange signals. One very subtle non exchange signal is simply to act as though nothing happened. Those teachers who are able to do so effectively and consistently can, over time, establish non response as an unobtrusive, though profound non exchange signal. Also, a variety of other less subtle signals are used. For example, the teachers turn their head away. Others, particularly if they are sitting at a table working with a child who then misbehaves, simply rest their elbow on the table and place their forehead on their hand, thus shading their eyes from the view of the child until the child stops misbehaving. Others simply turn their backs, walk away, and start working with and reinforcing a child who is behaving well. This last strategy is particularly effective because reinforcement of others for behaving well provides the disruptive child an opportunity for vicarious learning.

These non exchange signals all work well in terminating offensive behavior that can be ignored. But some offensive behavior cannot be ignored: one child choking another, a child making such a loud noise that all other activity in the room is disrupted. In those instances the teacher is instructed to "time out" the child: that is, to place him in a corner, a hall or small "time out" room quickly, without explanation, and otherwise give him as little attention as possible. "Time out" means a recess from the opportunity to work the positive classroom exchanges. However, "time out" periods are usually short, only a minute or so. They too are supposed to be a non exchange signal used to help the child to learn rather than to feed the teacher's hunger for retribution.

In general, the frequent use of "time out" is symptomatic of a situation where the reinforcers are too weak to motivate the child to work the instructional exchange. In such instances, the proper thing to do is to increase the power of these exchanges by increasing the strength of the reinforcers, or by reducing the cost of the behavior required to work the exchanges.

Some may feel that the "time out" procedures do at least border on punishment. Perhaps they do, but in a strict sense, they do not involve the application of aversive or pain-inducing stimuli, the application of which is defined here as punishment. Rather, they involve the withdrawal of the chance to earn pleasure-giving stimuli. It is for this reason that the effectiveness of the time-out procedures depends entirely on the power of the exchanges which are structured in the situation.

The Importance of Implicit Structuring

In general, our teachers are trained to structure new exchanges and to terminate old exchanges with little if any verbal explanation. In other words, the teacher does not negotiate the nature or terms of exchanges by talking things over with the children. This does not mean that there is no negotiation between the children and the teacher, but it is all done implicitly, not explicitly via verbal discussion. Thus if the children are not satisfied with the terms of the exchange, that is, the amount of or the frequency of reinforcement, they register this quite naturally, simply by reducing the rate of their activity. This then is the signal to the teacher to increase the power of the exchange. If her classroom teaching is to be effective, she must react to the behavior of her students. When exchanges are properly worked, the teacher learns from the children just as they learn from her.

The first and most important reason for implicitly structuring exchanges is that all of the behaviors which are reinforced repetitively in exchanges become exaggerated. Therefore, in a classroom where teachers negotiate a contract every time they want a child to do something, or where the children nag their teacher for pay after they have worked, the contracting and the nagging as well as the working will become exaggerated. Under such a system children eventually will not do anything without negotiating and nagging for pay. (Parents who structure reward systems for their children frequently make this same error, and get the same discouraging results.)

Rather, in setting up a token exchange the goal is to establish a *gift* system where the exchange occurs without having to be requested by the other, where each is sensitive enough to the other's nonverbal cues to give him what he hungers for, where if anything, each tries to give the other a little more than he receives in return. This is done, as suggested earlier, simply by having the teacher become sensitive to the child's appropriate behaviors and reciprocate with gifts—tokens and backups—as though those appropriate behaviors were gifts the child presented to the teacher. The result of such an implicit gift exchange, then, is the child's repeated reinforcement, not only for the appropriate behavior, but also for his taking the initiative to produce such behavior. Hence, when an exchange is structured implicitly, the child is repeatedly reinforced for taking initiative. A child so acculturated is sensitive to others, constantly does things on his own which produce pleasant responses in others, and becomes a sheer pleasure to be around. Part of the pleasure of being around him is the fact that it is not typical in our culture to be sensitive to those things about the child that are pleasurable and to ignore those things about the child that are not so pleasant.

The second reason (if one were needed) for implicitly structuring social exchanges is that many people, even well educated people, go through life unaware of the many exchanges that are present in their environment which are never mentioned. Such exchanges if they could only spot them, could be worked to their own and others' benefit and enjoyment. Hence, the laboratory's classrooms are designed to give children practice in spotting and working implicitly structured exchanges if only to make them more sensitive observers of their social scene.

EXPERIMENTS

In an applied social science the reason for being is to produce reliable, understandable changes which remedy problems. Hence, the investigations in the more successful applied sciences almost if not always involve rigorous experimentation, application of the scientific method which involves the controlled manipulation of certain variables under controlled conditions in order to produce changes in other variables.

This does not mean that observational, survey, and other related methods are not useful. On the contrary, each has its important use, for example, in the pre-experimental phase of an inquiry when relevant variables are being isolated and theories about relationships among variables formulated. The Surgeon General's original report (1964) suggesting a causal link between smoking and lung cancer was based on a number of statistical surveys. The causal link between smoking and lung cancer was established five years later in experiments where lung cancer was actually *produced* in experimental dogs by having them smoke tobacco for long periods under rigorously controlled laboratory conditions and comparing the incidence of cancer with that of a control group of dogs who lived under identical conditions except they did not smoke. Those experimental results were necessary before noncausal explanations of the correlation between lung cancer and smoking could be definitely eliminated.

This does not mean that earlier theories of acculturation which were developed with the use of observational and survey data are not useful. On the contrary, theories like those of Freud, Mead, Piaget and Sutherland often provide theoretical leads that are essential to rigorous experimentation. In this book we rely mainly on the experimental method of testing theories about acculturation problems and their remediation. The scientific advantage of that method should be noted at the outset.

THE CHILDREN

Experiments with and case studies of various types of children are presented in the next several chapters. In Chapter 2 the subjects are very young children, usually from suburban families. While these children are generally not disturbed in the usual sense, they, like disturbed children, fail to develop to their maximum potential when put into the traditional classroom situation. Consequently, they are ideal subjects to use in working out and pretesting procedures to be used with disturbed children.

In Chapters 3 and 4 the subjects are inner-city children. Some inner-city children do not make normal progress in school because the traditional educational system is not designed for their educational and cultural backgrounds. Hence, the experiments included in these chapters test alternative educational systems which are designed specifically to capitalize on the strengths and remediate the weaknesses produced by their early learning environments.

The subjects in Chapters 5 and 6 are hyperaggressive children whose disturbance makes them almost impossible to educate, or even to live with. The experiments are designed to extinguish the hyperaggressive patterns and to replace them with cooperative patterns which allow the children to make normal academic progress.

In Chapters 7, 8 and 9 the subjects are autistic, the most severely disturbed of all psychotic children. Originally thought of as a type of schizophrenic psychosis, autism can result apparently when the normal acculturation processes break down (to a great extent, if not completely) during the first two years of life. Therefore the experiments with autistic children involve acculturation procedures to help them develop the behavior patterns that are generally learned in the family prior to preschool or kindergarten.

As suggested earlier, our purpose is to develop an adequate theory of the humanization processes. In the subsequent chapters the theory which began to be introduced here will be developed and elaborated. Experiments and cases will be discussed and interrelated until the theory is summarized in Chapter 10.

QUESTIONS OF ETHICS

Whenever science is used in the name of solving problems, there are usually possibilities of misuse. The question of ethics, therefore, is generally relevant in effective applications of science. We consider the following to be a minimal list of ethical constraints appropriate to our work.

As social scientists, we modify social exchange systems and thereby induce changes in habitual response patterns of individuals only with the informed consent of those legally responsible for such systems and those legally responsible for such individuals (for example, parents in the case of our work with autistic children and school officials and teachers in the case of our work in the public schools).

In addition, we will only proceed with system and habit modification if in our professional judgment such modifications produce long term benefits for *all* of the involved parties—the parents, the school officials, the teachers, and especially the children. This implies consideration, study of and, in some cases, original research on the long term effects of the presence and absence of various behavioral patterns and the acquisition and non acquisition of various skills.

In our scientific work, we attempt to develop procedures for inducing system and habit modification which are effective and which, at the same time, minimize pain to those involved in the change. In remediating a particular problem, we try to select that procedure, from among the known effective procedures, which is least painful to those involved.

In our scientific work, including the publication of our experiments, we take the usual steps to protect the privacy of those we involve. In particular, while it is essential to our scientific reports that we note unfortunate behavior patterns and their consequences, we try to do the writing in a way that will not get the person into trouble. In other words, we do not report the authorities, parents, teachers, or school officials whom we observe acting irresponsibly. We do not get misbehaving children into trouble with teachers or parents.

CHAPTER 2

The Young Child

The vast majority of children learn, without specialized training, to use language, to play, and to cooperate, and they are conditioned so that attention, affection, and so on are reinforcers.[1] All this occurs naturally and easily in interaction with parents, siblings and peers—in what Cooley called the primary group. In technologically advanced societies, however, participation in occupational, political, and cultural, and other types of organizations requires specialized repertoires of behavior which children ordinarily cannot acquire in the primary group. It is for this reason, perhaps, that between the approximate ages of five and twenty-five persons in such societies are turned over to other agents of acculturation, mainly teachers, to acquire a formal education. Depending upon the effectiveness or the ineffectiveness of his experience in school, the child will develop into a student, and later on into an adult who can read well or poorly, who can write his ideas or who cannot, who loves learning or who has an aversion for it, in short, who has actualized his potential or has been stunted. Over the years a large amount of theory and research has centered around the question of how to influence the academic achievement of young children. We will review this research briefly to provide a context for our experiments with young children.

RESEARCH ON ACADEMIC ACHIEVEMENT

Since the early 1900's educators have attempted over and over again to accelerate or improve the academic achievement of students by "improving" the educational process. Interestingly enough, the results of these experiments on any given approach have been mixed; in general, the successful experiments have been more than balanced by the unsuccessful ones. Table 2.1 is a summary of J. M. Stephens' (1967) review of this research. It should be understood that the conclusions in this summary are not the

[1] Hamblin took the major responsibility for writing this chapter.

Table 2.1. Summary of Stephens' (1967) Review of Research in Education.

Relationship Investigated	Reviewers	Conclusion
1. School attendance and academic achievement.	Heck (1950)[a]	Almost no relationship.
	Finch and Nemzek (1940)[b]	Almost no relationship.
2. Televised instruction vs. instruction by teachers and academic achievement.	Schramm (1962)	Of 393 studies: 255, no difference; 83 favored TV; 55, personal instruction.
	Barrington (1965)	30 studies: mixed results, no overall difference.
3. Tape recorded lecture vs. live lectures and test performance.	Popham (1962)	No difference.
4. Independent study vs. classroom instruction and academic achievement.	Bittner and Mallory (1933)	Independent study results in slightly higher achievement.
	Childs (1952)	Independent study slightly better.
	Stephens (1967)	Independent study slightly better.
	Marr, et al. (1960)	With students randomly assigned to treatment, class achievement slightly better than independent study.
5. Size of class and academic achievement.	Marklund (1963)	281 comparisons: 222 showed no difference, 37 favored large classes, 22 smaller classes.
	Kidd (1952) Flemming (1959) De Cecco (1964) Powell (1964) Eash and Bennett (1964)	Mixed results; large classes have slight edge in academic achievement.
(Note: Both teachers and students prefer smaller classes.)		
6. Clinical interviews about school work and academic achievement.	Hoehn and Saltz (1956)	With clinical psychologists, slight improvement.

[a] With few exceptions the articles cited are review articles of as many as 450 empirical studies. For references see Stephens (1967).

[b] With IQ constant, r^2's ranged between .01 and .04.

Table 2.1 continued.

Relationship Investigated	Reviewers	Conclusion
	Hoehn and Saltz (1956)	With teachers, no improvement.
7. Tutoring by specialist and academic improvement.	Callis (1963)	Mixed results; no overall difference.
	Stephens (1967)	Mixed results; no overall difference.
8. How-to-study courses and improvement in academic achievement.	Entwisle (1960)	Mixed results; most such courses help some.
9. Special instruction vs. none and academic achievement.	Tilton (1947)	By teacher: mixed results, no net effect.
	Schoenhard (1958)	By parents: mixed results, no net effect.
10. TV with vs. without discussion and academic achievement.	Jacobs, et al. (1963)	No difference.
	Gropper and Lumsdaine (1962)	Discussion better, if carefully programmed.
11. Amount of time spent in study and academic achievement.	Strang (1937)	6 studies, almost no correlation.
	Jex and Merril (1959)	College level, almost no correlation.
12. Size of school and academic achievement.	Douglass (1931)	No correlation.
	Garrett (1949)	No correlation.
	Hoyt (1959)	18 studies: 6 found no advantage, 6 advantage large schools, 3 advantage medium size schools, 3 advantage small schools.
	Street, et al. (1962)	IQ constant: small positive correlation between size and achievement.
	Lathrop (1960)	IQ and type of high school program constant: no correlation.
	Kemp (1955)	IQ, social class constant: small positive correlation.
	Wiseman (1964)	IQ and social class constant: no correlation.

Table 2.1 continued.

Relationship Investigated	Reviewers	Conclusion
13. Qualities of the teacher and academic achievement.	Medley and Mitzel (1963)	Qualities judged by principals: no correlation with academic achievement of students.
	Ryans (1960)	Experience helps for a few years, then hurts.
14. Graded vs. ungraded classrooms and academic achievement.	Adams (1953)	No difference.
	Knight (1938)	No difference.
	Stephens and Lichtenstein (1947)	No difference.
15. Team teaching (where each teacher specializes in one or two subjects) vs. traditional teaching and academic achievement.	Stephens (1967)	No difference.
16. Homogeneous ability groupings vs. mixed ability groupings and academic achievement.	Pattinson (1963)	No difference.
	Stephens (1967)	No difference.
17. Progressive vs. traditional schools and academic achievement.	Chamberlin, et al. (1942)	A classic eight year study, no overall differences.
	Wallen and Travers (1963)	11 studies: no overall differences.
18. New vs. traditional science and mathematics curricula and academic achievement.	Stephens (1967)	Early trend suggests no significant differences.
19. Discussion vs. lecture and academic achievement.	Stovall (1958)	No difference.
	Wallen and Travers (1963)	No difference.
	McKeachie (1963)	Rough equivalence.
20. Pupil centered vs. teacher centered discussions and academic achievement.	Anderson (1959) Sears and Hilgard (1964) Stern (1963)	Mixed results: very slight difference in favor of teacher centered discussions.
21. Frequent quizzes and academic achievement.	Noel (1939)	No correlation.
	Stephens (1967)	No correlation.

Table 2.1 continued.

Relationship Investigated	Reviewers	Conclusion
22. Programmed instruction and academic achievement.	Stephens (1967)	About on par with other methods of individual study.
	Stephens (1967)	Saves time but not otherwise superior to classroom instruction.

present authors' but Stephens' and those of other professional educators whose research reviews Stephens quotes.

In general, of the twenty-two comparisons involving different learning environments or different styles of education, none made much difference in the academic achievement of the students. Included in the review, by the way, is a comparison of the effectiveness of progressive versus traditional education. Even these polar styles of education which were so hotly debated during the first half of this century produced no overall differences in performance in the three R's (this is where traditional education was supposed to excel) or in the so-called creative subjects, art, writing and music (where progressive education was supposed to excel). Eleven carefully done, relatively well-designed, long-term experiments together point inescapably to the conclusion that progressive education and traditional education result in no overall difference in academic achievement.

We might reasonably wonder about a "no difference bias" in Stephens' survey if it were not for two recent massive studies which, quite independently, lead to the same general conclusions. The first of these, sponsored by the U.S. Office of Education and directed by James Coleman, a distinguished sociologist, involved a very large, stratified probability sample of schools throughout the United States. In this survey Coleman and his associates (1966) measured a large number of variables which most educators suppose improve schools and hence improve academic achievement. Using modern computers and the most advanced statistical procedures, Coleman and his associates carefully analyzed the association between each of these variables and various standardized measures of academic achievement.

The report is a large book and it is impossible to do justice to the findings here. However, the following summary gives the overall picture. Coleman et al. used explained variance which, like r^2, may be thought of as predictive accuracy gauged in percentages. Thus 1 percent explained variance means that by knowing the magnitude of one variable a person can predict the magnitude of an associated variable with 1 percent accuracy; at the other extreme 99 percent explained variance means that one can predict the other variables with 99 percent accuracy.

Coleman's facilities and curriculum measures were:

1. The number of books per student in the school library.
2. The presence of science laboratory facilities.
3. The number of extra curricular activities.
4. The presence of an accelerated curriculum.
5. The comprehensiveness of the overall curriculum.
6. The strictness in promotion of slow learners.
7. The use of grouping or tracking.
8. The movement between tracks.
9. School size.
10. The number of guidance counselors.
11. Urbanism of school location.
12. Per pupil expenditure (the educator's Holy of Holies).

None of the above variables explained as much as 1 percent of the variance in academic achievement when the effects of other relevant variables were controlled, or held constant. In other words, Coleman and his associates found essentially no association between facilities, curriculum, and expenditure measures and the academic achievement measures. His results are therefore in essential agreement with the hundreds of small, individual studies included in Stephens' review.

Coleman's teacher variables were as follows:

1. Average educational level of the teachers' families (the mothers' education).
2. The average years of experience in teaching.
3. The localism of teachers, whether they had attended high school or college in the area and had lived there most of their lives.
4. The average level of education of the teachers.
5. The teachers' average score on a self-administered vocabulary test.
6. The teachers' preference for teaching middle class students.
7. The proportion of teachers that were white.

Even these teacher variables evidently have very little effect as may be noted in Table 2.2. In this multivariate analysis the family background, and student-attitude variables toward learning are by far the most important. Like Stephens, Coleman and his associates concluded sadly that the schools currently bring little influence to bear on the child's overall academic achievement, that is, independent of family background and general social context.

Table 2.2. Unique Percent of Variance in Verbal Achievement Accounted for by Characteristics of Schoolteachers and Student Body, in Regression With Two Family Background Factors and One Individual Attitude (After Coleman, et al. 1966, Table 3.231.1, p. 312).

	Grades			
	12	9	6	3
Unique contribution to variance accounted for by —				
School facilities	0	0	0	0
School curriculum	0	.2	0	0
Teacher qualities	0	0	0	.1
Teacher attitudes	.8	.9	.4	.3
Student body characteristics	4.7	4.9	8.2	1.4
Unique of all 5 jointly	9.6	8.1	10.9	2.5
Total by all 8	35.4	38.1	37.7	12.9

Similarly disconcerting results have obtained recently in a large scale experiment in New York City involving schools where initially students were, on the average, underachieving. If one had not encountered the above research, the More Effective Schools (MES) program which was evaluated in this experiment might look very promising. It involved the reduction of class size to a maximum of fifteen pupils in kindergarten and first grade, twenty in second grade and no more than twenty-two in grades three through six. In addition, the MES program had team teaching with four regular teachers available to every three classes. One of these was a mobile or "cluster teacher." In addition, there were specialized teachers for remedial reading, art, music and other curriculum areas. The program also included a large clinical team for placement testing, for diagnosis of learning disabilities, and for counseling, academic and personal. All of this was done at twice the usual per pupil expenditure.

The evaluation of the MES program was conducted by the Center for Urban Studies under the direction of David J. Fox, a professor at City College. Fox (1967 and 1968) reported that in most of the schools with MES the atmosphere among the staff was characterized by enthusiasm, interest and hope. (The teachers' union was enthusiastic enough to make the expansion of MES a prominent part of contract negotiations with the school board.) Moreover, parents and the community generally responded with interest and enthusiasm. Fox noted this was a major accomplishment in a period characterized by considerable stress in the schools and grave school-community conflict. However, Fox also suggested that the data were equally clear, that the MES program made no significant difference in the functioning of children as measured by observer ratings of how children performed in the classroom or by standardized tests on mathematics and reading.

Perhaps the most relevant data for our present purposes are those for reading achievement which are given in Table 2.3. Note that data from the two samples demonstrate that at the time the MES program was instituted there was a cumulative deficit in reading achievement which left the students at the end of the sixth grade approximately one year behind the national norms. (Remember the MES program was to erase that as well as other deficits in academic achievement.) Of the 20 changes in average reading achievement recorded after one to three years' exposure to MES, nine involved small improvements, four indicated no change, and seven represented greater deficits.

It was these and similar data that led Fox to conclude that the MES program—with its small classes, team teaching, specialized and remedial instruction, diagnostic testing and counseling—had no consistent effect on reading achievement. Certainly the data indicate that after two to three years of MES, the children were as far behind the national reading norms as were the children in the same classes before them who had never had MES.

Such consistent no-go results are, of course, extremely discouraging and they have had a profound effect in the field of education in keeping alive Gesell's theory that learning is primarily a function of maturation, or neurological ripening.

Yet these same results may be interpreted in another way. All of the instructional programs involved in these experiments have omitted one or more of the essential characteristics of learning environments which were outlined in the previous chapter. For example, all of them have specifically avoided the use of strong positive reinforcers. That omission alone might account for the failure. The rate of learning which is directly reflected in academic achievement is probably the result of a complex interaction, and the effects of manipulating lesser variables may be negated when the most important variable is ignored.

Had some of these educational programs been innovative enough to include all of the environmental characteristics which promote learning, then perhaps some of the other variables, which they did study—teacher training, class size, per pupil expenditure—might have shown some relation to achievement. In analogy, one cannot expect variables like the number of, the expertise of, or the expenditures for doctors to be related to the health of the community if the doctors are not using forms of therapy which actually produce health.

Table 2.3. Before/After Comparison of the More Effective Schools Program (MES) on Reading Achievement for Two Samples of Schools.

Fall Testing

		First Sample of Schools			Second Sample of Schools		
Grade	Nat'l Norm	Oct. 1964 0 years of MES	Oct. 1966 2 years of MES	Change	Oct. 1965 0 years of MES	Oct. 1966 1 year of MES	Change
2	2.1	1.8	1.8	0	1.6	1.8	+
3	3.1	2.6	2.5	—	2.4	2.4	0
4	4.1	3.0	3.3	+	3.2	3.2	0
5	5.1	4.0	3.8	—	4.1	3.7	—
6	6.1	4.9	5.1	+	4.6	4.6	0

Spring Testing

		First Sample of Schools			Second Sample of Schools		
Grade	Nat'l Norm	May, 1965 1 year of MES	May, 1967 3 years of MES	Change	May, 1966 1 year of MES	May, 1967 2 years of MES	Change
2	2.8	2.4	2.7	+	2.4	2.7	+
3	3.8	3.7	3.6	—	3.4	3.5	+
4	4.8	4.2	4.0	—	3.7	4.1	+
5	5.8	5.2	4.6	—	4.5	4.7	+
6	6.8	6.1	5.6	—	5.3	5.6	+

However, all educational research has not been this bleak. In some specific areas the innovations have been somewhat more consonant with social learning theory and consequently the results have been consistently better. In particular, research in the area of reading has been rather more productive. And, reading achievement is important, for it, better than any other variable including IQ, is predictive of academic achievement.

READING RESEARCH

In the early 1900's children enrolled in the first grade at the age of six and began to learn to read. About that time, school surveys became popular, quite numerous, and they consistently turned up a very disturbing fact. Large numbers of children were failing in the first grade generally because of inadequate achievement in reading (Durkin, 1966). There were two reactions. One, reminiscent of Head Start, was to establish kindergarten, the primary purpose of which was to provide the training and experience which would prepare pupils for reading. The other was to research the relationship between intelligence and reading achievement of first grade children.

The reports of the latter research, which showed strong relationships between end-of-the year measures of intelligence and reading achievement, prepared an atmosphere for the quick and uncritical acceptance of a study by Morphett and Washburne (1931) in which the suggestion was made that a mental age (MA) of 6.5 is prerequisite for success in beginning reading. Although many questions might have been raised, the Morphett–Washburne research which implied the need to postpone the teaching of reading, won the quick acceptance of professional educators and psychologists. Professional texts, written for reading methods courses, were soon proclaiming that school instruction in reading should be postponed until a mental age of 6.5 is reached.

There were some who were skeptical of the Morphett–Washburne finding. Among them were Arthur Gates, a professor at Columbia Teachers College, and his students who together launched a 5 year research program on the matter. In their first report (Gates and Bond, 1936) they concluded that the overall predictability (r^2), of reading achievement measured at the *end* of the first grade year by mental age at the *beginning* of the first grade was about .05. Thus, the predictive accuracy of the *beginning* of the year MA for *end* of the year reading achievement is only about five percent, which is hardly the basis for an academic policy.

However, their most provocative results (Gates, 1937) involved first grades in four different schools whose beginning reading programs varied on four significant dimensions: (1) the adequacy of the basic readers, (2) the amount of easy, interesting supplementary reading materials, (3) the amount of test and/or self-diagnostic materials, and (4) the quality of the teaching. In the first grade class judged best on these variables children with a mental age of 5.5 and above were able to learn to read at criterion level. In the first grade judged worst on these variables only children with a beginning mental age of 8.0 or above were able to learn to read at criterion level. (These results are summarized in greater detail in Table 2.4.) Such strong results in a Stephens' sea of non results are fantastic and the implications for the teaching of children, important. However, Gates and his associates buried their reports in an obscure journal and cautiously concluded "the optimum time for beginning reading is not entirely dependent upon the nature of the child himself but is in a large measure determined by the [nature of the] reading program." Thus the unusually strong research findings had little impact.

Perhaps one reason for this tragedy is that Gates' research and findings did not fit into any of the current theoretical paradigms and thus seemed irrelevant. As an illustration, Gates and his associates reported an r^2 of .71 between reading expertise at the end of the first grade and the number of books read during the year. Without a theory that expertise learning increases as a function of reinforced practice, a robust finding such as this could be passed off as meaningless, a curiosity to be forgotten. The temper of the times was to interpret all such strong correlations as associations between different measures of the *same* variable. An alternative interpretation which obviously should be investigated empirically is that the children should be given reinforced practice in reading; therefore, they should be provided with a large number of easy, supplementary reading books, with the incentives to motivate them to read these books. The effects on reading achievement and, in turn, academic achievement could be enormous.

Nevertheless, Gates and his associates' research findings fingered one of the crucial weaknesses of the genetic theories of child development. From other lines of research, it had by this time become increasingly clear that what is "natural development" for a child in one social or cultural environment is not "natural development" in a quite different social or cultural environment.

Cultural anthropologists, under the leadership of Franz Boas at Columbia University had established this point beyond reasonable doubt in their battle with a group of biological determinists, the instinct psychologists such as McDougall, Woodworth and James. Their cross-cultural studies demonstrated an extremely wide range of "natural" behavior. Obviously, Rousseau's "noble savage" behaved "naturally" according to the norms of his culture. Although theirs tended to be an extreme environmental position, anthropologists nevertheless scored a useful point because the differences in

Table 2.4. Summary of Gates (1937) Research.

Gates' characterization of the beginning reading programs in first grades in four schools.	Average size of classes	Number of classes	Number of teachers per class	Lowest beginning mental age group able to learn to read at criterion level[a]	Coordination between beginning MA and reading score at the end of the year (r^2)
1. Usual basal reading books. Ample supplementary practice, and teach-and-test materials. Large amount of supplementary easy reading and self diagnostic materials. Better than average teachers closely supervised by the person who developed the curriculum.	39	2	1	5.5–5.9	.38
2. Usual basal reading materials. Various types of practice and seat work, teach-and-test materials, and supplementary easy reading material. Gates and his associates developed and furnished curricula materials and presumably some supervision. Better than average teachers. N.Y. City school system.	48	1	2	6.0–6.4	.30
3. Better than average amount of typical classroom reading matter. Not much teach-and-test materials. Very good teacher. Class located in superior urban public school.	43	1	1	6.5–6.9	.19
4. Basal and supplementary reading materials inferior. Class taught by mass methods, just oral instruction; little attempt to adjust instruction to individual needs. Teachers adjudged below average for metropolitan school system where the classes were located.	40	2	1	8.0–8.5	.12

[a] In constructing this table we used a slightly different criterion than Gates used in his article. We calculated from Gates' data the percentage of the students in each beginning mental age group who at the end of the year failed to score 1.95 on the Gates Reading Test. Beginning mental age groups where 15 percent failed to score 1.95 were considered here not to meet the criterion.

culture are pronounced enough to produce sharp differences in "natural" response patterns. A more modern and, perhaps, a more accurate view suggests that there are physiological capabilities influenced by both heredity and environment. The interesting task is to learn how to structure an environment in order to facilitate optimal development.

There have been a number of animal studies which have illustrated the crucial importance of early environment on later development. For example, Cruze (1935, 1938) has shown that the early lack of reinforced practice permanently retards the development of a chick's pecking ability. Kuo (1932) has shown that over 80 percent of those chicks who were born permanently crippled occurred in instances where the yolk sac failed to move into its usual position and thereby failed to force the legs to fold on the breast and thus be exercised. Also, Riesen (1958) has found that chimpanzee babies who are kept in the dark for as little as seven months apparently develop atypical retinas which ultimately fail, resulting in permanent blindness.

Finally, Thompson and Heron (1954) studied adult problem solving of Scotty pups, comparing a sample of pups which were reared as pets in human homes for eight months with a sample of litter mates which were reared in isolation in laboratory cages for the same period. Later, when the animals were adults (18 months old), their problem solving ability was measured using Hebb–Williams' (1946) test of animal intelligence. The animals reared in isolation scored much lower on intelligence than the animals reared as pets in human homes.

These animal studies are relevant because earlier ones which yielded quite different results formed the basis of some rather strongly held attitudes about the treatment of children, especially young children. Furthermore, the Thompson–Heron study raises a question about the concept of genetically fixed intelligence. In particular, this study suggested that intelligence may not be genetically fixed but somewhat variable depending upon certain possibly yet undiscovered characteristics of an organism's learning environment.

THE DEVELOPMENT OF INTELLIGENCE

Actually intelligence tests are made up almost exclusively of symbolic or cognitive problems. Mental age, as measured by these tests, is determined directly by one's expertise in giving or discovering the solutions of these problems. In other words, MA divided by CA—chronological age or the amount of time the individual has had to acquire this problem-solving expertise—times 100 equals IQ, a measure of cumulative learning rate which has been presumed to reflect learning ability (cf. Jensen, 1967).

If IQ is a valid measure of learning ability, one should expect a high correlation between IQ and the learning rate on the standard tasks used by the experimental psychologists. This, in fact, is exactly what several investigations have shown. However, the correlations are much higher for middle than for lower class children (Jensen, 1961, 1963). Such results have led Arthur Jensen to the theory that a child's environment acts as a threshold variable. According to Jensen, when certain environmental influences are present, the individual's genetic potential for the development of IQ will be more or less fully realized and variations in the extent of these influences beyond this minimal threshold will make only a slight contribution to IQ. Jensen (1967) suggests that the situation is analogous to diet and physical stature. Once diet is up to a certain minimal standard with respect to vitamins, minerals, and proteins, the addition of more of these elements will make no appreciable difference in physique. Jensen (1969) has estimated on the basis of a large body of rather consistent evidence that for the white American and Northern European populations the genetic component accounts for 78 percent of the variance in IQ.

Other psychologists have taken stronger environmentalist positions; for example, Piaget (1952), Hebb (1949) and Hunt (1961, 1964) have argued that rich sensory experience *in the early years of life* is the essential environmental variable in the development of intelligence. A similar but more specific hypothesis has been suggested by other theorists. George Herbert Mead (1934), a social philosopher who has had great influence in sociology, stated quite explicitly that intelligence increases as a person develops his ability to interact symbolically with other people. If so, the development of spoken language would theoretically produce an increase in IQ.

More recently Bereiter and Engelmann (1966) have taken a position that the early development of verbal language is crucial to the optimal development of intelligence. Actually there is some evidence for this theory. For example, Bereiter and Engelmann have developed a rather elaborate curriculum to help inner-city children develop verbal language for obtaining and transmitting information and for carrying on verbal reasoning. The average increase in IQ of children who go through their program is 9 points (cf. Bereiter and Engelmann, 1966 and Bereiter, 1969).[2] Also, Durkin's (1966) evidence suggests that reading training prior to the first grade may have a substantial effect on intelligence. Durkin's is a longitudinal study of children who were successfully taught to read when they were three to five years of age by their mothers or by older siblings. A number of interesting

[2] The reported increase is 15 points, but 6 of these are apparently due to acclimation in the classroom which occurs with or without language training.

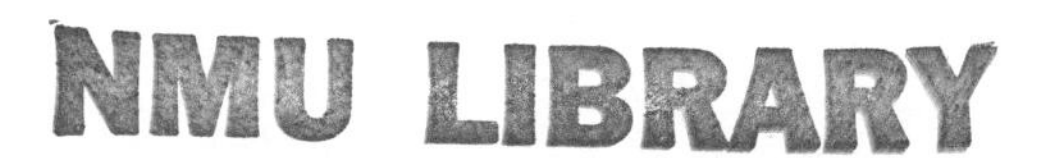

facts emerged. (1) The early readers scored on the average 24 IQ points higher than the non-early readers who had continuously attended the same school. (2) The early readers were so accelerated academically that 30 percent were double promoted, mostly in the primary grades. (3) While the very bright early readers did not maintain their lead past the sixth grade over the very bright non-early readers, the less than very bright early readers (whose first grade IQ measured 120 or less) progressively increased their lead over their controls. This result obtained in Durkin's original study and in her replication.

Missing in Durkin's analysis are before/after measures of IQ for early and non-early readers obtained under relatively well controlled experimental conditions. Only such data, which we will begin to supply later on, can clarify the nature of the relationship between IQ and early reading. However, Durkin's finding, that the less than very bright early readers progressively increased their lead in subsequent years over their controls is crucial in and of itself. As noted earlier, reading achievement is more predictive of academic success than any other variable, including IQ. Hence, any procedure that produces a cumulative increment in reading achievement has important educational implications. For these several reasons, then, we decided to experiment with early reading.

In the experiments which follow we will illustrate a number of ways of structuring instructional exchanges for young children to develop, among other things, expertise in reading and we will begin to have the opportunity to see the effects of early reading on IQ. In addition, some of the basic propositions outlined in Chapter 1 will be experimentally illustrated. In fact, the first experiment deals simply with the relationship between attention and strength of reinforcers used in the instructional exchange.

EXPERIMENT 1: INSTRUCTIONAL EXCHANGES

The purpose of this experiment, conducted in a preschool at Webster College by Bushell, Stoddard, and Hamblin, was to compare preschoolers' academic work patterns under conditions of two different instructional exchanges, (1) where the teachers reciprocate with both approval and backed-up tokens, and (2) where they reciprocate with approval alone.

Sixteen children, nine boys and seven girls, were enrolled in the class used for this experiment. At the beginning of the academic year, they ranged in age from 35 to 59 months. All had been enrolled in the class two months or more when this experiment was begun so they were experienced with the token exchange which had been in force from the beginning. All had become involved to some extent in reading, writing and arithmetic which were taught during the experimental hour.

At the beginning of the experimental hour, each of the three teachers sat at a table with either reading, writing or arithmetic materials. The children could choose to sit at one of the three tables working with a teacher on one of the subjects, or they could play with various educational toys, either alone or with other children. In the B conditions, the teachers attended the children and gave approval and tokens to the children when they were engaged in learning one of the three academic subjects at the appropriate table. In the A condition, the teachers gave attention and approval but no tokens. In all conditions, when half of the children chose to play or were otherwise continuously "out" of the study activities for two minutes, the study period was terminated. Otherwise it continued for the full hour.

In Figure 2.1 notice that the children averaged 45 minutes in attending lessons, and that a relatively steady state obtained from the beginning of B1, the baseline period.[3] Next, during A, the teachers reciprocated with approval, saying, "Good," "You're doing fine," "Keep it up!" They still prepared very interesting lessons. However, they did not have those little plastic tokens to pass out as the children worked, tokens that could be used to buy a nature walk, a snack, a movie, etc. The children continued to receive these backups during A, but, as in a usual classroom, they were exchanged for the children's being at school rather than for working at lessons.

What happened? The data in Figure 2.1 showed that the children continued to attend their studies for a time, almost at the same level as before. One would predict just this, that the conditioned reinforcers—e.g. teacher approval and those intrinsic to studying—should maintain attendance at lessons until extinction occurred because of the lack of backup reinforcers. Note that after seven days, toward the end of A, attendance at lessons did drop off, as expected, to about eighteen minutes per day (the median for the last five days in the period).

During B2 the token exchange was reinstituted. Note that the initial recovery was quite sharp from about eighteen to about forty-five minutes in the first three days. From that point the mean time attending study activities increased gradually until, toward the end of B2, the students were studying

[3] A 20 channel Esterline-Angus event recorder was used to record the amount of time each child attended lessons. The recorder was operated by a single observer who pressed self-illuminating switches on and off as the children started and stopped attending their lessons. The definition of attendance was whenever a child was physically present, facing the materials involved in an assigned learning task. No attempt was made to define whether or not the child was actually studying. Reliability checks were made by a second observer with the aid of a stop watch starting on day 32. Unknown to the regular observer, the second observer would take data on one of the children, a different one each day. The Pearsonian correlation squared between the two series of measurements was .98.

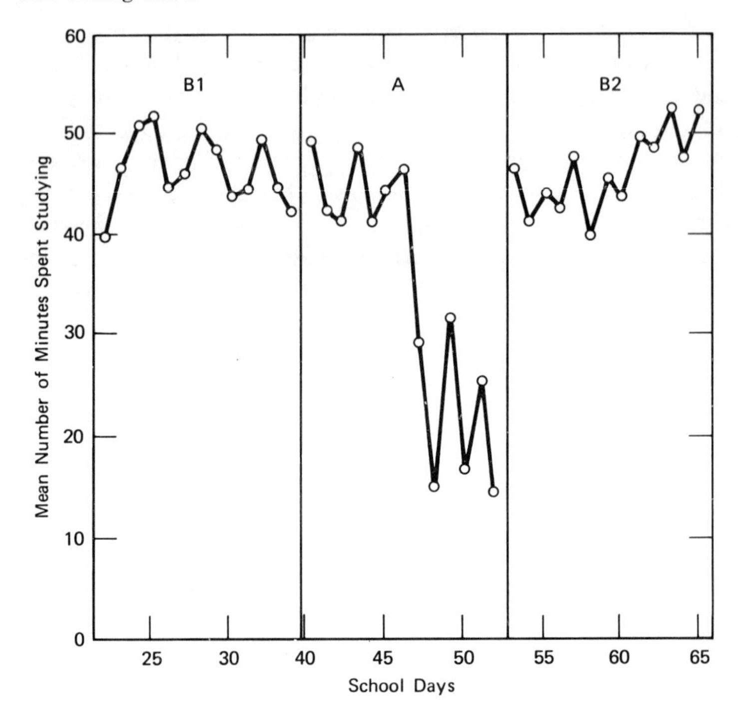

Figure 2.1. Mean time sixteen preschoolers spent in study period over three experimental conditions. In the B periods the teachers structured a token exchange for studying; in A an approval exchange. Experiment by Stoddard, Bushell, and Hamblin.

on the average of over fifty of the available sixty minutes. Hence, the cultural problem of developing the preschoolers' interest in academic materials is rather easily solved given a well-managed, moderately well-run token exchange.

At a more theoretical level the results illustrate the acceleration-deceleration principle: the equilibrium level (the relatively steady state rate at which an instructional exchange is worked) increases as the strength of the reinforcers used in reciprocation increases and, conversely, the equilibrium level decreases as the strength of the reinforcers used in reciprocation decreases.

Note also that the equilibrium after the reversal is at a higher level than that which was obtained before. This is known as the intensification-by-reversals effect. This effect is at work in most experiments because the subjects are apparently both unclear about the exchange contingencies and ambivalent about the exchange itself. Taking the exchange out and then reinstating it apparently clarifies the contingencies and at the same time provides a *contrast* which reduces ambivalence, that is, makes the subjects feel even better than before about working the exchange.

Reversals are generally done in experiments like this to test the causal assumptions in the theory. If the factor thought to produce a change when it is put in does not produce a reversal when taken out, then any causal assumptions must remain suspect. Needless to say, the first reason for using reversals in experiments is to test such causal assumptions. Secondly, because of the intensification-by-reversals effect, it is therapeutic.

EXPERIMENT 2: READING AND THE YOUNG CHILD

In designing an environment in which young children (some circa 33 months, others circa 55) could and would learn how to read, we tried to provide all of the conditions which promote learning: immediacy and consistency of feedback, self-pacing, and strong, positive reinforcers. To provide strong reinforcers we used, as before, a token exchange, which is by its nature self-pacing—that is, the teacher responds to the child's behavior, the child initiates the exchange. The two major problems which required innovations were consistency and immediacy of feedback.

Consistency

The major problem in teaching reading is that traditional English orthography (T.O.) is simply not consistent. The symbols take on varying sounds in different words. Furthermore, there is more than one symbol for a given sound. In fact Jaquith (1968) has recently likened English orthography to cryptography where much used sounds are assigned several symbols and where the same symbols may be assigned to one or more sounds to make the code more difficult to break. The result is confusion, a substantial impediment to learning.

In a phonetic alphabet, in contrast, each symbol has but one sound and each sound has but one symbol. Because of this, a phonetic alphabet is considerably less difficult to learn to read than is traditional English orthography. The initial teaching alphabet (i.t.a.), a phonetic alphabet for beginning reading invented by Sir Isaac Pitman, is designed for easy transition to traditional English orthography (see reprint of the original *London Times* article, 1961). Thus, it makes the initial task of learning to read and to write less difficult, while at the same time it prepares the child for the more difficult task of reading traditional English.

Experiments by Downing (1965) show that children learning to read with i.t.a. do, in fact, learn much faster and much better than do control children with T.O. By the third year the experimentals were well ahead of the controls *in reading T.O.* in spite of the fact that during the second year they had to go through a transition from i.t.a. Downing's experiment has been more or less "replicated" now many, many times. In two thirds of the replications the i.t.a. children show progress similar to that reported by Downing. In one third of the replications there is no difference in reading achievement between the children who learned to read using i.t.a. and those who learned to read with T.O. In no case, however, do the children trained in T.O. do better than those trained using i.t.a.

Most of the pre-primers available in 1967 in i.t.a. were relatively difficult. They were designed that way to give the child considerable experience in sounding out words (this is true even of the Downing readers). Consequently, one of our teachers, June A. Hamblin, developed a series of pre-primers in i.t.a. which are characterized by a simple, relatively repetitive vocabulary which is added to slowly enough to help the child develop a sight vocabulary as well as to give him practice in sounding out new words. While the story lines are not gripping to adults, they do involve common, everyday situations with which children are quite familiar and which generally hold their interest.

Feedback

To structure the environment so that it would be more self-pacing than the usual classroom and so that the children could get immediate feedback, we had them work together in pairs on a teaching machine, a Bell & Howell Language Master. The Language Master is a modified tape recorder which uses an IBM-like card on which is affixed a strip of dual track magnetic tape. Letters or words are written on the cards by the teacher and the associated phonetic pattern recorded on the tape. One child puts the card with a given symbol in the machine and the other child, pressing the appropriate button, then records what he thinks to be the correct phonetic rendition of the symbol. Then by flipping a switch and putting the card back through the machine, the children hear the instructor's prior rendition of the symbol. Thus the children look at the symbol, give its phonetic value, then immediately check their rendition against a phonetic value prerecorded by the teacher.

Teaching Children to Read

Once the children learned the phonetic values of the first ten symbols used in the primer series, their regular teacher, June A. Hamblin, started them on the actual process of reading, that is, of blending the sounds using a procedure which she developed. On the first day she helped the children to sound out three of the six words used in the first of the pre-primers. The children, in sub-groups of five, worked with the teacher, each taking turns blending sounds to obtain the three words. The teacher pointed from one to another in random fashion, back and forth, from child to child giving all reinforced practice until they knew the words by sight, that is, without apparent memory search. On the second day the first three words were reviewed, then in a similar manner the children learned the second group of three words. On the third day the six words were first reviewed and then the children were introduced individually to the first primer. To their pleasant surprise they could read! In a genuine book they could follow the story line which was illustrated by pictures! Each was able to finish his first book and to take it home that evening to read to his parents. It was a great day for these young children.

From the third day on the children spent four minutes each day individually with the teacher reading in the pre-primers and sounding out the words they did not know. During these times they were given backedup tokens and M&M's for reading or sounding out the story line correctly. When he finished a primer with the teacher, the child took it home to read to his parents that night. The parents were coached to give the child approval for reading progress. Rather than bother with the sounding out process, the parents were asked to prompt the child just by giving him the word if he were unable to sound it out within fifteen seconds or so.

From the beginning, as noted, the children worked in pairs on the Language Master where they were supposed to learn new sounds and the new words that they would encounter in the primers. Each day each pair was given about a dozen cards, some old, some new. The new cards were added as the children demonstrated that they had learned the symbols or the words on the old cards, i.e. had rendered each within about three seconds of presentation three days in a row.

The Experiment

During this daily fifteen minute period at the Language Masters, the children were put through an ABABC series by Pfeiffer, Shea and Hamblin which constitutes Experiment 2 (see Figures 2.2 and 2.3). In all of these conditions, the children were on a delayed exchange; the tutor-pupil pairs were given tokens at the end of the learning period for the number of cards the two could sight read.

In addition, during the A periods, a male teacher sat in the room with the children and the Language Masters as a non-person. That is, he did not attend to or otherwise reinforce the children. The purpose for this procedure was to reduce to zero teacher reinforcement for peer tutoring during the A periods. In the B periods the teacher walked around the room from one pair of children to another, warmly praising them and handing out tokens if he found them teaching each other on their Language Master but ignoring them if they were not.

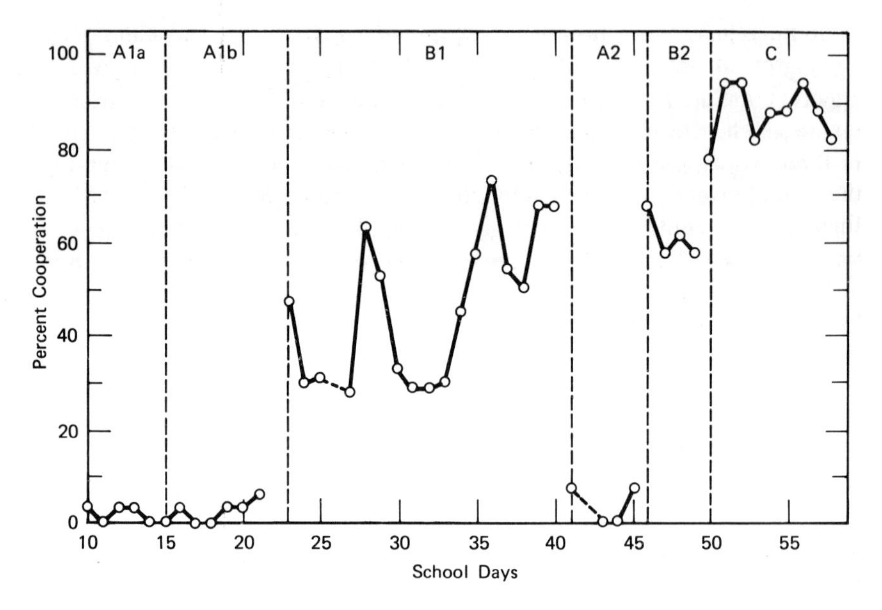

Figure 2.2. Median percent of scheduled time spent cooperating at Language Master each school day. (After Pfeiffer, 1969.) During A1a wage reinforcement was given for individual vocabulary gains; A1b and A2, for mutual vocabulary gains of cooperating pairs. During B1 and B2, wage reinforcers as in A1b and A2 plus tokens and approval intermittently while cooperating at Language Masters. During C, wage reinforcers as in A2 plus intermittent social approval by instructor while cooperating at Language Masters.

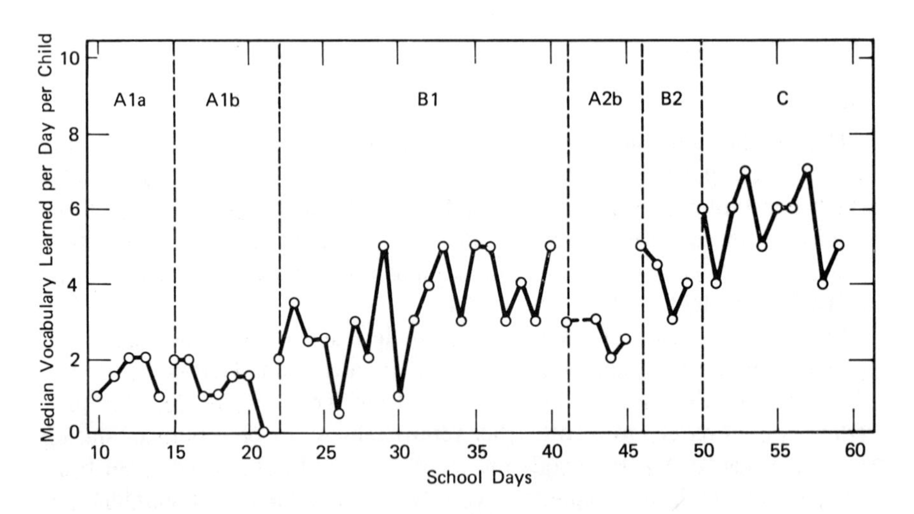

Figure 2.3. Median number of words learned to criterion per child each school day. (After Pfeiffer, 1969.)

The Results—Tutoring and Words Learned

During Ala and Alb, with just the delayed exchange in operation (see Figures 2.2 and 2.3), the children spent almost no (3 or 4 percent of the total) time tutoring one another at the Language Masters.[4] They did learn a few words, less than 2 per day on the average, but this was through individual effort. In B1, when the somewhat continuous approval and token exchange for working together at the machine was added, the amount of time spent in working with one another increased dramatically, until toward the end of the period when it leveled off at about 60 percent of the total time available. The number of words learned increased, eventually to almost 4 per day. In A2 using only the delayed exchange, the time spent in tutoring dropped precipitously again to almost a nothing level (4 percent). The number of words learned also decreased from the number learned in B1; 2.6 words per day. In the B2 period when the token exchange for working at the machines was again introduced, the time spent in tutoring increased and ultimately leveled out to around 63 percent of the available time, and the rate of learning new words stabilized again during the last ten days at approximately 4 per day.

Thus, all seemed to be going well, as predicted. However, toward the end of B2, it was noticed that the children were playing with their tokens much of the time and that this token fondling was apparently decreasing the time they spent teaching one another. This may have been due to the teacher's having fallen into the habit of telling them to put their tokens away whenever he observed them in such play. It was decided to try to eliminate the problem by gradually doing away with the tokens and using the teacher's approval as the only reinforcer during the learning periods.

Accordingly, during the first half of C the teacher phased out the tokens, giving them only half as often as he gave approval. During the last half, tokens were dropped altogether. From that point on, the teacher simply walked around from one tutor-pupil pair to another, giving them approval and encouragement but no tokens. Then as in all previous conditions at the end of the fifteen-minute work period, the children were tested and given backup reinforcers proportional to the number of words they both had learned.

[4] A 20 channel Esterline–Angus event recorder was used in recording the data. The definition of cooperation was that the children be at the Language Master working together, responding to each other as they attended the vocabulary cards. To check reliability, several persons were at different times given the definition of cooperation and with a stop watch they took data simultaneously with the regular observer but on just one cooperating pair, unknown to the observer. The mean agreement of these various checks was 89 percent.

What happened with this change in C? Something very interesting. The time spent in tutoring and the rate of learning words increased, stabilizing during the last four periods at about 87 percent and 5.5 words per day respectively. Theirs was an awe-inspiring performance.

Discussion

As we saw in Experiment 1 in this chapter, it is possible for a time to get a high rate of desired behavior using an approval exchange. However, approval is a conditioned reinforcer which is subject to the limitation of all conditioned reinforcers; that is, without being at least intermittently paired with backups, they become impotent. This happened in Experiment 1; a precipitous decrease in learning activity took place seven days after the token exchange had been terminated and teachers were left with an approval exchange.

However, it may be that *frequent* backups are not necessary, that delayed backups, such as were used in this experiment during C are sufficient once approval has become a conditioned reinforcer through numerous pre-pairings with established reinforcers such as tokens. Thus, since the students were on a delayed exchange for the number of words learned, the work pattern might have been maintained for a much longer period, if not indefinitely. It is too bad that the school year ran out requiring the experiment to be terminated before this could be determined.

It will be recalled that in the first experiment the attendance data conformed to the acceleration-deceleration principle, so also the data in this experiment. The children were not reinforced in some conditions for helping one another to learn words at the Language Master, but in other conditions they were. The equilibrium rate at which they finally tutored one another increased substantially during the reinforcement conditions and decreased almost to zero during the non reinforcement conditions. Since such tutoring at the Language Master was roughly related during the various conditions to the amount of reinforced practice the children had in associating the graphic and phonetic value of the criterion words, the number of words learned followed a similar but not quite as exaggerated pattern.

More Results—Reading Comparisons by Age

Now it is time to compare the progress of the two and a half year olds with that of the five year olds. Curves picturing the cumulative number of words learned by each child through time are given in Figure 2.4. How did the children of different ages do? Note that the younger children did about as well as the five year olds. Their sight vocabularies were almost as large.

Learning to associate the phonetic value of the words with their graphic representation is a special case of contingency learning. The data in Figure

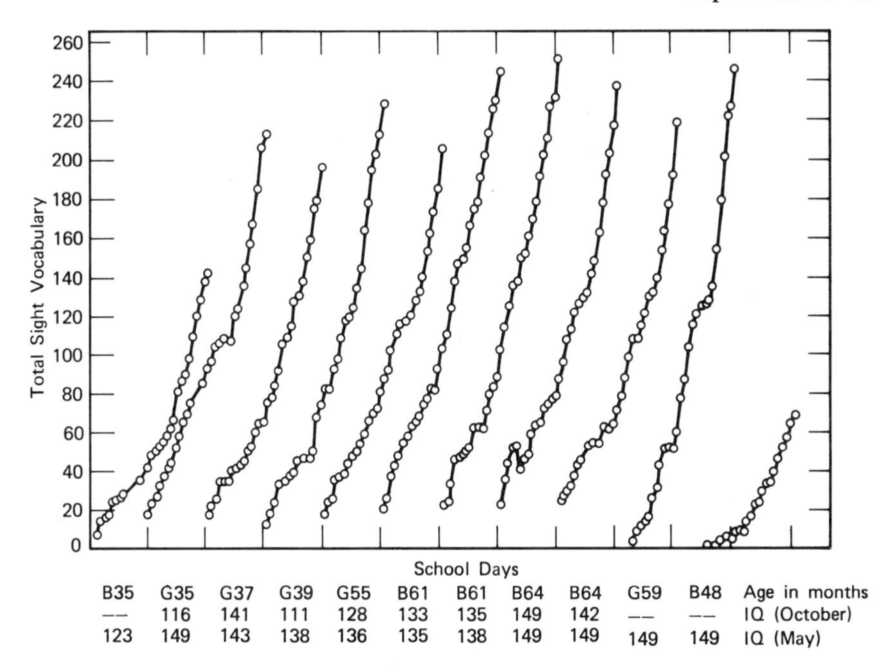

Figure 2.4. Cumulative Individual Sight Vocabularies for each child as a function of school days. B and G refer to sex of the child and the number, to the child's age in months at the beginning of the experiment. October and May Stanford-Binet IQ's are given where available. Note: the two right-most plots are of children who were introduced into the experiment when it was about half over. (After Pfeiffer, 1969.)

2.4, therefore, show that the cumulative rate of this kind of contingency learning increases at an increasing rate with reinforced practice. In other words, the data indicate that expertise at contingency learning, specifically the phonetic-graphic contingencies involved in reading, is apparently described by the same laws which describe expertise learning generally. As we shall see later, this is an important finding.

What happened with the before-after IQ measurements of these children? As may be noted in Figure 2.4, Carol (G 39) scored 111 in the fall and 138 in the spring, an increase of 27 IQ points, and Beth (G 35) scored 116 in the fall and 149 in the spring, an increase of at least 33 IQ points. In contrast, those who scored higher initially, in the 135–149 range, experienced almost no increase in IQ. These results are at best suggestive and they will be followed up in the next chapter. They did, however, sensitize us to the possibility that early reading promotes the development of IQ and to the idea of what will be called the comparison effect.

We first noticed the comparison effect when Joan (G 59) was introduced into the preschool while the other children were in the midst of this experiment. Joan, who had not as yet learned to read, expressed disbelief mixed with considerable consternation when she saw Jim (B 35), at the time an unusually small thirty-eight month old boy, reading fluently. This comparative deficit between Jim's and her own reading ability apparently threatened Joan's image of herself. In any event, progress in learning to read became an extremely powerful reinforcer for her. It was obvious that as she learned her symbols, how to blend them into words, and then how to read the primers, she experienced great pleasure and relief. She took advantage of every moment she was scheduled with the teacher. In fact she asked the teacher to spend extra time with her after class. Her parents reported that she would read each book that was sent home two, three, as many as four times in order to master the words. This continued for about three weeks during which time she learned her symbols, learned to sound out the words, and, in fact, could read the first eight primers. This was enough to catch up with the others, all of whom had been reading for four months. At that point Joan relaxed and began to work at a lower rate, just fast enough to keep up with or a little ahead of the fastest of the five year olds (the B 61 twins).

According to the comparison effect, then, individuals attempt to match or exceed the performance of certain other individuals in their environment. Because of this, performance at the comparison level becomes a reinforcer. The comparison effect, apparently integral to the operation of status systems in groups, evidently occurs in social situations whenever reinforcers reflect the value of performance.

It is possible that in a traditional classroom the value of the usual reinforcers, correct answers and grades, is determined in part by backups, such as parents' and teachers' approval, but also in part by comparisons with other's performance. This does not mean that classrooms are necessarily competitive in the zero-sum-game sense.[5] As may be recalled from Figure 2.4, all of the children who were there from the beginning learned to read almost equally as well as the others. It does mean, however, that the best students typically set performance standards.

Also, it is apparently not accidental that the two girls who experienced the largest increase in measured IQ were the ones who initially scored the lowest. They were the ones who, like Joan, were in a position to increase their performance to where it would equal that of others in the class. They were apparently enabled to score these gains, in part, because they could compare their performance against that of other children who were operating at the 135–150 IQ level. Had these children been in an environment where the other children were operating at 110–120 IQ level, one would predict

[5] A zero-sum-game defines true competition: that which one party wins is lost by another. Hence, the sum of the winnings and losses of such a game equals zero.

on the basis of comparison effect that Carol and Linda would not have experienced such a marked increase in IQ. Instead of 28 to 35 points they may have increased perhaps 5 or 10 points.

EXPERIMENT 3: PEER TUTORING

This experiment does not flow out of the theoretical interests which initiated this chapter but rather it began with a perplexing, intriguing, but unanticipated problem which we encountered while running the first experiment.

While the results from that experiment indicated a well designed and operated token exchange helps in educating very young children, we found that the best teacher-pupil ratio which we could obtain was 1 to 10. In that experiment, and our subsequent informal experience, we found that this is all one can expect with a semi-continuous token exchange. However, there appear to be other designs for instructional exchanges which may be more practical.

One basic design by Birnbrauer, Bijou, Wolf, and Kidder (1965) for teaching the mentally retarded involved programmed learning materials (with or without a teaching machine) which the children worked through themselves. Thus the teacher did not teach in the usual sense, rather she answered questions and checked the answers. Correct answers were awarded points which could be redeemed for backup reinforcers at the end of the classroom period. With such a system a teacher can generally handle a normal classroom, about thirty students. There is, however, a problem with programmed learning materials, in fact any instructional materials. When they are given in a large, steady dose, the children become bored. In the interest of variety, then, it may be important to develop other alternatives.

The system used in the second experiment (students working in pairs on teaching machines) is one possibility. It is probable that a teacher could handle fifteen such pairs, particularly if the children were a little older. The system does have the advantage of immediate feedback while allowing the children to work in an enjoyable social or cooperative situation. An extension of this system, which could have interesting educational possibilities, is a peer tutoring arrangement without a teaching machine, where the tutor teaches his pupil materials which he, the tutor, has already learned. This kind of peer tutoring arrangement was used in Experiment 3 by Stoddard, Bushell and Hamblin.

The Experiment

During a standard forty-five minute study period, seventeen children, the same subjects used in Experiment 1 plus one, could choose in all conditions (A, B and C) to work on individual lessons in one area of the classroom with one of two teachers, or they could team up in pairs and work in another area of the classroom with a third teacher. Careful records were kept on the progress of each individual child from the beginning, and a child who knew a subject was asked to tutor another child who did not.

Throughout the A and B conditions, the children had a choice; they could receive teacher approval and tokens for working either individually or in pairs. Furthermore, as they were completing a lesson they were given tokens proportionately to the amount of work correctly done, e.g. the number of symbols, words, numbers, etc., learned to criterion. However, in the B conditions, the children who were working together as tutor-pupil pairs were reinforced differentially—that is, both received a special token each time the pupil answered a question correctly on the assigned lesson material. This special token was larger and was made out of a more attractive plastic; more importantly, it was worth four of the regular tokens. C was similar to the B conditions except field trips were added to the backups, to the local fire station, police station, pet shop, and post office, for example.

Results

The children were put through a BABABAC series which terminated as the spring semester ended (see Figure 2.5). (We did so many reversals

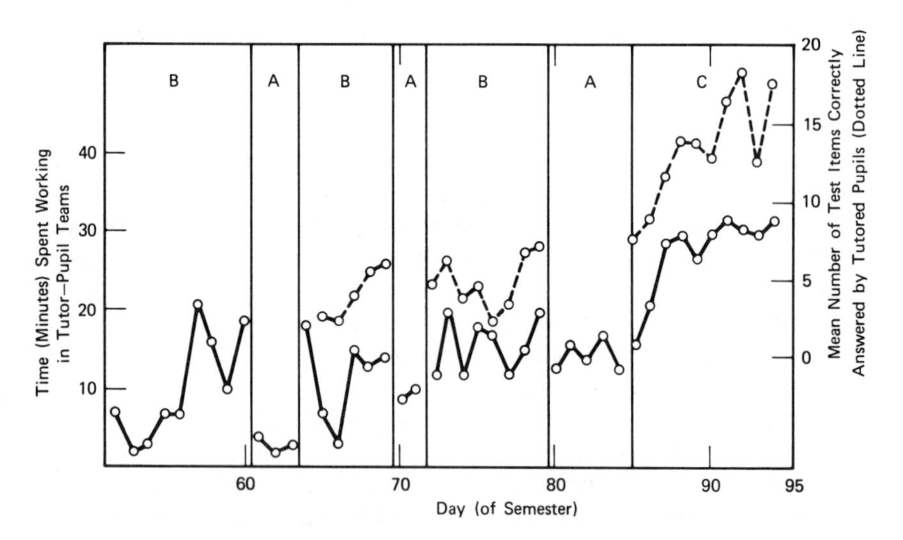

Figure 2.5. Mean time seventeen preschoolers spent studying in tutor-pupil pairs and the mean number of test items correctly completed by tutored pupils, by days through seven experimental periods. In the A conditions the teachers worked a token exchange for studying with a regular token for student-tutor pairs' correctly completing assigned tasks. In B, the token exchange was similar but special tokens worth four regular tokens were given to pairs for correctly completing assigned lessons. C was similar to B except field trips were included in the backups. (After Stoddard, 1970.)

to capitalize on the intensification-by-reversals effect.) What happened? Note that the average time which the children spent teaching one another was low at first, but by the end of C, the children were spending circa 33 of the 45 minutes teaching one another.[6] This represents about 73 percent of the available time. Since in any given class period some of the students continued to be instructed at the individual tables, in part to give input to the system, this 73 percent may be close to an ideal equilibrium. Also in Figure 2.5 note the remarkable increase in the average number of test items correctly answered by the tutored pupils, circa 17 per period! These tutors were teaching effectively!

Now, there can be problems with such a system of peer tutoring. For example, some children might always be the tutor, others, always the pupil. Therefore, in assigning lessons the teachers in this experiment attempted to give each child experience both as pupil and tutor. Since they kept a good record of each child's progress, this was not a difficult task, for the progress of any child is uneven, and every child does some things better than others. In fact, one child often taught a second child his numbers, and then later the second child helped the first child through a reading lesson.

There were great unanticipated benefits from this system. First, these children often developed into excellent natural tutors. The observers were continually amazed at the way they innovated effective teaching techniques. Second, in the process of tutoring the tutors themselves effectively mastered the material. This may not be too surprising since it happens to most of us who teach. Finally, the children and the teachers alike enjoyed working the system, perhaps more so than any system we have designed so far. This, of course, is crucial. To survive, a system needs to be more effective, more efficient than others, but also more enjoyable. In the long run, a system which does not yield intrinsic satisfaction, however efficient, is too costly to endure.

WHAT HAVE WE LEARNED SO FAR?

Nothing, in any firm sense. However, the above experiments do furnish a number of leads which if replicated in subsequent experiments could be important for acculturation theory and for the design of instructional systems. So for the purpose of establishing continuity with the findings of subsequent chapters, these leads will be outlined as a conclusion to this chapter.

1. The results of the three experiments show the importance of material incentives even for normal children. In particular, in the first experiment the teachers used social approval to reinforce attendance at lessons through-

[6] Data were taken by the same observer used in Experiment 1 on the same apparatus, and reliability checks were taken in the same way. Reliability was .94.

out all three experimental periods. (Recall they usually said "Thank you" or some other such phrase as they passed out tokens.) Yet when a token exchange was taken out during A, lesson attendance decreased gradually to a third of its prior level. Social approval is better than nothing, but its power with young children is generally only a fraction of that of the material reinforcers used in our token exchange.

2. It is obvious that non contingent rewards, be they movies, snacks, toys or whatever, do not sustain a high level of study activity. To be effective they have to be given in exchange for a high level of study activity.

3. The suggestion was made in Chapter 1 that the degree to which a person will attend to environmental features increases as the strength of related reinforcers increases. The first experiment was designed specifically to illustrate this, and it in fact did. As suggested, attention is crucial because it increases the rate of contingency learning. As one mother expressed it, "when the children are rewarded for doing their lessons, they pay attention to what the teacher says. This makes it so the teacher can actually teach them something."

4. In all three experiments we have seen the operation of the acceleration-deceleration principle. In any given experimental condition the children settled down to an equilibrium, a steady rate of working the instructional exchange (even though that rate was, at times, near zero). In general, the data indicate that the rate of working an instructional exchange increases as the strength of the reinforcers for working increases, and conversely, the rate decreases as the strength of reinforcers decreases. This principle apparently holds for the rates of a wide range of behaviors, such as attending lessons, learning symbols and words to criterion, and cooperating in peer-tutoring with or without a teaching machine.

5. Next we found that given an appropriately designed learning environment, 30–40 month olds learned to read about as fast and about as well as 50–65 month olds. This finding, while preliminary, supports Gates and his associates' earlier finding that success in learning to read is primarily a function of the learning environment. This would suggest that the Morphett–Washburne mental-age-of-6.5-prerequisite for learning to read is an artifact of a traditional educational environment which omits several characteristics important for optimal learning.

6. We encountered the intensification-by-reversals effect. The data from the three experiments, given adequate experimental controls, suggest that when the strength of reinforcement is decreased and then increased to its former level, the behavioral equilibrium is higher after the reversal than it was before. In other words we found that experimental reversals, designed initially to evaluate causal assumptions in theory, have an unanticipated therapeutic effect.

7. Finally, the data suggest a comparison effect. Comparison among peers apparently augments the value of the reinforcers used in the traditional educational systems—correct answers, grades, etc.

So much for young suburban children. Now we will turn to their counterparts in the inner city.

CHAPTER 3

Inner-City Children

In any school system one will find children who are learning at a rate that is above the norm (that is, above the average learning rate for the nation's school children as a whole), some whose progression is approximately at the norm and still others who are learning at a rate below, sometimes substantially below the norm.[1] While the faster rates of learning in school are not necessarily predictive of successful adaptations, there is, in fact, a substantial correlation, one that is generally interpreted causally (cf. Duncan, 1952, and Duncan, et al., 1968).

Although in almost any inner-city school one will find substantial numbers of children whose learning rates are superior to or approximately at the norm, the number of slow learners is unusually large (cf. Coleman, et al., 1966). This has been generally recognized for some time and there have been substantial efforts in St. Louis (the Banneker District) and other metropolitan areas to remedy the situation.

A number of theories have been developed to explain the initial and then the cumulative educational deficit of children, white and non white. The most popular current explanations appear to be the genetic deficit theory (Jensen, 1969), the expectation theory (Clark, 1965 and 1966; Rosenthal and Jacobson, 1968), the stimulus deprivation theory (Hunt, 1964, and Deutsch, 1967), and the language deficit theory. Of all explanations, the language deficit theory appears to be the most popular. According to this theory, the cumulative deficit in the educational achievement of some culturally disadvantaged children is supposed to be, among other factors, the result of a deficit in their early language training.[2]

[1] Hamblin and Buckholdt took the major responsibility for writing this chapter.

[2] Many have proposed variations in the language deprivation theory, for example: Bereiter and Engelmann (1966, pp. 28–43), Bernstein (1962, 1964), Cheyney (1967), Cohn (1959), Deutsch (1967), Henry (1967), John (1963), Newton (1960), Weikart (1966), and Wittick (1965). However, the research and supporting results are meager; for example: Bereiter and Engelmann (1966), Deutsch (1967), Weikart (1964).

From their work with black preschoolers, Bereiter and Engelmann (1966) have spotted several typical language deficits. For example, they report that some such children are plagued with an inability to deal with sentences as sequences of meaningful parts; some tend to drop out smaller connectives and other structure words. Many do not understand how connectives and modifiers such as, "or," "and" and "not," change the meaning of sentences. According to Bereiter and Engelmann, these are the deficiencies which prevent some children, in part at least, from using language as a medium for learning and which account for their apparent retardation.[3]

Consistent with their theory Bereiter and Engelmann have established preschoolers where "from the first day the children were given an intensive, fast-paced, highly structured program of instruction in basic language skills, reading and arithmetic." In evaluating their program they initially assumed that IQ scores of the children are an indicator of overall academic achievement. Consequently, they first tested their children using the Stanford-Binet two months after school began. (This two-month delay was to eliminate from the data the six point gain that is expected for such children merely from their becoming adjusted to the classroom situation.) At that time the average IQ was approximately 93. When the children were retested after seven months of school, the mean IQ had risen to slightly above 100. This probably occurred because of the use of intensive language training; at any rate, at the end of the year the children improved to the point where they tested normal on verbal ability.

Although we were unaware of Bereiter and Engelmann's research as we began experimenting with instructional systems for slow learners, we shared their view about the effects of verbal language deficits and about the importance of verbal language training. As a beginning we wanted to see how a well-designed token exchange might accelerate language acquisition.

[3] This is not to suggest that the dialect spoken by most blacks of the inner city is an inferior language. Recent work by linguists (cf. Aarons, Gordon, and Stewart, 1969) suggest that "black language" in the inner city is systematic, functional, perfectly adequate, in fact, no more deficient than any other dialect. The issue is not the dialect, but the allegedly inadequate training in or the acquisition of language by some children. Presumably the undeveloped ability of children to use verbal language would have the same intellectually inhibiting effect whether that language was the dialect or standard English. The other related issues are whether to teach in standard English or in the dialect. Some have suggested that the black dialect may make learning easier for the children. Others feel that the children, at least most of them, are quite capable of learning both, and to not teach them standard English, in addition to the dialect which they learn anyway, would severely limit their freedom later on in life, when language acquisition seems to be more difficult.

EXPERIMENT 1: LANGUAGE ACQUISITION CONTROLS

Arrangements were made to run the experiment at an inner-city preschool in St. Louis. Twenty-two black children, ages three to five, attended regularly. All lived in the Pruitt-Igoe Housing Project; the majority came from families on ADC. As in our other experimental classrooms, the teachers were instructed to ignore the aggressive, disruptive behavior and to reward attention and cooperation with social approval and plastic tokens, which later were exchanged for milk, cookies, admission to the movies, toys, etc. The children quickly learned the system and as they did the disruptions diminished and cooperation increased. Within three weeks most of the children were participating in the lessons; disruptive behavior had become only an occasional problem.

After the token exchange was well established and well understood by both teachers and students, our attention was focused upon seven children with verbal problems—those who, in spite of the introduction of the token exchange, were still talking and otherwise progressing far below the normal rate. These children seldom initiated verbal exchanges with the teachers or with other students, although they sometimes would answer appropriately with a word when queried directly.

As we observed the particular nonverbal children in our school, we became convinced that their problem was not so much that they were unable to talk as that they were too shy to talk to strangers, that is, to non family. In their homes, we heard most of them talking in broken sentences with their mother or with siblings. This suggested to us that the causes of their non talking were probably social and not hereditary. Consequently, we decided to put these seven children through an ABABA experimental series with a token exchange designed specifically to develop a pattern of talking with non family, particularly with teachers and other children in school. However, we had some bad luck. By the time the baseline (A1) period had been completed, three of the seven children had dropped out of school (for various reasons apparently not related to their performance in school, for example, one family moved to another area in the city, another child became ill), so the results reported in Figure 3.1 represent averages for four, not seven, children.

What happened? During the A1 baseline period, when a token exchange for attention and cooperation was in effect (as it was for the rest of the class), the four children said something in about 8 percent of the fifteen-second sampling periods in which they were observed. With this token exchange the children were reinforced for talking, specifically for answering a question correctly, but they received tokens for other things as well, for example, sitting quietly, listening attentively, doing art work.

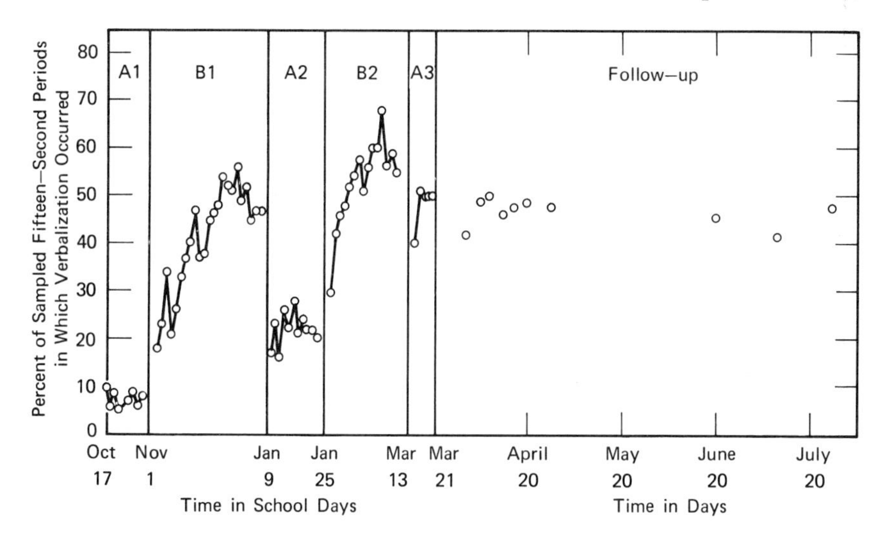

Figure 3.1. Percent of sampled periods in which talking occurred through time for four "nonverbal" children and through five experimental conditions. In each of the A conditions a new teacher was introduced who structured a token exchange for participation in lessons. In the B conditions the teacher then structured a token exchange for talking. The follow-up was similar to the A conditions. (After Buckholdt, 1969.)

In B1 the teacher was instructed to elicit talking in various ways. Primarily, however, she followed the imitation paradigm suggested by Bandura and Walters (1963). If the child responded appropriately when she asked a question, he would be reinforced with one or more tokens depending upon the value of his answer. If he failed to give even an approximation of a correct answer, she would ask the same question of another child in the group; or if none in the group could or would approximate a correct answer, she would ask a normal talker whom she called over from another group. Once another child had provided an accurate model, she would then go back to those children who had been unable to respond appropriately and ask them the same question. If they gave her a fair approximation of the correct answer given by the model, they were reinforced. In addition, the children were reinforced with tokens for any spontaneous speech with the teacher or with the other children. Head shaking, finger pointing and all other forms of nonverbal communication were no longer reinforced. Note in Figure 3.1 that the verbalization increased gradually until it finally leveled out at approximately 48 percent.

To reverse the experimental conditions beginning in A2, a second teacher, who was new to the school, took over the experimental group. She was trained to structure a token exchange for attention and cooperation, as used in A1. What was the result? As may be seen in Figure 3.1, the rate of talking dropped off immediately, then increased gradually, sporadically until talking was occurring on the average in 23 percent of the last eight fifteen-second observation periods.

When the new teacher reintroduced the token exchange for talking at the beginning of B2, the talking rate increased rapidly, much more so than the first time, until it stabilized at almost 60 percent.

In the final reversal, we again took out the token exchange for talking and gave the experimental group to a new teacher. This time, the reduction was smaller, to 50 percent. During the four months following the termination of the formal experiment, occasional checks showed that the equilibrium continued to obtain; there was no appreciable reduction in the average rate of talking.

These data illustrate the acceleration-deceleration principle discussed in the last chapter as well as the intensification-by-reversals effect. Also note that the equilibria which were obtained in the successive A periods gradually increased from 8 percent to 23 percent to 47 percent. This is the most substantial intensification observed to date in successive A periods.

The findings should be crucial for those who wonder if children on token exchanges must always be given material reinforcers to maintain the pronormal behaviors produced. This experiment suggests that behavior changes will be permanent if a normal level of expertise is developed during the course of the token exchange program and if existing exchanges in the culture reinforce the acquired pattern. Since there is substantial reinforcement for talking in our culture, it is to be expected that once a talking pattern is established, it will be maintained. This also appears to be true for reading, but not generally true for mathematics beyond the simple arithmetic which most people use and remember.

Controls

Be that as it may, how does the rate of talking of the experimental children compare with that of normal talkers? Throughout the experiment, measures were periodically taken on the speech patterns of two comparison groups: four ghetto children in the preschool who seemed to have no verbal problems and eight suburban children who attended our preschool at Washington University. These data, summarized in Table 3.1, show that toward the end of the experiment (during A3) the experimental children were talking at a slightly higher rate than the comparison groups. In addition, the experimental children, who at first directed almost all of their words to the teacher, gradually came to talk to their teacher and their fellow students in about the same proportions as did the comparison children (see Table 3.2). The observers also noted that the quality of the children's communication improved. In the early periods the children's responses were hesitant, usually

Table 3.1. Average Verbal Percentage[a] of Four Experimental Children, Twelve Comparison Children, Four Inner-City Preschoolers and Eight Washington University Preschoolers.

Experimental					Inner-City					Washington U.				
A1	B1	A2	B2	A3	A1	B1	A2	B2	A3	A1	B1	A2	B2	A3
8	48	22	58	50	46	51	43	44	40	40	46	44	38	42

[a] Percentages, for the experimentals and the other Mullanphy preschoolers were calculated for the last four days of each experimental period; percentages for the W.U. preschoolers were calculated for one day at the end of each period.

Table 3.2. Average Percentage[a] of Sampled Time Units in Which Speech Was With a Teacher or With Other Students for The Four Experimental Preschoolers, Four Inner-City Preschoolers, and Eight Washington University Preschoolers.

	Experimental					Inner-City					Washington U.				
	A1	B1	A2	B2	A3	A1	B1	A2	B2	A3	A1	B1	A2	B2	A3
Average Percentage of Sampled Time Units In Which Speech Was Directed At Teachers	83	75	63	50	46	42	42	40	45	48	46	50	48	52	57
Average Percentage of Sampled Time Units In Which Speech Was Directed At Student	10	20	31	44	47	53	50	53	50	46	50	45	44	43	38

[a] Measurements in Periods B1 and B2, A3 and Maintenance for "Experimental" and Mullanphy children are based on the last four days of the period; for Washington University Preschoolers they are based on one day at the end of each period. All percentages are based on 56 sampled 15-second time units. Percentages do not add to 100 because a verbal target could not always be identified.

single words or phrases. In contrast, toward the end of the experiment (during A3) and during the follow-up period the children talked in complete sentences 72 percent of the time. In comparison, the four preschoolers talked in complete sentences 74 percent of the time, and the Washington University preschoolers, 76 percent of the time.

While we were disappointed that three of the original seven experimental children dropped out of the preschool before language training began, each returned occasionally, a day here and a day there. During their infrequent visits, these children were allowed to join their old friends and to receive the same treatment their friends received. Also, the usual measures were taken of the frequency of their talking. The data are given in Figure 3.2. In general, the speech patterns of these children did not change from what they were in A1, the original baseline period. The major exception was Terri, who began to attend frequently during the beginning of B2. She began to talk more, presumably in response to the token exchange for talking which was in effect during that period. In fact, her verbal frequency reached a high of 42 percent before she became ill again and was forced again to drop out of preschool. She recovered from her illness quickly, however, and returned for a few days during the A3 and maintenance periods. Unfortunately, she had not been under the influence of the language exchanges long enough, for her B2 gains were not maintained. Her verbal frequency returned to the original baseline rate, varying between 0 and 12 percent, averaging about 5 percent.

Other measures taken in the A3 maintenance period showed that Terri's speech had not improved much during the year, even though she had participated briefly in the language exchanges. Of the few verbal responses she did emit, 93 percent came in the form of one-word answers or incomplete sentences. In addition, 74 percent of her speech was directed to a teacher.

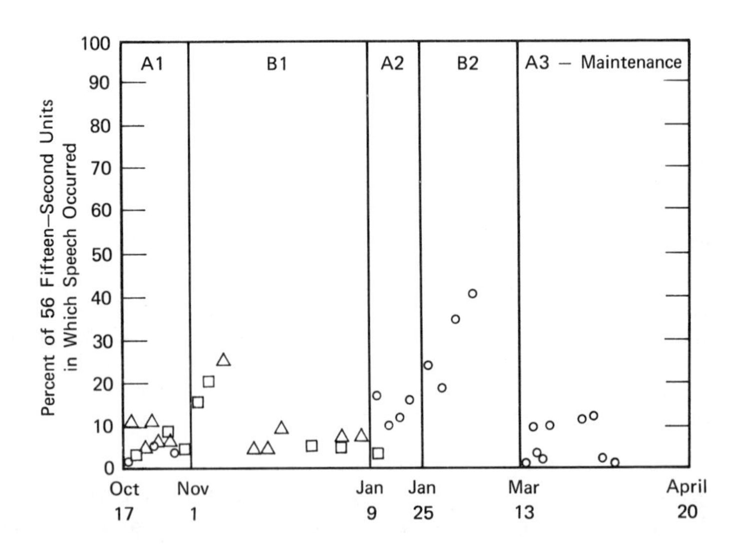

Figure 3.2. Percent of fifteen second intervals in which speech occurred for three non-verbal inner-city preschoolers as they sporadically attended class over the year. (After Buckholdt, 1969.)

In other words, at the end of the year, Terri's verbal behavior was similar to that of the experimental children before they had gone through the experimental series.

Generalization

The changes in behavior patterns observed in the classroom generalized to the home. In interviews with Buckholdt each parent noted a substantial improvement in the child's speech as well as other changes in behavior patterns.

Originally, Lou's mother worried that he "would never stand up for his rights," that he lacked aggressiveness, assertiveness, and self defense. She also observed that he "never did talk too much," but she did not see this as a particular problem. The following excerpt from the interview conducted at the conclusion of the experiment summarizes the changes which impressed her:

BUCKHOLDT: Does Lou ever talk about school when he comes home?

MOTHER: Oh boy! Constantly! You started him talkin', and now who's gonna stop him?

BUCKHOLDT: So you've noticed a change in him?

MOTHER: Have I! Yesterday Mike and I were wondering how we was gonna stop him from tellin' about Little Red Riding Hood and the Three Bears —he just goes on, and on, and on.

BUCKHOLDT: Have you noticed any other changes in him since he started school?

MOTHER: Yes, we have trouble with him talking to strange people; you know, people that he don't know on the street. This talkin', it's just . . . it's amazin' really, but he's talkin' so much to me, I can't take it.

Lou's mother felt that her boy had become too verbal! A boy whose verbal frequency was about average for the preschool! His increased verbal usage apparently conflicted with her values which evidently prescribed quiet, silently obedient children. No longer could she perform her household tasks without the questions, revelations, even the objections of an inquiring child. Perhaps her attitude and the actions she took to enforce it were initially responsible for the verbal problems which her son had when he arrived at preschool; she had evidently trained him to be a nontalker.

Although Ben had attended Head Start classes, he still had a severe verbal deficiency, a pattern of extreme withdrawal and a lack of aggressiveness. To make matters worse, other children were fond of bullying him. After attending the experimental preschool, however, his mother noted some changes:

BUCKHOLDT: Have you noticed any changes in Ben since he started school?

MOTHER: Yes, he comes home and starts countin' and saying different rhymes, and he helps his sister with the things he learned in school. He's talkin' quite a bit at home now, too. Even talks to other kids on the street. He seems to be growed up. If anybody says anything to him or does anything to him, he sort of talks up more than he used to. He really loves school and his teachers.

Similar changes were evident in the preschool. By the end of the B2 period, Ben began to make a number of friends in the preschool and he started to participate in group activities. By the end of the school year he was even capable of defending himself. The confidence he developed while learning to talk apparently generalized.

Joyce and Ruth were sisters who both seemed withdrawn, nervous, even anxious at the beginning of the year. At the end of the year, however, they appeared quite different to their mother.

BUCKHOLDT: Have you noticed any changes in your daughters since they started preschool?

MOTHER: Definitely! Joyce, she's learned her alphabet and colors very well. Ruth also. Both seem to have learned independency. They sort of help themselves and feel more confidence in themselves.

BUCKHOLDT: Have you noticed anything else?

MOTHER: Both girls were shy when they started, but they've gotten over it. They've gotten used to playing with kids and they're not so nervous with them now. They have more confidence in themselves and I think it worked good for them. They both talk a lot more now, too, especially in sentences. I have an older son who had talkin' problems—guess you might call him tongue tied. He was a very nervous kid. He failed, well actually, even though he was passing from grade to grade, I think he actually failed those first four or five years in school. Now he's beginning to pick up though. His not talking really made it hard for him and hard for the teachers; they didn't realize that he was really shy and afraid to express himself.

BUCKHOLDT: How old is he now?

MOTHER: He's fifteen.

BUCKHOLDT: Do you feel that your daughters will have these same problems?

MOTHER: Definitely not! They may have problems, but not these.

The behavioral changes that occurred in these children while they were attending the experimental preschool are congruent with George Herbert Mead's (1934) analysis of the nature and function of language. It would seem somewhat presumptuous to argue that our language training created more active minds, greater intelligences, and more acceptable self-evaluations in each of the four children, but that is what Mead would have predicted and the interview data seem to bear out his predictions.

EXPERIMENT 2: LANGUAGE ACQUISITION AND IQ

The first experiment was perhaps more successful than we had hoped. However, the preschool situation was rather special (one teacher to four or five children) and the language materials with which the children learned were rather *ad hoc*. Consequently two years later arrangements were made by the experimenters (Doss, Buckholdt, and Hamblin) to use a program designed for the acquisition of language and related conceptual skills by Carl Bereiter and his associates (Conceptual Skills Program, OISE). These materials were designed to help children to acquire standard verbal English as well as the ability to use rudimentary logic. The children learn to speak in sentences, while making the usual shape, size, and color discriminations. The materials also deal, among other things, with affirmations and negations. Toward the end of the year the children respond to questions involving prepositions, that is, relationships among objects.

In the six experimental kindergartens (each of which ran half a day, three in the morning and three in the afternoon taught by three teachers) a token exchange was structured, first to get children involved in academic work and then to reinforce them for correct answers. The usual backup reinforcers (milk, cookies, or toys) could be bought during two periods a day. Following the prescribed instructions of the program (which at that time was in its first year of field testing) the teaching strategy involved both teacher imitation and peer imitation. At first, the children were broken up into small groups (for example, the red group, the yellow group). In the beginning the teacher would address a question to one of the groups. If no one in the red group answered correctly, she would ask the yellow group. If no one in that group knew the answer, she would provide the answer which could then be imitated. The quicker individuals would be called on to answer questions, and then, the slower ones. Errors were signaled by no token and by having someone else attempt an answer, preferably a child from another group; if those failed, the teacher. Whenever the children as a group gave a correct answer, each received a token and whenever an individual gave a correct answer, he was given a token. In addition to language training, the children received instruction to help them acquire their prereading skills, for letter, sound and word recognition and some numbers. The children also had stories read to them and they were given periods for art work and for social play.

The Results

Note in Figure 3.3 that the children taught by the experimental teachers experienced rather substantial IQ gains over the year. The changes in the

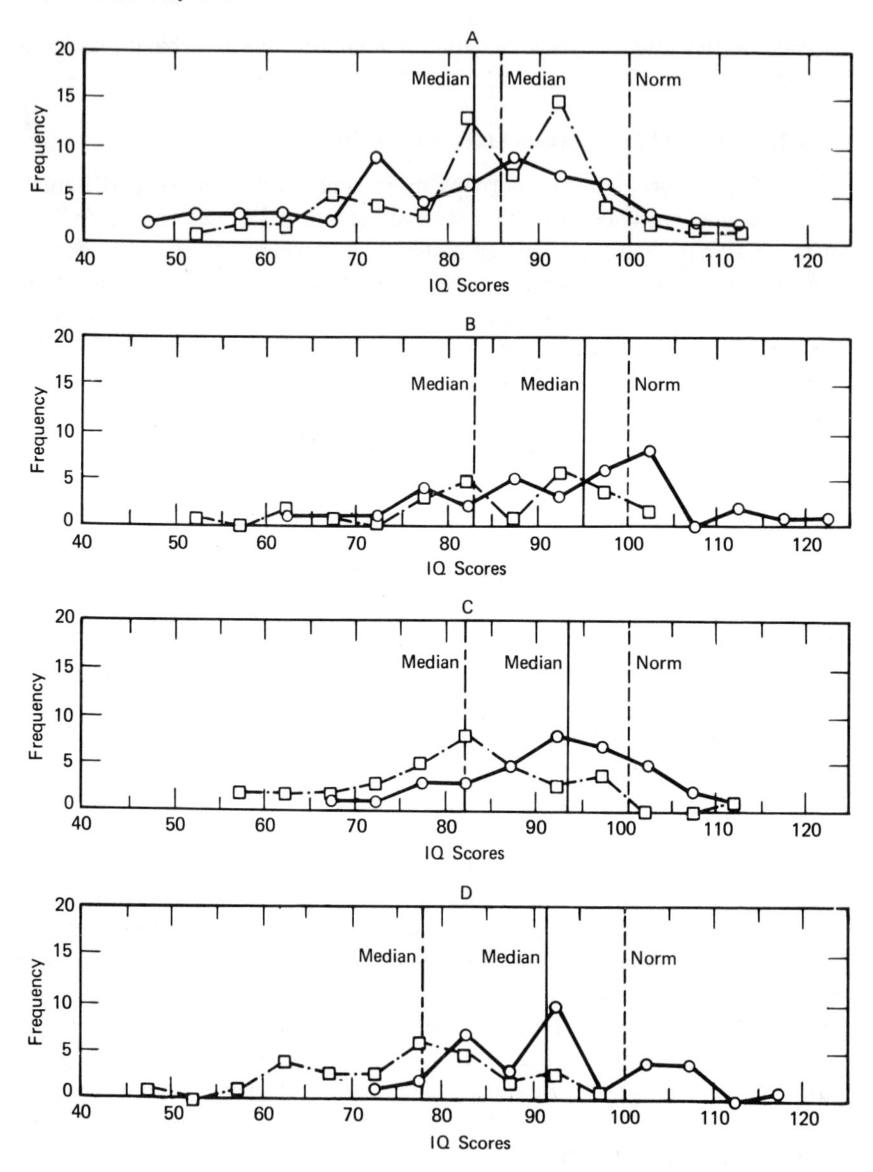

Figure 3.3. Frequency distribution of Otis–Lennon Mental Ability test scores administered in October, 1968 (□— — —□) and in March, 1969 (○———○). Figure A is pooled results from six comparison kindergarten classes (less thirty-two children with IQ's 79 and below who were used in an experiment not reported here). No reinforcement or curricula intervention was made. Figures B, C, and D are results from six experimental kindergarten classes (three teachers) which had a token exchange system and language training twenty minutes a day in groups of fifteen to twenty children.

medians were 12, 12, and 14 IQ points respectively. Thus the differences between teachers were small. The IQ tests involved were different forms of the Otis–Lennon.

These are rather substantial shifts but they are made even more remarkable in the context of what happened to the comparison classes. As may be noted in Figure 3.3 (A), the comparison classes started out with a median IQ of 86 points which was higher than the initial medians of the experimental classes of 84, 82, and 77 IQ points, respectively. Over the year the comparison classes on the average experienced a median decline in IQ of three points. Hence, the net median increase in IQ for the experimental classes was 12 plus 3 or 15 IQ points.

The frequency distributions of individual change scores are plotted for the experimental and the comparison children in Figure 3.4. While confirming the original analysis, these data illustrate further the basic difference in the response of the children to the experimental and comparison learning environments. The variation in response is much smaller among the children in the experimental environments who with four or five exceptions all improved to some degree. On the other hand, the children in the comparison environments fluctuated wildly, some making substantial gains, some making substantial losses but most making small losses. Although the comparison data may seem wild, they are not particularly atypical (cf. Skodak and Skeels, 1949).

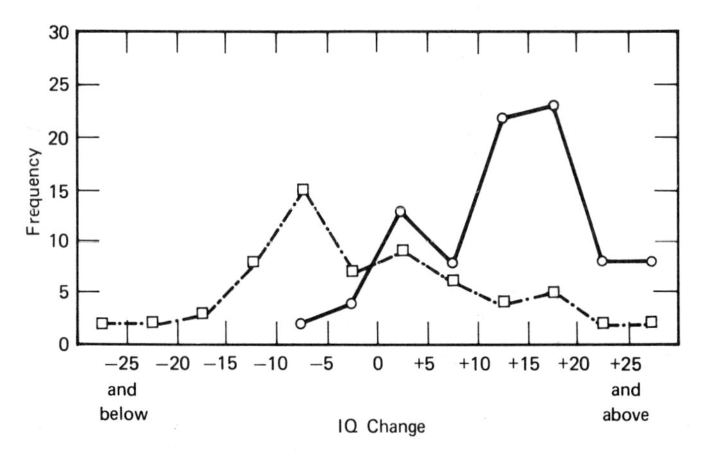

Figure 3.4. Frequency distribution of change scores computed from the difference between the Otis–Lennon Mental Ability IQ scores given in the Fall, 1968, and in the Spring, 1969. The tests were administered to children in the six experimental kindergarten classes (O———O) where the standard curricula was supplemented with Bereiter language training and a token exchange primarily for correct responses and in six comparison kindergarten classes (□— — —□) where the children received the standard curricula sans language training, sans token exchange.

EXPERIMENT 3: WORKING AT LESSONS

In the past preschoolers or kindergarteners have been used in experimental attempts to change IQ. So in this experiment we decided to investigate the possibility of using verbal and graphic language training including reading, writing, and arithmetic in an attempt to change IQ's of first graders (six- and seven-year-olds). At the same time, it was decided to investigate a related issue. We, as well as others, have observed that disadvantaged children find it difficult to get involved in academic studies, particularly reading and arithmetic. For example, Jensen (1967) has made the following suggestion: "Anyone who has observed disadvantaged children in the classroom, particularly in the primary grades, notes as one of their most outstanding deficiencies these children's inability to sustain attention. This deficiency becomes clearly manifest in the first grade, as soon as reading is introduced and other structured cognitive demands are made upon the child." In addition Jensen suggests that as school proceeds the situation actually deteriorates. "Some children begin actively to resist focusing attention on teacher-oriented tasks and activities. Normal attentional behavior gives way to a kind of seemingly aimless and disruptive hyperactivity."

Pursuant to these ideas, we approached a local school district and persuaded the superintendent to allow us to do a year-long experiment in one of his classes. He was skeptical, hesitant, but finally was willing to allow us to work with thirty-three black children who had completed kindergarten (many of them had been in the Head Start program), but who were ajudged not to be prepared for regular first grade work. Thus, they were placed in a special class in the hope that remedial training would improve their school performance. From a more cynical point of view, this was a remedial kindergarten class segregated to become the slow learners, the truants, the dropouts, the unteachables.

The teacher of this class, Mrs. Bailey, appeared to be dedicated, well-prepared and, in general, quite able. She was effusive in her praise of the children when they were doing well and she would, on occasion, reward the children with a piece of penny candy. However, she did not countenance any nonsense, she ruled the class with a sharp tongue when they got out of order and at times used corporal punishment.

During a one-half hour period each day data were taken on eleven of the thirty-three children in the classroom. The assistant teacher in the class had been hired the year before by our laboratory and trained by our staff. Each day at the beginning of the experimental period the teachers simply assigned the lessons and instructed the children how to do their assigned work. During ten of the thirty minutes, they moved from child to child in the group, helping them, answering their questions, and giving them individual instruction. During the rest of the time, the students were left first with the assistant teacher absent and Mrs. Bailey supervising all thirty-three students, and then with both teachers out of the room.[4]

The work assigned involved discrimination exercises, rhyming exercises and other such paper, pencil, and crayon tasks which required them to draw lines between objects which were alike or which rhymed, and then to color each pair a specified color.

The data in Figure 3.5 show that during this baseline (A) period when tokens were not used, the eleven experimental children worked about 75 percent of the available time when both teachers were present. However, it

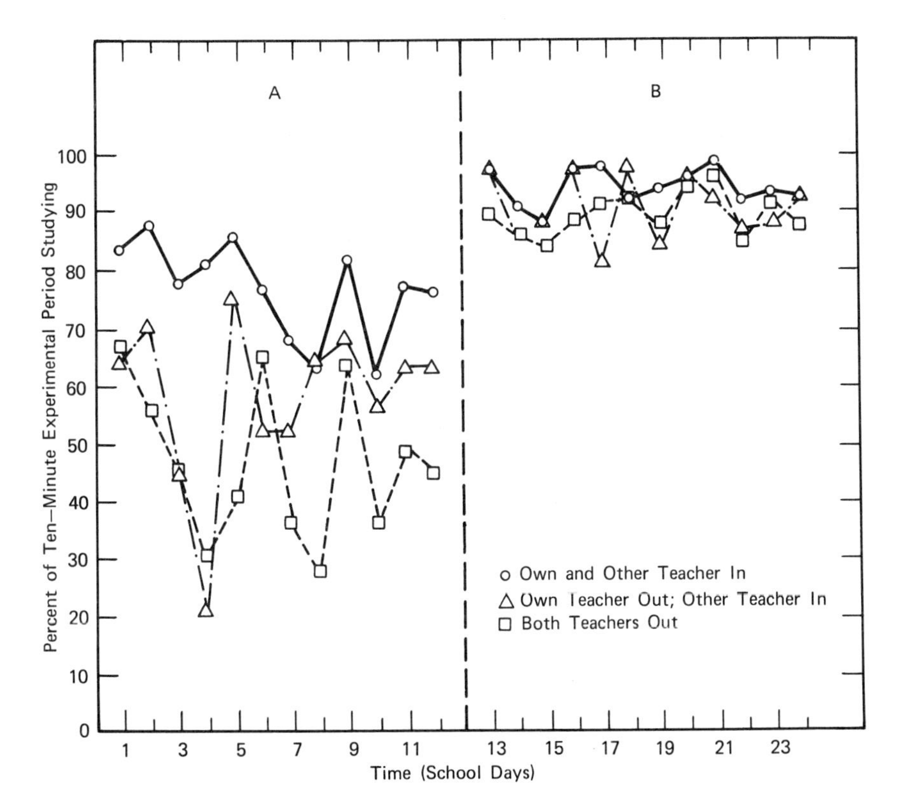

Figure 3.5. Comparison of percent of time children spent in independent work with their own and another teacher in the room, with their own teacher out and another teacher in, and both teachers out of the room during baseline condition A and during condition B with a structured token exchange system.

[4] The sequence of these three experimental periods was changed each day so that no one condition would be disproportionately affected by variables related to time.

is significant to note that, as Jensen suggested it might be, the trend line was downward from about 80 percent at the beginning of this baseline period to about 70 percent toward the end. When the assistant teacher was out of the room, the percentage dropped to between 65 and 55 percent, and when both teachers were out, to something less than 50 percent.

During B when the token exchange was instituted, there was a dramatic change in the children's work pattern. From almost the first day the children worked at their studies about 90 percent of the time, whether both teachers were present or one or both were absent. In other words, the data suggest that the incentive provided by the token exchange enabled the children to maintain a strong work pattern with or without teacher supervision. We had somewhat expected a substantial improvement but not the disappearance of such a differential work pattern.

This is a crucial result in the history of our research, for it was the first that suggested that a token exchange is easily adapted to a larger classroom. Our experience to this point had been with semi-continuous token exchanges which were too time consuming to be practicable in all but a special classroom. At best a good teacher can handle only ten students on such an exchange. However, with a delayed exchange where the rewards are given only for work correctly done, a teacher can manage the normal classroom. Even so, a delayed system will not work until a child is relatively well acculturated. Until this experiment was run with this class of so-called slow learners, we were unsure of the practicality of extending the use of a token exchange to the average size classroom.

EXPERIMENT 4: LEARNING TO READ

According to Mrs. Bailey's judgment of academic ability, the experimental group represented the top third of the class. The second group started the token exchange with Mrs. Bailey at the same time the first group started, and their response was similar, although we never took formal measurements. There were, however, eight children adjudged lowest in academic ability who did not respond to the delayed token exchange. They worked, or at least went through the motions, but did not learn. After watching them for a time, it became apparent that these children had certain learning disabilities. Like the children in Experiment 1, most of them were shy, inhibited talkers, and most had not learned to imitate, that is, to model their behavior after that of the teacher or of the other children who were working the environment successfully for reinforcers. Buckholdt structured a talking exchange for these children similar to that used in Experiment 1, using food for the reinforcer instead of tokens and backups. The response was similar to that which obtained before; after six weeks of two 20 minute sessions per day, most of the eight children were talking fairly well and were able to make the kind of discriminations that kindergarten children usually make.

Then there was the problem of teaching them how to read. For about a month the eight of them worked with Mrs. Bailey and their other classmates to learn the sounds of the different symbols. The other children did well enough, but the eight had no success whatsoever: none learned to associate a single sound with the appropriate symbol during this month. So again we structured a more powerful learning environment, this time giving the children individual instruction from peer tutors, fellow students who had been able to learn best in the usual teacher-student context.

For the purpose of the experiment we randomly divided the eight children into two experimental groups, A and B. In addition, a third group, C, four children who had been trying to learn sounds over a period of six weeks in the regular class setting also without success, was recruited from another classroom.

Every day each child and his tutor would go to a small room at the opposite end of the building from the classroom to work uninterruptedly without supervision on a Language Master for twenty minutes on thirty-three sounds. Alphabet symbols of the sounds (for example, "a" or "th") were pasted in the upper left-hand corner of a Langauge Master card. The sound itself, plus a word beginning with that sound, was recorded on one sound track of the card. For example, if a card had an "m" on the upper left-hand corner, when the child ran the card through the Language Master, he would hear "m, monkey, m." This procedure reduced the chance that the student might learn to associate the wrong sound with the symbol. As noted in Chapter 2, the second sound track on the card was available to the student to record the sound for himself.

After the scheduled twenty minutes our observer would arrive to test the student. She would hold up each of the thirty-three cards and ask the student to identify the sound symbolized on the card. If he identified the appropriate sound within ten seconds, he was given credit for knowing the sound. An exchange was structured for Group A where both the pupil and the tutor were rewarded according to the student's progress in learning the different sounds. Six tokens were given if the student correctly identified the sounds he had identified during the previous experimental session. Two additional tokens were given for each new sound he identified. Also, each day that the student learned two new sounds, both the student and his tutor earned a special prize—a cup of ice cream, a candy bar, or a popsicle.

In Group B, the tutors and students each received eight tokens at the beginning of each twenty-minute session which they attended, regardless of their progress. And as usual the tokens could be traded for material reinforcers. Group C received no tokens or other material reinforcers. Rather, the tutor-student pairs simply met every day for their twenty-minute period, during which the tutor tried to teach the student his sounds. However, the observer gave the tutor and his student approval when the student demonstrated progress.

What happened? The summary data for the three groups are given in Figure 3.6. While the differences among the three groups are substantial, it is obvious that peer tutoring itself had a powerful educational effect. Even C, the group which showed the least progress, learned the sounds of a significant number of symbols; their median at the end of twenty days was 13.5. Rachel learned twenty-seven sounds; Andrew, twenty-two; Linda, five; and Jerry, none. The individual attention, the patience of the peer tutors helped, but even so, theirs was a spotty performance which is to be expected when an instructional system for slow children relies on conditioned reinforcers. The children in Group B did better; the median learned in twenty days was twenty-three. However, predictably, the greatest effect obtained was with Group A; their median was thirty-three sounds learned to criterion. When the tutoring experiment was over, the children who had not learned all of their symbols were put on a token exchange with their tutors, as Group A, until they had learned to criterion all thirty three.

The training evidently generalized. A month before the experiment, the

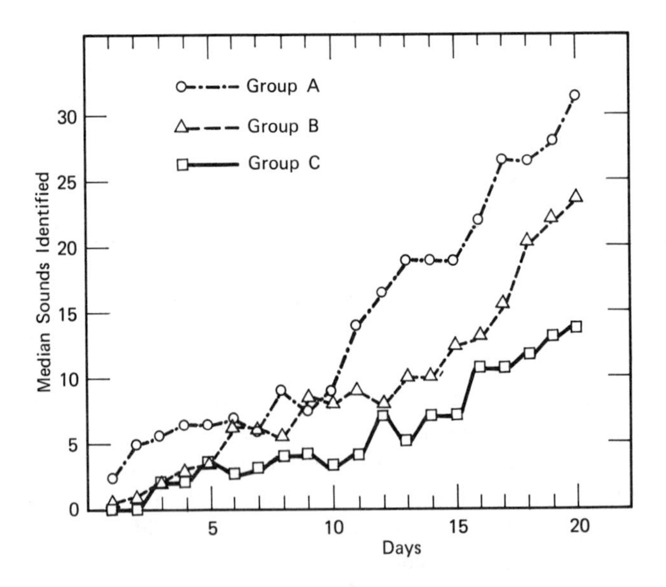

Figure 3.6. Effects of peer tutoring for Group A with material reinforcers for learning sounds, Group B with material reinforcers for attendance, and Group C with no material reinforcers.

eight had miserably failed the Metropolitan Reading Readiness Test. Afterwards, all passed with quite satisfactory scores as may be noted in Table 3.3. In tribute to such a performance, we now began to refer to them as the "famous eight!"

EXPERIMENT 5: IQ CHANGE

While some of the students were participants in the experiments reported above, the entire remedial kindergarten was used for a year-long demonstration. After the first month which was baseline, a delayed token exchange was instituted for the entire class where demonstrated progress in the usual kindergarten and the first grade curricula was reinforced with tokens which could be used to buy cookies and ice cream in the late morning recess, toys and other backups in the later afternoon recess.

The overall progress of the total class is indicated by the before/after IQ scores from different forms of the California Mental Maturity Test. These data are given in Figure 3.7 for the children who were in school all year. The median IQ in the fall was 82 points, in the spring, 100 points. Thus the class had an increase in their median IQ of 18 points.[5]

Table 3.3. Reading Readiness Test Scores for the "Famous Eight" Before and After Peer Tutoring Experiment.

	Test Scores[a]	
Child	Before Peer Tutoring (February)	After Peer Tutoring (April)
Ann	41	55
Howard	36	56
Dan	5	52
Terry	21	57
Bob	33	54
Tim	28	55
Ed	22	54
Susan	31	56

[a] Passing Score is 52; maximum, 58.

[5] In general, the "famous eight" and the other students who started out in the bottom half of the class did relatively better (with an increase in their median of 38 IQ points) than did those who started out in the top half (whose increase in median was 12 IQ points). Such differential improvement is typical of most classrooms, including the others reported in this chapter, and is in part, at least, due to the unreliability of the testing instruments which results in a regression toward the mean (cf. Diederich, 1956).

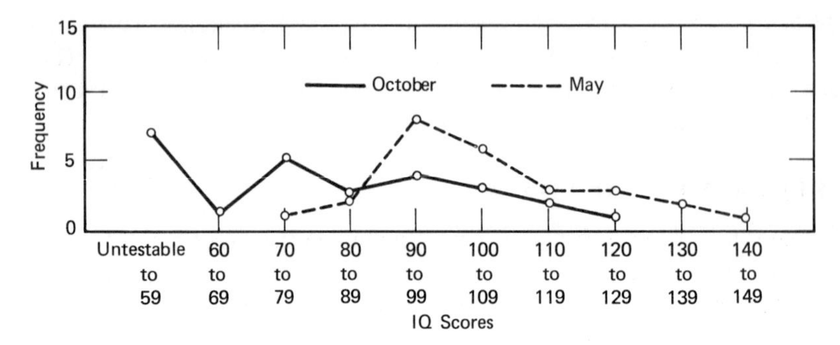

Figure 3.7. October–May IQ frequency distributions (California Mental Maturity); Mrs. Bailey's inner-city first grade class.

Three boys who initially scored in the upper half of the class also experienced substantial declines in IQ's over the year. They were among nine children whom Mrs. Bailey sometimes rattan whipped or otherwise punished during the half days when Buckholdt was at another school. While the other children seemed to withstand her punishment, these boys did not. They progressively withdrew as the year wore on. While Mrs. Bailey was excellent in many ways, she apparently could not avoid reverting occasionally to her old punitive ways and these boys unfortunately paid for her lapses.

DISCUSSION AND SUMMARY

The above series of experiments suggest that the early social learning environment of inner-city children is apparently such that many develop a language deficit which artificially depresses their IQ's. In any event, as we have seen, when put in an environment especially designed for the acquisition of language, even the most handicapped of these children acquired normal language expertise within a few months time. Data from two subsequent experiments further suggest that language training results in an increase in measured IQ. A median improvement of 15 points (12 points plus 3, the median loss of the comparison children) obtained when a language program developed by Carl Bereiter and associates was used in six kindergarten classes and an 18 point increase obtained when a verbal and graphic language program (including reading and arithmetic) was used with six- and seven-year-olds in a remedial kindergarten. If, as suggested in the second chapter, MA is interpreted as a cumulative rate of learning of certain rather general intellectual abilities, then the increment in that rate is approximately double that of previous years. In the kindergartens, for example, the median MA increased from fifty-five months to sixty-six months, or eleven months; their previous average increase in MA was a little less than six months for a similar seven month period.

The experimental data suggest that the slower MA related learning for inner-city children (.85 MA levels per year on the average) may be primarily the result of the weak, conditioned positive reinforcers used in their traditional school and home environments. At least, when strong material reinforcers were used for correct work in the instructional exchanges in our experiments, MA related learning rates increased from well below to well above normal. Similarly, the "aimless hyperactivity" so characteristic of some inner-city children in the traditional educational system was replaced by an intense work pattern.

Consistent with the results of the last chapter, the data in this chapter indicate that behavior rates accelerate as the strength of the related reinforcers increases; and conversely, the rate decelerates as the strength of related reinforcers decreases. In the last chapter the experiments with young suburban children suggest that this principle held for attending lessons, cooperating in peer tutoring with or without a teaching machine, and indirectly in the rate of learning symbolic contingencies (reading, arithmetic) to criterion. It would seem that the results of the experiments described in this chapter—adding material reinforcers to increase the total strength of reinforcers for correct work—accelerated the rate of talking (by a factor of six), the rate of attending lessons (from between 40 percent to 70 percent of the available time to 95 percent) and the rate of acquisition of MA related abilities as measured on standardized IQ tests (by a factor of two). These results then are consistent with our earlier findings.

However we also encountered some situations in which the acceleration-deceleration principle failed to obtain. In the case of some children it was necessary to strengthen component patterns by having them work learning environments designed for the acquisition of the component skills before they were able to work more complex tasks for reinforcers regardless of their strength. Thus in the first experiment the non talkers were unable to work the academic exchange for tokens and backups, since these children were verbally inhibited. Consequently, for remediation it was necessary to structure a special learning environment to accelerate talking *per se* and thus allow the children to increase their talking skills. In such an environment the rate of talking did increase and in three or four months the children had acquired normal talking expertise as measured on several criteria. Then, when put into the regular learning environment where the material reinforcers were exchanged for correct academic work they were able to make normal progress. The normal talking skills apparently were an essential component of correct academic work. Similar results were obtained with the "famous eight."

In general, educational environments should be designed to accelerate component behaviors and develop component expertise which are then synthesized at a later stage with other component behaviors and expertise for the acceleration of more complex behaviors and the acquisition of more complex expertise. If the scheduling is done appropriately, all of the component patterns are accelerated and the component skills are acquired before an attempt is made to accelerate the more complex patterns and acquire the more complex expertise.

Also, as we have seen, the repetitive reinforcement of the more complex pattern indirectly maintains the original equilibrium of the component pattern. Thus, in the case of speech in Experiment 1 the equilibrium was maintained in the four month follow-up via indirect reinforcement. The speech patterns were components of correct academic work which was being reinforced during that follow-up period. As we will become increasingly aware, the problem of maintaining behavior patterns once they are acquired is considerable. Most patterns of behavior, although they are not reinforced directly, are maintained indirectly because they are essential to the production of other criterion behaviors which are, themselves, reinforced repetitively. In subsequent chapters we will come back to the maintenance problem time and time again and will find that indirect reinforcement is a major strategy for maintenance. It is, perhaps, the most effective of all strategies.

We will not pretend that the experimental results presented in this chapter are definitive—much remains to be learned about structuring optimal learning environments in inner-city and other classrooms. Nevertheless, the data suggest that the defect which results in the cumulative deficit typical of many children in inner-city schools lies not with the children, but with their educational environment. In fact, the data suggest that given an appropriate learning environment, inner-city children may be educated for the more technical, the more demanding jobs which in our society seem to grow in number faster than they can be adequately filled by the graduates of the present educational system.

EPILOGUE 1: THE FATE OF MRS. BAILEY'S CLASS

Mrs. Bailey's class was inherited by Mrs. Ward. She was competent enough when she made an effort to be so, but during this second grade year she moonlighted on a second full-time job. As a consequence, she was generally tired, without a teaching plan, very disorganized. While she gave her children the usual academic fare, she made her assignments ineffectually and slowly. The children, therefore, were reinforced primarily for quiet, busy-work. The results were catastrophic.

As may be recalled, before they went into Mrs. Ward's class their median IQ was 100. The following spring, after being in Mrs. Ward's class a full academic year, the median was 86, a decline of 14 IQ points! We did not fully anticipate such negative results, but wondered, nevertheless, what would happen if these children were placed, if only for one period a day, into a more favorable learning environment. Consequently, the staff conducted a special arithmetic experiment with these children for eight weeks toward the end of the academic year. This training apparently resulted in approximately one half levels median improvement in arithmetic. In that particular experiment the children were repeatedly reinforced for correct answers for simple addition and subtraction problems during ten-minute periods, morning and afternoon each day for the last eight weeks of spring term. By simply reinforcing their correct performance, that is, giving them a penny for every two problems correctly worked, most of the children, using their counting frames, were able to develop a working knowledge of the borrowing and carrying principles. Toward the end several were getting over fifty of a possible sixty problems correct in ten minutes. During those eight weeks they covered the work in three notebooks, more than twice as much as they had done in the previous seven months. These were not stupid children!

EPILOGUE 2: TERRY HOLDER, A CASE STUDY

When Terry Holder entered Mrs. Bailey's first grade, adults terrified him. Whenever a teacher approached, he trembled and often covered his face with paper or his hands. When his teacher was not nearby, he would sit quietly, rocking back and forth, sometimes humming, smiling to himself but usually in complete silence. Other children did not disturb or frighten him, but they were unable to talk with him or interest him in any way. If they tried, he completely ignored them. He had erected a silent, rocking shell around himself that was virtually impenetrable. Most clinicians would probably have diagnosed him as moderately autistic.

His parents, constantly drunk, paid little attention to him except for whippings and tongue lashings. He was rarely allowed to play outdoors with friends. A neighbor observed that his parents never "paid him no mind unless he was messing up."

His ability to communicate verbally had been so inhibited that it was difficult, if not impossible, to teach him anything at school. He could not identify shapes, he could not name the colors, he could not count; he simply did not have the basic skills which kindergarten children need and are expected to have mastered. At first the teachers believed that he was merely shy. "In a few weeks he will come around." But after two months, while not quite as frightened of adults as he had been, he was still practically mute and virtually unteachable.

In December, with the rest of the "famous eight," Terry worked food exchanges with Buckholdt twice daily for twenty minutes a session. As may be recalled, they were reinforced with cookies, ice cream, soda and candy for following simple directions, for counting, for identifying colors and the like. Although Terry progressed a little, he remained considerably behind the other children in his group. The teachers now believed he was "retarded." One suggested that we would be wasting any further time spent with him and recommended that we concentrate exclusively on the more promising children.

However, we were not ready to abandon Terry. We sensed an untapped intelligence. He appeared to understand what was happening in the classroom even though he was not participating. On numerous occasions, he tried to answer the teacher's questions. Sounds would perch and twist on his lips but he usually could not make words of them. When tested in late October he earned a 57 IQ score, evidence that he was able to do some work.

In early February, the experimenters tried a new approach. Terry's verbal skills had not developed through imitating other children so we decided to work directly on them. First, we had to teach him to respond to questions from the teacher. He had occasionally tried to answer Mrs. Bailey's questions, but was able to respond only after long delays and with much prodding. To correct this, Mrs. Bailey structured an exchange that rewarded only prompt answers.

Terry loved chocolate M&M's so these became his first reinforcers. Twice a day the teacher called Terry to her desk and displayed eight to ten M&M's in her hand. If he named the color of each she pointed to within five seconds, he received it. If he did not, it was put back in a can. Since Terry had shown earlier that he knew all the colors, reward was contingent only on his prompt, correct answers. For the first two or three sessions he was able to earn only a few M&M's. But by the fifth session he responded quickly enough to earn all of them; and he kept this up for the last five sessions. The requirements were then escalated. M&M's were still used as rewards, but they were acquired by prompt naming of familiar objects (book, pencil, eraser, chalk, etc.) which the teacher presented to Terry. The verbal skill developed in the previous sessions increased rapidly and Terry was usually able to give the correct names as he learned them.

Although within a week and a half Terry was responding promptly and consistently to the teacher's questions, he still had a verbal deficiency. He responded with one word answers or with broken phrases; he still lacked the free verbal style and the ability to use syntax of most of his classmates and he still refused to talk to his classmates.

Therefore, with Mrs. Bailey's help two strategies were designed to continue his development. First, he was reinforced with praise and tokens whenever the teachers noticed him talking with other children; and if he responded to a question in class or initiated conversation with the teacher, he was immediately rewarded. However, the pressure of thirty-three other children in the class prevented the teacher from providing a more effective continuous exchange. Second, a new, more demanding exchange was structured especially for Terry. For two fifteen-minute periods each day, Mrs. Bailey taught him how to tell a story. She would first show him a picture of farm animals, birds, jungle beasts or perhaps Indians and then make up a story about them. When she finished, she would ask Terry to retell the story or preferably to make up a new version. Terry was reinforced with praise, tokens, and M&M's every twenty seconds that he was able to talk, relating his story.

At first he talked for only fifteen to thirty seconds per period, but by the second week he was able to continue telling a story without stopping for two minutes. By the end of the third week he reached a maximum six minute period without interruption. His stories were not smooth; he often told the same part over and over, but he talked in sentences most of the time and continued his monologue for a full six minutes—more than twelve times what he could do in the beginning.

By the end of this three week period, Terry had become quite verbal—too much so in Mrs. Bailey's opinion. As though trying to compensate for those years of silence, he talked to anyone who would listen and often to those who would not. He answered any question asked of him, and often returned with a question of his own. His speech was now spontaneous and free, at least by the standards of the usual classroom.

We had noted similar rapid speech development the previous year in the preschool experiment, so what surprised us most was the improvement in Terry's school work. He gradually began to do the assignments along with the others, and before long he was making amazing progress. Shortly before speech training and the aforementioned peer tutoring experiment began, he scored a miserable 21 points out of a possible 58 on the test on prereading skills. But after speech training and after the tutoring experiment, he earned a retest score of 57. Only one child in the whole class had ever earned a higher score!

Terry's new-found skills and motivation continued to propel him throughout the rest of the school year. Via peer tutoring, he quickly learned and was soon able to identify complete words, then groups of words. In the last weeks of school, the teacher gave the children a list of words they were required to know if they were to complete the series of introductory readers before the end of school. On the last week, a contest was held to determine who had learned the most words. Terry was the only one in the class who knew them all.

Terry had become a completely different child by June. The previous

September, he seemed dull, autistic. His IQ score of 57, if anything, overestimated his classroom performance. He seemed to be unteachable. Six months later, after working a series of appropriately designed instructional exchanges, he was bright, spontaneous, and motivated. Furthermore, his new IQ score of 131 mirrored his progress. Terry had made a remarkable change from the bottom to the top of his class! Terry and we had seemingly won.

However, there are no cheap victories. Permanent modifications of behavior patterns come only with permanent changes in the learning environment. In Terry's case we had not changed his home environment. His parents were still alcoholics, and they still alternately neglected and brutalized him. So we wondered what would happen to him over the summer.

Actually, very little seemed to have happened. The following fall Terry continued to talk at a slightly higher than normal rate. He continued to be outgoing, continued to be friendly with his teachers and with his peers. However, like many children his age, he seemed to find it difficult to settle down to the everyday routine in school. In particular he had difficulty making progress in the larger classroom situation. In a small group or with peer tutoring he learned quickly and well, but not in the larger class. Also, he began to show an aggressive pattern towards his peers; he sometimes threatened a beating after school for those who outshone him in classwork. We thought this was a good sign, evidence that Terry continued to care about school achievement—an antithesis of his earlier, more serious, seclusive autistic pattern. Besides, we felt we knew how to work with Terry to help him overcome his developing hyperaggressiveness and his newfound academic difficulties.

Then a genuine tragedy happened. Terry's parents moved out of the school district and, although they could have made arrangements to have Terry continue with us, they evidently chose not to do so. In the ensuing months we had several reports. We were told Terry was continuing to talk freely and well. Then we lost track of him until two weeks before the end of the school year. One morning the principal brought him to our experimental class to enroll him once again.

The first reaction of those of us who had known him, had grown to appreciate him and even to love him, was one of elation. Terry Holder was back! But that elation was quickly replaced by deep grief for this was no longer the Terry Holder that we had known. He had regressed in those months away from us; he no longer talked to anyone except almost inaudibly to the assistant teacher who had worked with him some the year before. Again, he was the frightened little boy, unable to sit still, unable to concentrate, unable to learn.

We have not had a direct report about what happened to Terry Holder during those eight months he was away. However, in addition to an unhealthy home situation, he could have been exposed to the rattan whip, used by some teachers in the school system in question to bring into line those children who are hypertalkative and/or hyperaggressive. When he left us, Terry Holder was both to a degree, but more hypertalkative than aggressive, and so a likely candidate for the rattan. As with some children who are so punished, Terry could have withdrawn again into that impenetrable shell. And, of course, in a pathogenic classroom once he had withdrawn to the point where he would fit in quietly without bothering his neighbors or teacher, he could have been left alone, if only to vegetate.

The depth to which Terry had regressed was gauged during the last week of school when the children were again given an IQ test. Terry was unable to sit still long enough to concentrate well enough to make one correct response. He was untestable. Terry had certainly followed a roller coaster course. In twenty months his IQ performance, as measured on different forms of the California Mental Maturity Test, had changed from 57 to 131 to untestable. This is one reversal which we did not plan, nor are we certain that the damage can be repaired. We can only try. Oh, God, when will such tragedies stop happening to little children!

SUMMARY

These two cases were included as an epilogue because they represent important data which qualify the effectiveness of our work. These two cases make it perfectly clear that the gains so painstakingly made in our experimental work can easily be destroyed. Some will say that these regressions in IQ show that we have not really changed the mental functioning of these children.

To us the data alternatively suggest that learning environments can vary tremendously in value and in potency. Some are orthogenic, that is they help the child acquire pro-normal patterns; others are pathogenic, they cause the child to lose pro-normal patterns and they foster withdrawal or the development of bizarre, disruptive patterns. Furthermore, the various orthogenic and pathogenic environments apparently vary in potency. Some foster a higher rate of learning than others.

The orthogenic environments which we have structured to accelerate the acquisition of MA related abilities were evidentally fairly potent; at least the acquisition rates increased approximately by a factor of two. Thus, the mental age (MA) increments during the seven month period covered by the experiments when added to previous increments apparently increased measured IQ from 15 to 18 points on the average. In our view MA learning rates are precisely like any other learning rates—if they are to be maintained the learning environment must be maintained; if they are to be accelerated further or decelerated the environment must be changed accordingly. In the two instances described in the Epilogue cases the environments were not held constant but changed radically, actually in value from being orthogenic to being more or less pathogenic and the results were catastrophic, as we have noted.

There are other cases on record where massive IQ changes were induced (Skodak and Skeels, 1949; Skeels, 1966). In those instances massive IQ changes were observed when children were introduced into qualitatively better learning environments and the induced changes were maintained because the improved environments were maintained. The changes, 15 to 30 IQ points on individual Stanford-Binet tests, were if anything larger than those reported in our experiments.

The implication is, it may not be enough to provide powerful orthogenic learning environments for children whose progress is slow during their preschool, kindergarten, or even their primary years, that for such children the entire educational system may have to be strengthened.

CHAPTER 4

Inner-City Classes: Problems and Procedures

THE ACADEMIC ACHIEVEMENT EXPERIMENTS

In the experiments with inner-city children in the previous chapter the instructional environments were designed in detail by Buckholdt, Doss, and Hamblin and the teachers were coached and supervised on a daily basis to insure that the systems were put into effect as designed.[1] In the following series of experiments we took a quite different tack, in part, to see how well teachers with minimal training and supervision could do with a token exchange.[2] We had two reasons for this. (1) We wanted to test the limits of our exchange procedures to see, in effect, if teachers and their students could benefit from them with minimal training and without major changes in the curricula. (2) We wanted to learn how our instructional exchange system might be subverted or misused when teachers and others began to adopt them to their own purposes with little supervision. In both these respects the year's work was at least partially successful.

In six experimental classes the teachers were trained by our staff and were given the resources required to run a token exchange. In addition,

[1] Hamblin, Buckholdt and Ferritor took the major responsibility for writing this chapter.

[2] Instead of spending three to four hours every day in each class, Buckholdt spent three to four hours every week and in two cases where the classes were located in Tennessee only six days during the entire school year. In general, as before, the teachers were all taught to structure learning environments using token exchanges, primarily via the case study method. Also, all were given the opportunity to read and discuss expositions of the principles of operant conditioning as well as the preliminary exposition of exchange theory and procedure as described in the early reports of our experiments. All were coached and their problems discussed.

there were five comparison classes.[3] The overall achievement results are given in Table 4.1. Note that in every instance the experimental classes did better than did their comparison classes. The data indicated, however, that two of the six experimental teachers benefited their classes minimally by having them on a token exchange. They did just slightly better than their comparison classes, and that slight edge would probably not have been obtained in Mrs. Ward's class had we not intervened with our arithmetic experiment. However, in the other four classes the differences are substantial. On the average by the end of the year these four classes were approximately on level—i.e. at their norm—whereas their comparison classes averaged six months behind the norm.

A more detailed picture of the results and of what the experimental teachers did to get their results is both interesting and informative, even if it is tentative, essentially *post factum*. We will start with the most successful of the two fourth grade classes.

Mrs. Allen's Class

Mrs. Allen created an ingenious learning environment for her fourth grade class. She used workbooks, worksheets, games and tests which allowed her to reinforce correct work in every area of the curricula with tokens and other more subtle reinforcers. Although she sometimes reinforced children for behaving well, for starting to work the minute an assignment was given or for being at work in the seats when she returned from being out of the room, at least 90 percent of her tokens were for work correctly completed.

Because the school system used the Iowa Basic Skills Test scores to gauge progress, and in effect, to decide their later fate as students, Mrs. Allen felt it was important to help her students do well on this test. First, she isolated those materials in the curricula which corresponded to the areas to be tested by the Iowa Basic, and taught those first. In addition, the slower children were tutored during recesses, lunch hours, or after school by peers and by Mrs. Allen.

Before starting with us, Mrs. Allen had been using an exchange system which she had developed by trial and error over her teaching career. Our training simply helped her to refine, to strengthen an already effective learning environment. In prior years she had been able to develop her charges to the point where they progressed 1.0 to 1.1 levels on the Iowa test. Although our experimental system was in effect for only five months, Mrs. Allen's class showed an average improvement of 1.9 academic levels (see

[3] There were supposed to be six, but in the spring the teacher of one of the fourth grade comparison classes declined to allow us to give the second set of achievement tests. The experimental teachers were selected in part because of their interest in our instructional exchanges. Hence, our results may be tinged because of "self selection."

Table 4.1. Before/After Achievement Data for Six Experimental Comparisons.

	Norm	Before/After Achievement Data	
		Experimental Classes	Comparison Classes
Mrs. Allen, 4th grade	4.9	1.9 levels to 5.3	.6 levels to 4.1
Mr. Smythe, 4th grade	4.9	1.4 levels to 4.7	
Mrs. Johnson, 1st grade	1.8	1.8	1.3
Mrs. James, 1st grade	1.8	1.7	1.3
Mrs. Ward, 2nd grade	2.8	.35 levels to 1.7	.35 levels to 1.5
Mrs. Easton, 1st grade	1.9	1.3	1.2

Figure 4.1). The children were tested first in late November; they averaged 3.4, .8 levels behind the norm which was 4.2. By June their median was 5.3, 4 months above the norm, 4.9. The comparison class showed an average improvement of .6 levels.

Mr. Smythe's Class

The results of the second experimental fourth grade class were not as spectacular; yet they are important because they involve a completely different way of organizing a class for peer tutoring. In the peer tutoring experiments we have reviewed thus far, the teacher assigned specific students to tutor other specific pupils on particular subjects; the tutor and pupils were rewarded according to the pupils' demonstrated progress. Such a formal system, while effective, requires a great deal in the way of thought and organization from the teacher. The alternative is to restructure the instructional exchange so that students are reinforced not for individual progress but for the progress subgroups make on the tests. Thus, reinforcers could be given on the basis of the group average, the average of the top three students or of the bottom three students. The advantage of most group reinforcement arrangements is that they provide an incentive for students to help one another master the academic materials in question without the elaborate organization and attention required in experiments with individual tutoring and individual incentives.

Over the academic year, each of the five subgroups into which the class was broken were on group or individual exchange contingencies at least eight months.[4] They were given tokens daily for correct work done on

[4] Each subgroup was equated on initial ability, represented the actual range of ability found in the class so that within each subgroup there were high and low achievers. This experiment was done by Craig Hathaway who is presently analyzing the data in detail for his Ph.D. dissertation at Washington University.

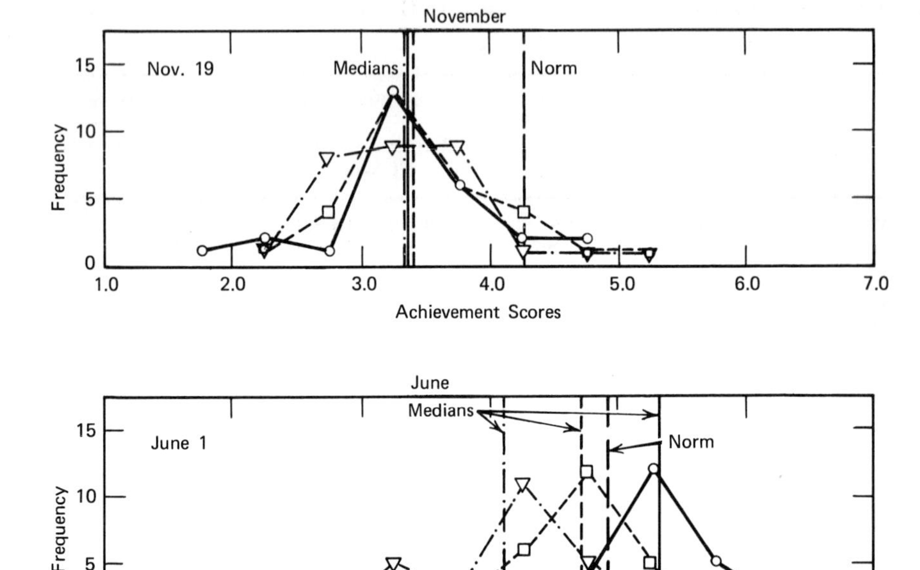

Figure 4.1. November and June frequency distributions for three fourth grade classes—Mrs. Allen (O———O), Mr. Smythe (□— — —□) and comparison (△----△)—on the Iowa Basic Skills Test.

assignments and on Monday-Friday tests. As may be noted in Figure 4.1, the class scored on the average 3.3 when they took the Iowa Basic Skills Test in November, and they scored on the average of 4.7 when they took an alternate form of the test during the first week of June. Although they were not quite up to the norm, 4.9, this class made very substantial progress from testing a full academic level behind the norm in November.

Mr. Smythe's greatest difficulty was in giving assignments with which the children could help one another. He, like most reared in our culture, was individually oriented and it took him some time to learn how to give assignments that did not preclude mutual help. There was one notable bonus which we did not anticipate. Mr. Smythe found it difficult to tolerate talking when the students were on individual contingencies. However, when his class was on group contingencies he learned to relax and to ignore their talking; during the study periods they were "supposed" to help one another.

At this juncture the performance of the fourth grade comparison class should be noted. From November to June, the comparison class progressed on the average from 3.4 to 4.1 on the Iowa Basic Skills Test. This means that by the end of the year the controls were performing at a level normal for a beginning fourth grade class so they were .8 levels behind. Nevertheless they had progressed .6 academic levels in eight months.[5]

Mrs. Johnson's and Mrs. James' Classes

As may be recalled from Table 4.1, Mrs. Johnson's and Mrs. James' classes were, over all, about on level at the end of the school year. However, the performances on arithmetic and reading were quite different, and the evident reasons for the differences are interesting. These two first grade classes located in Tennessee had been designated by the school system as "Follow Through" classes.[6] Because of this, the room was furnished with a number of rather interesting mathematical games, but most significantly from our point of view the children were furnished with a series of consumable arithmetic workbooks which they could work through at their own speed. The teachers gave the children tokens in proportion to the number of problems they did correctly and as a result most of the children made rather remarkable progress. The median scores on the Metropolitan Achievement Tests by Mrs. Johnson's and Mrs. James' experimental classes on arithmetic as pictured in Figure 4.2 were 2.0 and 1.95 respectively. These levels are in excess of the norm 1.8 (since the tests were given in early May). In contrast the two comparison classes did miserably, although one was also a "Follow Through" class. Both scored on the average 1.0. This is a very substantial difference in relative and in absolute terms.

The experimental results on reading were, in comparison, not nearly so good. In fact, they were no better on the average than those obtained by the comparison classes as may be noted in Figure 4.3. Why? As in the comparison classes the curriculum involved reading in groups with the teacher and reinforcement for progress as they read. This teaching procedure might have been effective but the pace set by the teachers may have been too slow. They were hesitant about "pushing" the children, about expecting too much.

[5] The teacher, Mrs. Green, told our tester that she had tried very hard to do a good job, that she wanted her class to do well in comparison to the two experimental classes. In retrospect, she did do well, better than our comparison teachers have done on the average. In eight months of instruction the average comparison class fell behind two to four months; hers fell behind one month.

[6] The "Follow Through" program is sponsored by the U. S. Office of Economic Opportunity as the continuation of their Head Start program into the primary years of school. The classes benefited by the "Follow Through" program were given money, on a per student, per year basis, to enrich the educational environment. In this school system most of the money was spent on teacher's aids, experimental curricula, various types of teaching machines, and other classroom equipment.

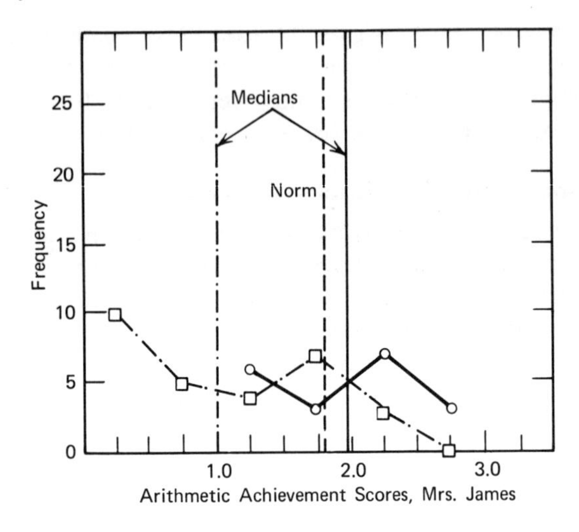

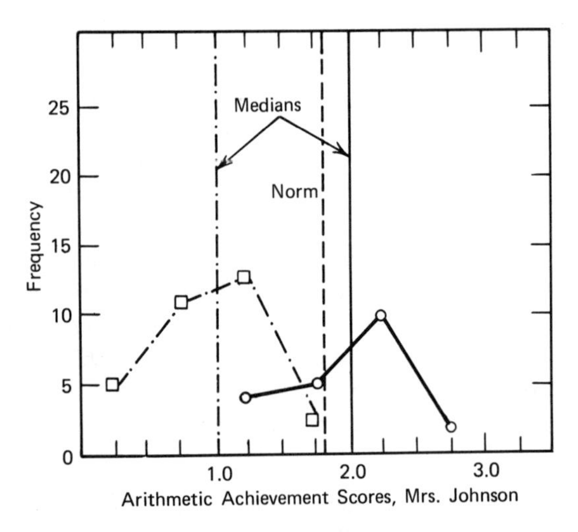

Figure 4.2. Frequency distribution for Mrs. James' (top) and Mrs. Johnson's (bottom) first grades (○———○) and the comparison classes (□— — —□) measuring arithmetic concepts and skills administered in the Spring, 1969.

Missing also were assignments to learn vocabulary words via peer tutoring or via the Language Master which was furnished each room by "Follow Through." Absent were the easy, interesting readers which the children could read and be tested on for comprehension. Missing were workbooks and work sheets to give the children interesting games to work for correct answers. Had these curricula materials been used together with the token exchange for correct work, the children's progress in reading theoretically would have been in excess of level.

Mrs. Ward's and Mrs. Easton's Classes

It may be recalled that Mrs. Ward's rather special problems were discussed toward the end of the last chapter (she moonlighted on a second

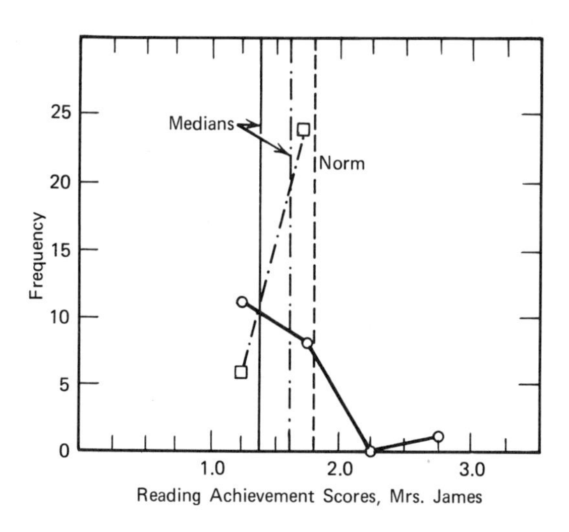

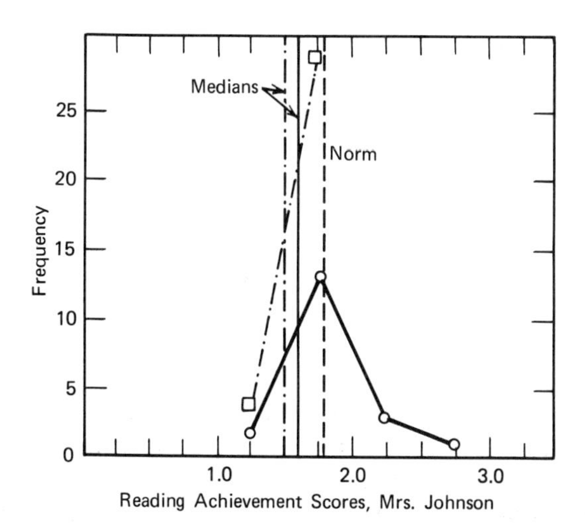

Figure 4.3. Frequency distribution for Mrs. James' (top) and Mrs. Johnson's (bottom) experimental first grades (O———O) and the comparison classes (□— — —□) measuring reading on the Metropolitan Achievement Test Administered in May, 1969.

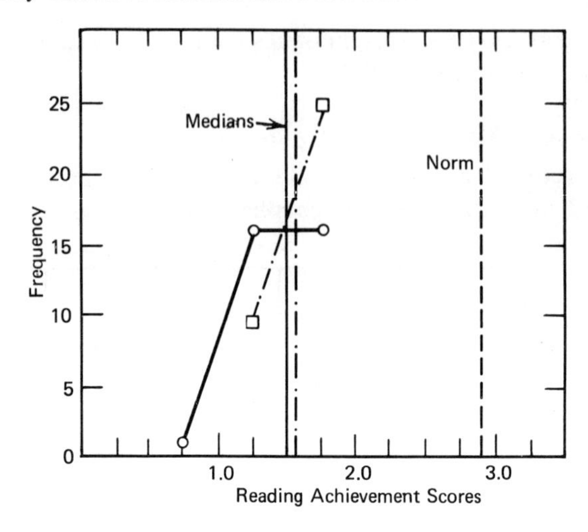

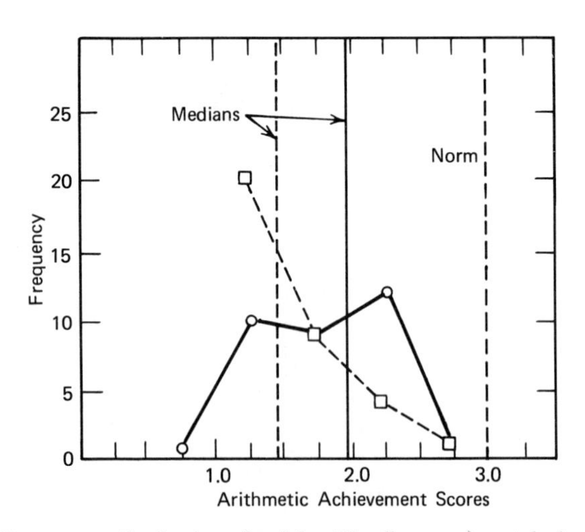

Figure 4.4. Frequency distributions for Mrs. Ward's experimental class (O——O) and the comparison class (□— — —□) measuring reading and arithmetic skills on the California Achievement Test administered in the Spring.

full-time job which made her tired and disorganized). The data from her second grade class along with those of the comparison class are given in Figure 4.4. In reading her children made one month's progress as measured on alternate forms of the Metropolitan Achievement Test given in early October and early June. This compared to four month's improvement in reading registered in the comparison class. In arithmetic the gains were six and three months respectively which put Mrs. Ward's class ahead of the comparison class. However, that gain, it may be recalled, was largely due to an eight week experiment by the staff which was done at the end of the year, during which time the experimental children worked through the problems presented in three workbooks.

The data for Mrs. Easton's first grade class and the comparison class are given in Figure 4.5. There the picture is somewhat similar to the one obtained in the previous figure. The experimental class did somewhat better than the

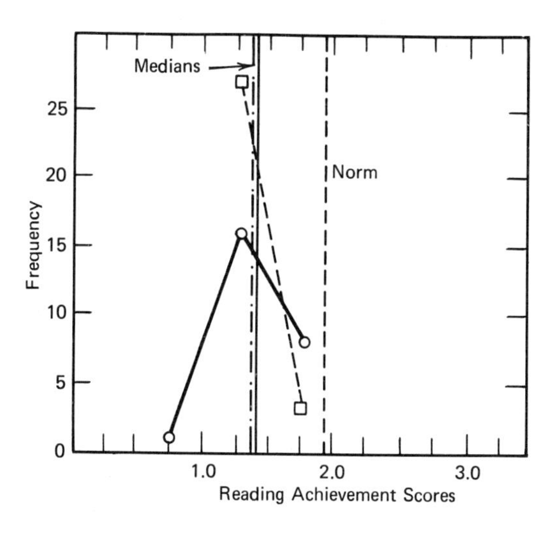

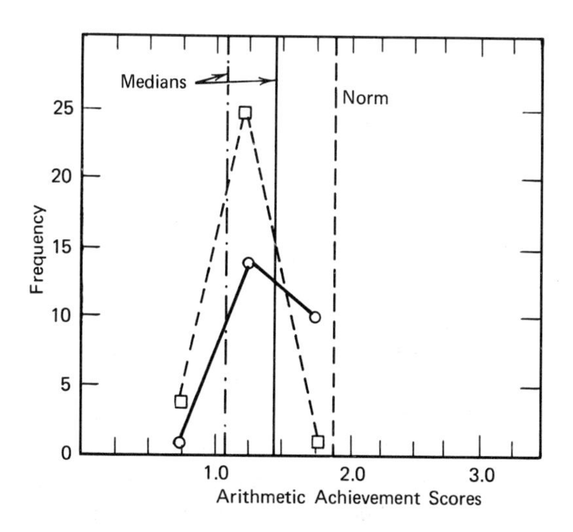

Figure 4.5. Frequency distributions for Mrs. Easton's experimental first grade class (O——O) and a comparison class (□– – –□) on reading and arithmetic skills on the California Achievement Test, June, 1969.

comparison class with progress in arithmetic being greater than the progress in reading. Actually Mrs. Easton did rather a good job, given what she had to work with. In her particular school the children in the primary years are graded and promoted according to reading ability. The A1 children are those who, like the remedial first grade in the previous chapter did not pass kindergarten, are adjudged too immature to begin learning materials to pass the prereading test. Children classified A2 are adjudged mature enough to begin learning the material required to pass the prereading test, and B1 is assigned to those first grade children who have passed the test; thus there can be a great difference between A1 and B1 children. They generally represent the extremes of the inner-city continuum of six-year-olds. It so happens that the class assigned Mrs. Easton included no A2 and B1 students; all were A1's. The comparison class, on the other hand, was composed almost entirely of B1 students; there were a few A2's. Thus, Mrs. Easton did fairly well. In fact, at the end of the year her class was almost as well off as was the second grade comparison class (whose data were given earlier in Figure 4.4). The composition of that second grade class at the beginning of first grade was one half A1 and the other half A2.

This is not to imply that there were no problems in the way Mrs. Easton conducted her class. She, like the other experimental teachers, did some things and failed to do others which resulted in her students' not making the progress they might have otherwise made. In fact, our thousands of hours of observation in these and other experimental and comparison classrooms have led us to the conclusion that most teachers in one way or another fail to help their students progress. However, rather than personalize these problems in the discussion of a specific teacher, we will now turn to problematic teaching procedures in general and contrast them with the recommended procedures. It is to be recognized at the outset that some of the problematic and recommended procedures have been evaluated more adequately than others.

PROBLEMATIC AND RECOMMENDED PROCEDURES

Behavioral Objectives

As mentioned in the last chapter one of the main theories which has been proposed to account for the underachievement of inner-city children is the expectation theory (Clark, 1965, 1966; Rosenthal and Jacobson, 1968). According to the expectation theory teachers in inner-city schools simply do not expect enough of their students and, therefore, accept a performance much below their capacity. This, in turn, results in the cumulative deficit documented by the Coleman data. While the expectation theory may not be adequate to explain the general cumulative deficit of inner-city students, it does apply in our experimental classrooms with the use of a token exchange. The token exchange, if at all well designed and managed, essentially solves the motivational problems that beset inner-city students. The result is that the children are enabled to do with pleasure two to three times more work than they were formerly able to do. However, many of our experimental teachers have found it difficult to change their expectations, that is, to expect and then plan for two to three times more work than formerly. The usual result is that such teachers do, in fact, waste their students' and their own time by giving them forty-minute time allotments for lessons that could be completed in fifteen minutes; they settle for much less progress than might be obtained. To correct this situation teachers using a token exchange are advised to develop a clear set of ultimate behavioral objectives which are realistic for the students in their classes.

In the teaching of complex skills, such as those involved in verbal language, reading, writing and mathematics, it is helpful to identify the hierarchy of component skills which in turn define a set of intermediate behavioral objectives. With respect to reading, for example, the hierarchy may involve: the ability to use syntax rather competently, the ability to see similarities and differences in a large number of graphic patterns, the ability to follow a series of lines of graphic symbols from left to right, from the top to the bottom of a page, the ability to produce the sounds that go with the various letters of the alphabet, singly and in combination, the ability to sound out words, etc.

Most curricula materials provided for teaching by a school system have been designed on the basis of an appropriate hierarchy of behavioral objectives. Thus, theoretically, all the teacher has to do is to follow faithfully the curriculum and the hierarchy problem will be solved. However, curricula materials vary considerably in their adequacy. The adequacy of the analysis of the hierarchy of skills, and hence the specification of intermediate behavorial objectives, varies and is at some times much more adequate than at others. Therefore, it is possible that the teacher will be saddled with curriculum materials which are more or less inadequate, which omit materials for the development of several of the essential component skills. Thus, to be effective the teacher must be informed about the essential component skills and the implied intermediate behavioral objectives, enough to recognize the deficiencies of the curriculum that either she, or her school system has chosen, and to provide the appropriate supplementary material.

All of this may sound terribly difficult, terribly complicated. However, the remedial procedure is straightforward. The secret: analyze each student's errors on assigned work. The pattern of errors will generally indicate the component skills in which the student is weak. For example, most students who are having difficulty with reading in the early grades will make certain phonetic errors. In such instances the curricula materials may be particularly weak in phonics and the teacher may have to obtain some supplementary materials which will help the children acquire the phonetic skills that they are missing. A summary of problematic and recommended procedures for setting behavioral objectives is given in Table 4.2.

Table 4.2. Behavioral Objectives.

Problematic Procedures	Recommended Procedures
1. The teacher fails to set ultimate behavioral objectives which allow the children to develop to capacity. The usual result: a much less than optimum rate of academic progress, the inadvertent structuring of pathogenic exchanges.	1. The teacher sets ultimate behavioral objectives including the development of the universally expected skills. The result: accelerated progress on verbal language skills, reading, writing, and mathematics. She supplements these objectives with others which she, the children, the parents, the school system may feel are important.
2. The teacher fails to use incorrect work to determine which component skills students have not yet acquired, and hence fails to prescribe the appropriate remedial work. The result: children without component skills required for a task will fall farther and farther behind their peers.	2. The teacher reviews the errors of each student on assigned work and on tests; spots weaknesses in component skills; designs remedial instructional exchanges to strengthen weak component skills. The usual result: students whose previously weak component skills are strengthened through remedial instruction will later acquire the more complex skills with minimal errors, frustration and discouragement. In fact, such remedial work sometimes turns them into excellent students.
3. The teacher sets up several intermediate behavioral objectives to work on simultaneously, that is, in one time period. The usual result: confusion and failure.	3. The teacher tests for and lists behavioral deficits, orders them in terms of an appropriate learning sequence. Chooses curricula materials appropriate to the acquisition of each. Helps her students work through the curricula materials, acquiring each component skill to an optimal level, as gauged by an exit test. Thus, each student works on only one behavioral objective at a time and continues the acquisition of each component skill until he passes the exit test.

The first three sets of procedures in Table 4.3 perhaps more than any others account for the differences observed among the experimental classes. Mrs. Allen, Mr. Smythe, and with respect to arithmetic, Mrs. Johnson and Mrs. James all selected curricula materials that allowed their students to answer questions and work problems and all assigned two to three times as much work as the students not on the token exchange normally cover. Our own staff ran into the quantity of work problem in their arithmetic experiment in Mrs. Ward's class. They started out providing the students

Table 4.3. Curricula.

Problematic Procedures	Recommended Procedures
4. Teacher relies on various "time-fillers," for example, using worksheet or similar material will have one child answer question #1, another child question #2, and so on. The usual result: students have much less practice obtaining correct answers than they might and hence, they make minimal progress.	4. Teacher selects curricula materials, i.e. workbooks, work sheets, that will allow students to answer a large number of questions, etc. The teacher uses correctly answered questions as criterion behavior for reinforcement.
5. The teacher provides curricula materials which allow the children to make correct responses but fails to provide enough work for the children. The usual result: less than optimal progress. Children who have no acculturating exchanges to work after they have finished the assignment in less than the allotted time, will often find pathogenic exchanges to work.	5. The teacher assigns two to three times as much work as students not on a token exchange are normally able to cover in a given period. Reinforces them for progress as determined by their daily record. The result: correct work and the learning which accompanies it is accelerated, often by a factor of two.
6. The teacher fails to provide intrinsically interesting curricula materials. The result: students will be bored, much of the power of the token exchange will be lost.	6. The teacher provides new experiences, change of pace, variation, in curriculum. She uses aesthetically pleasing visual aids, includes a large number of educational games.
7. The teacher fails to reinforce creativity, i.e. originality in response patterns.	7. In the acquisition of any complex ability there comes a time when children start making original response patterns, i.e. talking in original sentences, writing original descriptions, thoughts, etc. The teacher is attentive to such originality and systematically accelerates it by repetitive reinforcement.

with twenty problems to work in a ten minute period and ended up having to provide them with sixty.

Some teachers are hesitant to assign so much work since they have been taught not to push children. We are not suggesting that teachers push children, but once they have motivated them *positively* that they cease to put artificial limits on their progress. Thus by increasing the number of problems that Mrs. Ward's students could work from twenty to sixty, the staff were simply allowing those students who could and wanted to do more, to do so and to be reinforced for it.

Mrs. Allen, perhaps better than any of the other teachers, provided her children with a curriculum characterized by change of pace, variation and new experience. Mrs. Allen also provided her students with a large number of educational games, most of which she invented. Mrs. Johnson and Mrs. James, because theirs were "Follow Through" classes with a special budget, were able to provide aesthetically pleasing visual aids and a large number of educational games. These were effective in arithmetic because they provided a large amount of material for the children to work in addition to variety. Mrs. Allen was the only teacher who effectively reinforced creativity. Hers were the only students doing "creative writing." She also gave her students the opportunities of teaching and tutoring, essentially creative activities, and they were reinforced for their effectiveness in these activities.

Classroom Management

At first we wondered if it might be possible for a teacher to manage a normal size class using a token exchange. Our experience indicates that it is possible, but to do so most effectively certain procedures are required. The teacher must move more and more to delayed reinforcement procedures. She must reinforce correct work rather than good behavior and utilize her students as helpers. In order to do this effectively she must bring her organizational abilities into play. She must manage her classroom in a way that will allow the students to be much more actively involved in the teaching-learning process. Our summary for the problematic and recommended classroom management procedures is given in Table 4.4.

Some of the items in Table 4.4 require comment. The tendency of some of our experimental teachers was to give most of their tokens to maintain quiet behavior. As mentioned in the last chapter, one of the major problems of inner-city schools is a kind of disruptive, hyperactivity which makes inner-city teachers especially sensitive to the problem of maintaining order, of reducing noise. Thus, it is understandable that when given the opportunity to structure a token exchange in a classroom, they use it to solve what they consider to be their greatest problem. However, we feel that using a token exchange to maintain quiet behavior at the expense of academic achieve-

Table 4.4. Classroom Management.

Problematic Procedures	Recommended Procedures
8. The teacher does not work out a tight schedule for the day. The usual result: long transition periods, the assignment of non-productive busy-work.	8. For each subject, using the intermediate objectives as guides, the teacher works out a tight schedule of activity usually keeping several days ahead of the class. This schedule is not rigidly held to, but is designed to allow the children to progress at rates which are faster or slower than she initially schedules. The usual result: the children will make optimal progress and the teacher will have time in class to manage the learning environment effectively.
9. The teacher gives most of her tokens to maintain quiet behavior, few for correct work. The usual result: the class will be quiet and orderly, but academic progress will be minimal.	9. After the first month when more tokens are used to maintain good behavior, the teacher gives 90 to 95 percent of her tokens for correct work. The usual result in all the classes but for the very young or the very disturbed children: the students will settle down to working at an optimal rate, i.e. 90 to 95 percent of the time. The students will make some work connected noise, i.e. talking to one another, walking to get paper, sharpening pencils, etc., noise that most teachers easily tolerate.
10. The teacher fails to use the better students as graders, assistant teachers, and tutors. The usual result: the teacher will be unable to run an effective token exchange in a normal size classroom. She will overwork herself, cut down the academic progress of all students, particularly the slow ones.	10. The teacher corrects papers of students who finish first. Those with perfect or near perfect papers are assigned to correct the others' papers: gives out tokens in proportion to progress. The best students are assigned to be student teachers, to put other students through drills, to run educational games, and to tutor slow students during school, before and after school, during lunch or recess. Tutors are given tokens in proportion to the demonstrated progress of the students they work with. With tutors and graders, the teacher will be able to manage the usual size classroom on a token exchange more easily than

Table 4.4. continued.

Problematic Procedures	Recommended Procedures
	if she had an adult assistant teacher. The students who teach and tutor will master the curricula materials better than they would otherwise. Slow students will typically double progress they otherwise would have made.
11. The teacher fails to have daily progress recorded. The usual result: cannot reinforce students for day-to-day progress; underestimates long term progress, does not catch her errors in structuring her learning environment. Also, in the absence of reinforcing progress, the teacher ordinarily sets universalistic performance standards, e.g. giving tokens out to just those children who do 90 percent or even 70 percent or better. The usual second order result: (a) For those unable to perform at criterion level: frustration, eventual reticence to do schoolwork. (b) For those able to exceed criterion, less than optimal progress.	11. The teacher has each student keep a daily record of scores on written work and on tests; maintains a graph for each subject. The teacher or student checker checks the graph to determine daily progress for the student before deciding how many tokens to give him. The result: the student is reinforced for progress, the teacher is able to gauge accurately each student's long term performance and be aware early of any problems that the student might be encountering.

ment is unwise, if not an abdication of responsibility. A teacher's responsibility is not to be a caretaker assigned to keep the inmates quiet, docile, but by definition, to educate, to help the children to acquire those skills which will allow them eventually to take with some satisfaction productive, contributing roles in adult society.

In practically all of the experiments in this book which involve the acceleration principle a very simple rule of thumb is followed. The behavior to be accelerated is specified as the criterion behavior, the behavior which is reinforced to the extent that it occurs. However, the interesting thing is that in almost all instances behavior other than the criterion behavior is also accelerated by increasing the strength of reinforcement. We saw in the last chapter in Experiment 3 that when tokens with material backups were given in proportion to the number of correct answers, time spent studying went up from between 40 and 70 percent to between 90 and 95 percent of the available time. Studying appears to be an essential prerequisite, a component of producing correct answers. Hence, such behavior was reinforced indirectly and, therefore, accelerated when the strength of reinforcement was increased for the production of correct answers. Thus, a precision principle appears to be in effect: whenever the strength of reinforcement is increased for criterion behavior the component behaviors are also accelerated.

However, this principle must be qualified. Whenever an individual is particularly deficient in the skill required to produce the component behavior, indirect reinforcement may be inadequate to accelerate the component behavior. Thus, the talking of children in Experiment 1 in Chapter 3 did not accelerate during baseline when talking was indirectly reinforced as a component of correct academic work. However, it did accelerate when talking itself was made the criterion behavior, and thus, was directly reinforced by the tokens and material backups. Also, after these children had acquired the normal talking skills, talking was maintained via indirect reinforcement as a component of correct academic work.

Some teachers hesitate to use the better students as graders, assistant teachers, and tutors, in part because they feel their students will be incompetent, and in part because they feel that such duties are detrimental to the better students' academic progress. In fact, however, the exact opposite is true, as is shown in the results of tutoring experiments in past chapters as well as in the following experiment by June A. Hamblin for her doctoral dissertation.

The subjects were thirty-two inner-city preschoolers (twenty-six white and six black). These children whose ages ranged from 44 to 71 months (median 59 months) were randomly divided into four experimental groups and put through a beginning reading program. The treatment was identical in that: (1) the children in all of these groups were introduced to reading via the method outlined in Chapter 2. (2) All were subjected to the same i.t.a. primers (prepared by the experimenter) with the stories and illustrations appropriate to the social and visual world of the inner-city. (3) All received teacher attention and approval contingently for working, for making progress on tests, and for good behavior. (4) All received tokens, and the same material backups for tokens. (5) All had the opportunity of spending twenty minutes per day for eight consecutive weeks in reading sessions. (6) All spent half of that time in tutorial with Language Masters, learning their symbols and words (after which they were tested). (7) All spent the other ten minutes reading the primers aloud to an adult. However, in two of the groups the tutoring was done by adult teachers or by teenage Job Corps workers who had been trained to tutor the slower children and in two of the groups the brighter students tutored the slower students. Finally, two of the groups received tokens for reading, one per page read aloud correctly in the primers and one for each symbol or word recognized correctly within five seconds during the daily tests. It turned out that our regular tester was unable to get IQ scores on half of the children and that the testable children learned to read much more quickly than the untestable ones.[7] Hence, the data in Figure 4.6 are given for the testable (designated as the high to medium IQ children) and the untestable groups (designated as the low IQ children).

Note that the high and medium IQ children read to criterion, on the average 1.4 books over the eight week period when reinforcers were for attending and when tutored by the adults, (in this experiment the closest approximation to the traditional learning situation). If such children were involved in peer tutoring, their reading achievement better than doubled to 3.0 books or if given tokens for reading (with adult tutors) their reading nearly tripled to an average of 4.15 books. However, the high to medium IQ children's reading performance quadrupled to 5.5 books when involved in peer tutoring and given tokens for reading.

Note in that same figure that the low IQ children with adult tutoring and with tokens for attending read no books to criterion. In the words of one of the teachers, "They just fooled around; they never settled down to try to learn to read, although the adults tried to teach them." However, the low IQ children did read on the average 1.39 and 1.1 books respectively if peer

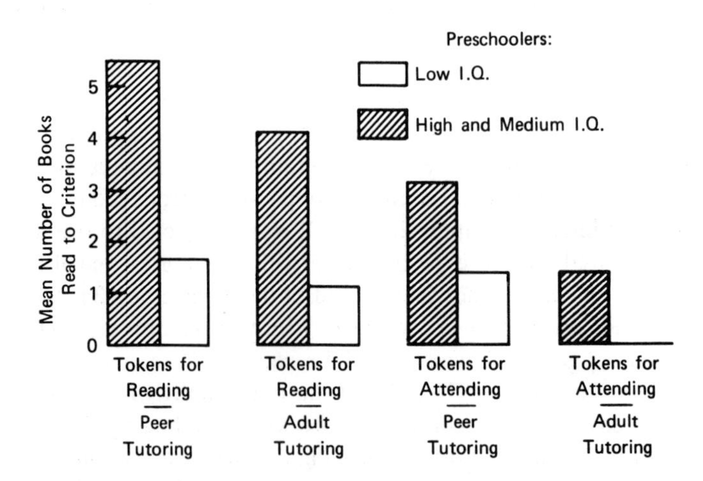

Figure 4.6. The relationship of books read (attendance controlled) to tokens and tutoring by IQ levels. (After J. A. Hamblin, 1970.)

[7] The reason was that the California Mental Maturity Test which was used was designed for first graders. Hence these children were "untestable" only because the test was inappropriate for them.

tutored, or if given tokens for reading. If both peer tutored and given tokens for reading the number of books read increased further to an average of 1.65. Hence, under favorable conditions (peer tutoring and material reinforcers for reading) even these low IQ children learned to read, and at a rate substantially higher than that of high and average IQ children in the traditional system.

In other words, the data suggest that even these very young students, when given the opportunity to tutor often turn out to be gifted, natural tutors, creative in helping their peers who cannot learn in the usual classroom situation. Why do they succeed so well? For one thing, they aren't as big, and hence, they apparently do not frighten or inhibit their peers as much as adult teachers do. Also, they use a language that their peers understand. Jules Henry, after observing in inner-city classrooms over an extended period, suggested that teachers often talk over the heads of their children. (In fact, he characterized some teachers' language as anticognition.) Children, when tutoring their peers, simply do not have that problem. Some may be clumsy at first, but given practice and tokens equal to the number the tutored children earn when later tested, they ordinarily become adept.

Also, the data from this experiment suggest that the better students who do the tutoring learn more during the tutoring sessions with another child on the Language Master than they do during a like session with an adult tutor. This may be difficult to understand, but to teach effectively any teacher has to first master the material himself. In this instance the tutors' own mastery of the material raced well ahead of that of the children being tutored.

Furthermore, tutors get invaluable training in the teaching skills which seem to be a component of most high level occupations. It is not just the professional teacher who teaches. The best salesmen teach their customers; the best leaders, the led; the best physicians, their patients; the best lawyers, their clients, the jury; and so on. Thus, teaching and tutoring provide the better students with a rare opportunity to develop their skills in verbal communication, in verbal explication, and in helping other human beings. For these and other reasons, we feel that the use of peer tutoring is an attractive alternative to the use of adult assistant teachers. It also makes instructional exchanges with material and other backups financially feasible. The annual salary of an assistant teacher is much more than the annual cost of both the backup reinforcers and the curricula changes which we recommend.

Finally, it is difficult for almost all teachers to see the wisdom of keeping daily progress records, for on the face of it such records seem to be unusually tiresome. However, scores on written work and tests, which the students graph for each subject, allow the teacher to reinforce the student for demonstrated academic progress, rather than for some universalistic performance standard. The tendency of almost all of our experimental teachers is to give out tokens to just those children who perform at a certain level, say 90 percent or above, or 70 percent or above. While such uniform criteria are easy for the teacher to manage, it makes unequal demands upon students of different abilities. It puts great pressure on the slow students and almost none on the better students. This is also the situation in most classrooms where grades rather than tokens are the reinforcers. The universal result: those students who do least well in the beginning log the greatest progress on any before/after tests. The data in Table 4.5 (American Council on Education, 1954) show how pervasive this tendency is. We found a similar situation in all of our experimental classrooms. For example, in Mrs. Allen's class those students who started out in the bottom half of the achievement distribution registered a gain of 2.1 levels during the year, whereas those who started out in the top half registered a median gain of 1.6 levels. This differential improvement has had various interpretations. The most popular explanation: regression toward the mean which results from the unreliability of the standardized tests. While some regression undoubtedly occurs because of the unreliability of the measuring instruments, the effect may be much smaller than it is generally thought to be. Let us suggest that the differential progress of the initially low and the initially high students is mostly the result of the tendency of teachers to take their students lock step through curricula materials and thus hook the rate of progress to the capacity of the low group to move through the materials. Theoretically, then, with individually prescribed instruction, where the students move through the curricula materials at their own pace, the picture would change. Those who initially scored high should show the greatest progress. To do that, however, it is necessary to grade students on their

Table 4.5. Average Gains of Students on Post Tests, Classified According to Pretest Standing.[a]

TEST	Low Group	Low Middle Group	Middle Group	High Middle Group	High Group
Critical thinking in social science	6.89	5.48	3.68	4.20	2.26
Science reasoning and understanding	6.26	5.16	2.93	2.04	0.31
Humanities participation inventory	18.00	5.05	4.94	1.39	−2.07
Analysis of reading and writing	5.33	2.89	1.81	1.22	0.25
Critical thinking	6.68	4.65	3.47	2.60	1.59
Inventory of beliefs	9.09	5.31	4.65	3.32	1.01
Problems in human relations	3.19	1.67	1.31	1.51	−0.36

[a] Adapted from the American Council on Education (1954).

progress and that requires individualized records, exit tests which allow students to stop working on certain materials when they have reached a certain level of competence, and arrangements for individual or small group instruction in relation to new materials.

The Provision and Management of Backups

Our basic finding has been that when the backup reinforcers are appropriate children will work approximately 95 percent of the available time. If children choose to work less than that, it probably means that they are not really interested in the backups. Thus, the selection of and the use of backup reinforcers is crucial in structuring an effective learning environment in the classroom. While the problem may seem complex, there are guidelines that may be followed in the provision and management of backup reinforcers, which are not that difficult to effect. These are summarized in Table 4.6. In Table 4.7 a list of backup reinforcers which are usually available in schools is given to the prospective teacher. Most teachers usually find it necessary to supplement these backups with ten to twenty-five dollars worth of toys and candy per month.

On Avoiding Pathogenic Exchanges

Based mainly on the experimental work to be presented in Chapters 5 and 7 but based also on our informal observations and experimentation in inner-city classrooms, we have come to the sad conclusion that most of the troublesome, bizarre behaviors that children engage in in the classroom are of the teacher's own doing, the consequence of the teacher's own behavior toward the children. The general theory of pathogenic exchanges will be developed in some detail in subsequent chapters, but an exposition of the problematic and recommended procedures for teachers would not be complete without those that are relevant to the management of disruptive behavior; see Table 4.8. The reader will probably not fully appreciate this list until he has read the subsequent chapters. The experiments, the research, the discussions there should provide the background which will make these statements meaningful.

It is recognized that the research in the subsequent chapters involved children who are not generally considered to be normal. Is it fair to apply the principles generated in experiments with such children to normal children in their regular classroom? Becker and his associates (1969) have done a similar series of experiments to see, in fact, if the principles do generalize to so-called normal children. His evidence suggests that such children when put into a pathogenic social learning environment tend to develop disruptive patterns although these are not usually as severe as those of the hyperaggressive, the psychotic children described in subsequent chapters. Thus the dynamics appear to be similar.

Table 4.6. The Provision and Management of Backups.

Problematic Procedures	Recommended Procedures
12. The teacher has a small number of backups, and does not vary them. The usual result: the children satiate, i.e. become uninterested in backups, reduce drastically the rate of working the instructional exchange.	12. Has a large number of backups, uses any given backup well below satiation frequency. Note: satiation frequency will vary. Children will eat ice cream, candy every day without satiating, but other things may interest them perhaps once a week, or once a month. For example, in preschool playing with Playdoh is a good backup reinforcer, if the opportunity does not come more than once a week. When satiated the children will appear to be uninterested in that which formerly interested them.
13. The teacher selects those backup reinforcers which she likes. The usual result: the children will work for some of the things that she picks, some will not interest the children.	13. (a) In buying items to sell in her store the teacher has the children do the selecting. (b) The teacher watches children for clues as to what *they* enjoy and provides those as backups.
14. Teacher has (a) fixed prices for backups, (b) fixed periods between backups, and (c) a fixed number of tokens for various criterion behaviors. The usual result: children will work at a much less than optimal level, an implicit contract develops and children will come to resist any changes in the terms.	14. Teacher varies one or more (a) prices, (b) intervals between opportunities to purchase backups, (c) the number of tokens for various criterion behaviors. The resulting uncertainty, which does not need to be great, will keep children working at an optimal level, will allow children to learn to tolerate change, to avoid rigidity.
15. The teacher fails to use backup reinforcers already available in her classroom. The usual result: she will spends an excessive amount for material backups.	15. The teacher observes the children, carefully noting what they enjoy, lets them buy the privilege of doing or having what they enjoy as long as it does not bother others, or hurt themselves.

Table 4.7. Backup Reinforcers That Cost "No Money," i.e. Were Readily Available in the School, Which Mrs. Allen Used in Her Fourth Grade.

Note: Mrs. Allen's students had the opportunity of earning about 100 tokens per day. Thus, hers might be termed a "rich" economy. She referred to her tokens as dollars and printed up $1, $5, and $10 bills. In a rich economy it is necessary to have large denomination tokens to facilitate the counting. There were a number of things that the children obviously enjoyed doing which Mrs. Allen sold. The prices quoted are approximate averages.

1. Free time for studying, reading, playing educational games: each ten minutes = 5 tokens.
2. Having one's hand stamped with indelible ink with one of several rubber stamps (i.e. Airmail, First Class Mail) which the school furnished Mrs. Allen = 2 tokens.
3. Program in the auditorium = 25 tokens.
4. Having a party in the classroom = 60 tokens.
5. Having a movie = 30 tokens.
6. Talking with a friend = 3 tokens.
7. Going on a field trip = 100 to 200 tokens.
8. Taking a nature walk near school = 10 tokens.
9. Opening a charge account = 10 tokens.[a]
10. Opening a bank account = 10 tokens.[a]
11. Looking in the mirror = 2 tokens.
12. Listening to a record = 5 tokens.
13. Looking at television = 10 to 20 tokens.
14. Listening to the radio = 5 to 20 tokens.
15. Having the first seat in a row = 10 tokens.

Note: Mrs. Allen found that her students enjoyed helping her, so generally she sold the opportunity as follows:

16. Sweeping the floor = 3 tokens.
17. Dusting the room = 5 tokens.
18. Emptying the trash outside = 3 tokens.
19. Passing out or putting away books = 2 tokens.
20. Passing out or taking up papers = 1 token.
21. Being the room supervisor = 5 tokens.
22. Operating the tape recorder = 5 tokens.

Note: Mrs. Allen sold school supplies for tokens. These were furnished by the school.

23. Pencils = 8 tokens each.
24. Erasers = 5 tokens each.
25. Extra paper = 3 tokens per sheet.
26. Art supplies = 10 tokens each.
27. Rubber bands = 3 tokens each.
28. Weekly newspaper = 10 tokens.

[a] Mrs. Allen established charge accounts and bank accounts as part of her social studies curriculum.

Table 4.7. continued.

Note: Finally, Mrs. Allen sold certain privileges that teachers ordinarily like to keep at a minimum.

29. To be excused during class period to go to the toilet = 10 tokens.
30. To be excused during class period to go for a drink of water = 10 tokens.
31. To be excused during class to take a message, money, a gym suit to a friend or relative in another class = 10 tokens.
32. To chew gum for one half day = 10 tokens.
33. To eat candy for one half day = 10 tokens.
34. Looking out the window at events = 3 to 15 tokens (one token per minute).

Table 4.8. On Avoiding Pathogenic Exchanges.

Problematic Procedures	Recommended Procedures
16. The teacher talks to her children, tells them to stop every time they disrupt, gives long lectures about misbehaving, does not reinforce good models. The usual result: over time the frequency of disruptions will increase.	16. The teacher ignores disruptions, periodically rewards one or more students with a token and a "thank you for working, Bill, Carol." The usual result: the disrupters will realize they are not working and will therefore stop disrupting and start working to earn tokens and the teacher's approval. Over time disrupts will decrease.
17. The teacher feels the need for retribution against children who misbehave, takes pleasure, satisfaction in their punishment. The usual result: one or more of the following (a) uses time-out punitively, i.e. rough handling on the way to time out room, leaves child for long periods in the room; (b) withholds or "forgets" to give tokens for correct work by children who have misbehaved; (c) excessive use of fines, levies more than a minimal fine, and fines more than once or twice a day. The second order result: she destroys the warm friendly quality of the teacher-pupil relationship and the classroom situation degenerates into an aggressive teasing exchange.	17. Teacher feels the long term remission of children's problems is more important than her feelings. Develops her ability to set up and manage counter exchanges where she (a) identifies what she is doing that is repetitively reinforcing her children's misbehavior; (b) terminates that exchange; and (c) structures an alternative exchange to reinforce pro-normal behavior which is functionally an alternative to the misbehavior. (Counter exchanges will be illustrated extensively in succeeding chapters.) Result: the children's behavior problems disappear. The teacher-pupil relationship is not sacrificed. In fact, a mutual fondness develops and the teacher escapes the pain of getting continually angry, or being continually mean.

Table 4.8. continued.

Problematic Procedures	Recommended Procedures
18. The teacher repeats requests several times, if necessary, until the child responds. The usual result: the child will get to the point where he has to be asked several times before he will do anything.	18. The teacher treats her requests as an implicit opportunity to learn, to earn reinforcement (implicit because she never explains that to the children). If the child does not respond the first time, without rancor she simply gives another child the opportunity. The usual long term result: the children will respond almost always the first time a request is made.
19. The teacher negotiates, makes deals with the children to get them to do things. In other words, she turns the token exchange into a contractual relationship. The usual long term result: the teacher will be unable to live up to 25 to 35 contracts without making errors, and hence, without frustrating some of the students' expectations, also the children will get to the point where they will do nothing without negotiating a contract for payment.	19. Instructional relationships between children and teacher are patterned after a gift exchange. The teacher waits until the child performs the criterion behavior and she treats that behavior as a gift, showing her appreciation verbally and by giving him something he values in return. Hence, the terms of the exchange are not discussed, rather each learn to be sensitive to the other, to provide the other that which will keep the exchange being worked at a high frequency. The usual long term result: mutual trust, respect, liking. Also, if the teacher is somewhat variable in her response pattern, the relationship will be quite flexible.
20. When interacting with the class as a whole the teacher makes the probability of reinforcement unequal for students, i.e. predictably reinforces only (a) those models of good behavior who are near her, (b) those students she likes, (c) those who get above a certain score. Alternatively she calls on students in some predictable order, i.e. goes up and down the rows. The usual result: only those students who have a large probability of reinforcement will attend work and get the right answer; the others will give up.	20. The teacher makes the probability of reinforcement approximately equal at all times for all students. The result: students will attend work and give the correct answer at a level at or near capacity.

Table 4.8. continued.

Problematic Procedures	Recommended Procedures
21. The teacher (a) follows a medical model, expects acquired behaviors to be self-maintained, (b) shifts from continuous to intermittent reinforcement too quickly. The usual result: her hard won behavioral changes will be temporary. The children will regress to old disruptive patterns which were maintained at least via periodic reinforcement.	21. The teacher provides maintenance reinforcement for all pro-normal patterns using one or more of the following procedures: (a) moving to intermittent reinforcement, gradually reducing the frequency, (b) making the behavior in question a component of a more complex pattern which is repetitively reinforced (this provides indirect reinforcement), (c) bringing skill level up—i.e. reducing the costs of the behavior to the point where the behavior can be maintained by conditioned reinforcers such as approval, the indication that one's message (verbal) has been received, getting the right answer, etc. (d) bringing skill level up to where the behavior can be maintained by delayed reinforcement, i.e. a weekly or monthly pay check, college degree, a yearly raise, etc.

SUMMARY

This chapter began with a series of experiments conducted in public school classrooms with the cooperation of the teachers and the school system. The experiments were designed to test the limits of our exchange procedures and to see if the teachers and the students could benefit from them with minimal training and with minimal changes in the curriculum. We found that four of the six experimental teachers were relatively successful. They brought their classes' achievement levels up to normal or thereabouts. In other words they were able to correct the cumulative deficit that characterizes classes in inner-city schools. (The comparison classes were on the average, still six months behind.)

Yet the focus of the chapter is less experimental than applied. Outlined are a series of procedures, some of them problematic, others recommended. As noted, not all of the recommendations were based on solid experimental evidence. In fact, many rest on informal but extensive observations of teachers in actual classrooms and informal experimentation with our teachers as we have tried to help them with the problems they were experiencing in our experimental classrooms over a period of four years (1966 through 1969). Hence, in a way, the recommendations can be taken as an outline for formal experimentation, in order to see if, in fact, the procedures do usually produce the results we have attributed to them. Even so, our informal experimentation usually allows us to forecast the results of formal experiments with considerable accuracy so we have some confidence in the recommendations as they are made here.

We should also note that all of the twenty-one recommendations picture more accurately than our experimental work the complexity of the problem of structuring effective learning environments for children. Earlier impressions to the contrary, creating effective learning environments for children is not an easy task. Children are capable of far more learning than most teachers ever guess. However, accelerated rates of learning will only be obtained when the environmental conditions are exactly right, when they capitalize on the operating characteristics of the human biological learning mechanisms.

Even so, there is a danger involved in the complexities of these recommendations: teachers who could become very effective in structuring learning environments for children might well be frightened away. A more appropriate response for such teachers: their recognition of the complexities and their willingness to spend the time, the energy necessary to develop the requisite competence. It is our feeling, however, that few teachers working alone from the kinds of materials we are providing in this book, will be successful in structuring maximally effective learning environments. Teachers, it would seem to us, would have a much better chance if they worked in pairs, or in groups where, in addition to the reading, they could discuss the principles involved, where they could coach one another using essentially the same procedures outlined in Chapter 8. Learning to use curricula appropriately, spotting deficient component skills and providing remedial curricula materials is a tricky business. Also the avoidance of pathogenic exchanges is very difficult when one tries to go it alone, but with discussion, with coaching, the difficulties are surmountable. Hence, our advice: make it a cooperative endeavor, and gather the evaluation data via students' records.

CHAPTER 5

The Hyperaggressive Child

The hyperaggressive child is a serious problem.[1] He is miserable, and he makes life miserable for those around him. He gets categorized as a bad boy. With or without "therapeutic" drugs he does not progress well in school. He typically cannot or will not concentrate, complete academic projects, or learn effectively. In grade school he falls behind as much as three or four years and becomes the discipline problem of the class. Thus, in a very special sense, the hyperaggressive child is a retarded child, who, at best, often ends up in special education classes.

The traditional treatment for aggressive children is punishment—often harsh punishment. This is not only of dubious moral value, but it does not help the worst offenders particularly. But if punishment is not desirable and does not work, what is better? Alternative approaches have come from the various theories or concepts about what causes hyperaggression.

FRUSTRATION AND AGGRESSION

Freud saw aggression as a basic drive of the organism, analogous to other physiological drives such as those for eating, drinking, and sleeping. In our inhibiting civilization, this aggression presumably accumulates as frustrations accumulate until it threatens or actually bursts forth through the defenses of the ego and the superego—the long term effects of hardly remembered training, of parental example and control. Freud suggests these outbursts may be avoided only by more or less regular "cathartic drainage." As Baruch has expressed:

> When pus accumulates and forms an abscess, it must be opened and drained. If this is not done, it may destroy the individual. Just so with feelings. The hurts, fears and angers must be released and drained. Otherwise, these too may destroy the individual. When enough fear, anger

[1] Hamblin and Buckholdt took the major responsibility for writing this chapter.

> and hate have been released, they diminish. They stop pushing from within. After enough of the "badness" comes out, the "goodness" appears. (Baruch, 1949)

Another group of authorities (Dollard et al., 1939) explains the effects of catharsis this way: "The occurrence of any act of aggression is assumed to reduce [temporarily] the instigation to [further] aggression." Frustration produces aggression,[2] which may be expressed immediately and overtly (resulting perhaps in violence but allowing quick catharsis without which it would accumulate and threaten later in greater aggression).

The control of aggression might then be obtained by (1) avoiding anything that might cause frustration; (2) allowing the individual to express aggression freely in a way that would not cause serious damage. These strategies have been embodied in several therapeutic designs—group therapy sessions and schools in which frustrating stimuli were systematically removed, and constant opportunities for catharsis prevailed (cf. Redl and Wineman, 1957; and Neill, 1960). However, in laboratory tests the catharsis hypothesis has not fared well (Tables 5.1 and 5.2). The results have been weak and inconsistent, not worth the serious attention of scientists or therapists. And without catharsis, Freudian therapy for hyperaggression falls flat.

Other authors including ethologist Konrad Lorenz (1966) and psychologist Nathan Azrin and his associates (1965) seek to demonstrate that aggression is a basic instinct or reflex in animals and that man cannot escape his animal inheritance. But to draw conclusions about instinctual or reflex behavior in animals—even when those conclusions are accurate—and then to assume that they apply even to other similar species (to say nothing of man) without the proper experimental evidence is an extremely dubious enterprise.

A third biological theory, unfortunately largely ignored in the behavioral sciences, but based on the work of a number of pediatricians, holds that much hyperaggression in children comes from a more general hyperactive syndrome caused apparently by a chemical imbalance in the brain (cf. Stewart, et al., 1966; Signor, 1967). Strangely enough, the use of common sedatives aggravates the condition in these children, but amphetamines have a calming effect, and are widely used today. As Stewart observes: "We do know that there is not another condition in psychiatry that responds so

[2] The evidence suggests that interference and the frustration it produces does in turn lawfully produce aggression at least in some people (cf. Hamblin et al., 1963). We will suggest later that these relationships involve conditioned reflexes not genetically determined reflexes.

Table 5.1. Tests of Catharsis Hypothesis—Direct Formulation.[a]

Author	Date	Independent Variable(s)	Dependent Variable(s)	Subjects	Results[c]	Explained Variance (%)[b]
Kenny	1953	Doll play	Projective test	Children	Negative	. . .
Feshback	1955	(a) Insult (b) TAT cards	(a) Questionnaire (b) Sentence completion test	Male-fem. college students	Positive	6.3 2.3
Pepitone, Reichling	1955	Insult	Questionnaire	Male adults	Positive	18.7
Thibault, Coules	1952	(a) Angered (b) Communication to frustrator	Description of frustrator	Male college students	Positive	4.2 4.7
Feshback	1956	Doll play	Projective test	Children	Negative	. . .
Worchel	1957	Frustrated	Digit symbol test	Adults (not college)	Positive	5.1
Kahn	1960	Insult	Questionnaire	Adults	Negative	. . .
Thibault, Riecken	1955	(a) Personality rating scale (b) Angered (c) High/low status condition	(a) Verbal responses (b) Rating scale	Adults (male)	Negative	23.3
Horwitz	1954	Angered	Questionnaire	Adults	Negative	. . .
Magaziner	1961	Angered	Restoral of self-esteem	Adults	Negative	. . .
Hokanson, Shetler	1961	(a) Angered (b) Electric shock	Systolic blood pressure levels	Male-fem. college students	Negative	3.6 2.8
Hokanson, Burgess	1962	(a) Angered (b) Electric shock (c) Verbal aggression	(a) Systolic blood pressure (b) Heart rate	Male-fem. college students	Negative	9.0 9.2

[a] Source: Ellis, 1967. Formulae enabling one to convert t and F scores into measures of explained variance are contained in Hays, (1963).

[b] Where percentages of explained variance are not presented, the reader may assume that the reporting in the original has not permitted transformation of results into a measure of explained variance.

[c] Negative results mean that the angered subjects become more and not less angry after being aggressive to others in contradiction to

dramatically to drugs. It happens in about half of the children, but it is an obvious change. The children simply turn into different beings."

Three or four of every 100 children are hyperactive (Stewart, et al., 1966). But what percent of hyperactives are hyperaggressive? Stewart's data in Table 5.3 show the major behavioral characteristics of the hyperactive syndrome. Note that about 50 percent show the characteristics of hyperaggression, that is, temper tantrums, fights, teasing, destructive behavior. Stewart, who has done extensive work with hyperactive children, has noted that the 50 percent or so who respond favorably to stimulants are not the hyperaggressives. Those who do respond so dramatically to drugs tend to be relatively puny, physically underdeveloped; hyperaggressive-hyperactives tend to be robust and well developed. Thus, there must be two hyperactive syndromes: the first involving underdeveloped children, who to a large extent can be helped by the use of the stimulant family of drugs; the second involving hyperaggressive children, who are unresponsive, to date at least, to any specific biochemical therapy.

THE EXCHANGE THEORY OF AGGRESSION

However appealing, interesting and logical any or all of these theories may be, none have led to a therapy demonstrably effective with hyperaggressive children. And, however they differ, they have one element in common: they ignore the role of social learning. To put it mildly, this is a significant omission. Of all animals, man is the most adaptable, the most teachable, the one whose behavior is least rigidly programmed at or before birth. We know that his response patterns—even those that seem the most automatic, the most habitual—are in almost all cases learned or conditioned. What if aggression, too, is a *learned pattern,* which survives and even flourishes (at least in some people) because it is repeatedly reinforced?

Unfortunately, society does often reinforce aggressive behavior. Some cultures and some families are open and brazen about it—they systematically and consciously teach their young that such behavior is desirable, even virtuous. In our own society the child who can beat up the other kids on the playground is often respected by his peers, and perhaps by his parents. The soldier achieves glory in combat. The status, the booty, or the bargaining advantages that come to the aggressor in almost any society can become reinforcement to continue and escalate aggression. In more civilized cultures, however, the young are taught not to use aggression, and there is an attempt to substitute less harmful patterns. But even so, aggression is sometimes reinforced unintentionally—and the consequences, predictably, are the same as if the teaching were deliberate.

Table 5.2. Tests of Catharsis Hypothesis—Vicarious Formulation.[a]

Author	Independent Variable(s)	Dependent Variable(s)	Subjects	Results[c]	Explained Variance (%)[b]
Bandura, Ross, Ross	(a) Exposure to aggressive models (b) Frustrated (mildly)	Aggressive doll play	Children	Negative	. . .
Lovaas	Exposure to aggressive cartoon	Aggressive doll play	Children	Negative	22.7
Mussen, Rutherford	(a) Exposure to aggressive cartoon (b) Frustrated	Balloon popping	Children	Negative	28.4
Siegel	Aggressive cartoon	Aggressive doll play	Children	Negative	. . .
Walters, Thomas	Aggressive film	Delivering electric shocks —duration and intensity	Adult males	Negative	14.2 8.5
Berkowitz, Rawlings	(a) Angered (b) Aggressive film (c) "Justified" aggression	Questionnaire responses	Male and female college students	Negative	7.6
Feshback	(a) Angered	Word association test	Male and female college students	Positive	2.3

[a] Source: Ellis, 1967. Formulae enabling one to convert t and F scores into measures of explained variance are contained in Hays, (1963).

[b] Where percentages of explained variance are not presented, the reader may assume that the reporting in the original has not permitted transformation of results into a measure of explained variance.

[c] Negative results mean that the angered subjects exposed to models being aggressive to others become more and not less angry in contradiction to the catharsis hypothesis.

Civilized cultures are not kind to hyperaggressive children. A recent survey in England, for instance, found that the great majority of teachers felt that aggressive behavior by students disturbed more classrooms than anything else and caused the most anxiety among teachers. At least partly as a result, the dropout rates for the hyperaggressives was two and one-half times as great as for "normals," and disproportionate numbers of hyperaggressives were treated in mental clinics.

In our research with disturbed children we have taken seriously the theory that aggression is a learned habitual pattern of behavior; that people, specifically children, become aggressive because they get something for it and they continue to be aggressive because the reinforcement is continuing. In investigating this hypothesis we gathered two types of data. First we observed ongoing exchanges between teachers and hyperaggressive youngsters in the classroom. We recorded sportscaster-like descriptions of these ongoing exchanges and made detailed analyses of their structure, particularly of what it is that seems to reinforce aggression. In addition, we did a series of experiments where we attempted to substitute a cooperative, academically productive pattern for hyperaggressive behavior patterns. What follows is a report of these investigations and experiments, and the implications of the results for aggression theory as well as for the remediation of hyperaggression.

EXPERIMENT 1: HYPERAGGRESSIVE PRESCHOOLERS

Our subjects were five extraordinarily aggressive four-year-old boys, all referred to the laboratory by local psychiatrists and social workers who had been able to do very little with them. All had been diagnosed as hyperactive; none had responded to amphetamine therapy. The experimenters, Desmond Ellis and Hamblin (Hamblin, et al., 1969), hired a trained teacher. She was told about the boys and the general nature of the experiment and then was given her head. That is, she was allowed to use her previous training during the first period (A1) to provide a baseline comparison with what followed. It was hoped she would act like the "typical teacher." We suspect that she did.

Let's Play "Get the Teacher"

The teacher was, variously, strict disciplinarian, wise counselor, clever arbitrator and sweet peacemaker. In each role, however, she failed miserably. After the eighth day, the average of the children was 150 sequences of aggression per day! Here is what a mere four minutes of those sequences were like:

> Mike, John and Dan are seated together playing with pieces of Playdoh. Barry, some distance from the others, is seated and also is playing with Playdoh. The children, except Barry, are talking to each other about what they are making. Time is 9:10 a.m. Miss Sally, the teacher, turns toward the children and says, "It's time for a lesson. Put your Playdoh away." Mike says, "Not me." John says, "Not me." Dan says, "Not me." Miss Sally moves toward Mike. Mike throws his Playdoh in Miss Sally's face. Miss Sally jerks back, then moves forward rapidly and snatches Playdoh from Mike. Puts Playdoh in her pocket. Mike screams for Playdoh, says he wants to play with it. Mike moves toward Miss Sally and attempts to snatch the Playdoh from her pocket. Miss Sally pushes him away. Mike kicks her on the leg, kicks her again and demands the return of his Playdoh. Kicks her again, picks up a small steel chair and throws it at Miss Sally. She jumps out of the way. Mike picks up another chair and throws it more violently. Miss Sally cannot move in time and chair strikes her foot. Miss Sally pushes Mike down on the floor. Mike starts up, pulls over one chair, then another, another; stops a moment. Miss Sally is picking up chairs. Mike looks at her. She moves toward Mike. Mike runs away. John wants his Playdoh. Miss Sally says, "No." He joins Mike in pulling over chairs and attempts to grab Playdoh from Miss Sally's pocket; she pushes him away roughly. John is screaming that he wants to play with his Playdoh; moves toward phonograph, pulls it off the table and lets it crash onto the floor. Mike has his coat on; says he is going home. Miss Sally asks Dan to bolt the door. Dan gets to the door at the same time as Mike. Mike hits Dan in the face. Dan's nose is bleeding. Miss Sally walks over to Dan, turns to the others and says that she is taking Dan to the washroom and that while she is away, they may play with the Playdoh. *Returns Playdoh from pocket to Mike and John.* Time: 9:14 a.m.

Wild? Very. These were barbarous little boys who enjoyed battle. Miss Sally did her best but they were just more clever than she, and they *always* won. Whether she wanted to or not, they could always drag her into the fray, and just go at it harder and harder until she capitulated. She was finally driven to their level, trading a kick for a kick and a spit in the face for a spit in the face.

What she did not realize is that she had inadvertently structured an exchange where she consistently reinforced aggression. First, as noted, whenever she fought with them, she *always lost.* Second, more subtly, she reinforced their aggressive pattern by giving it serious attention—by looking, talking, scolding, cajoling, becoming angry, even striking back. These boys were playing a teasing game called "Get the Teacher." The more she showed that she was bothered by their behavior, the better they seemed to like it, and the further they went.

These interpretations may seem far-fetched, but they are borne out dramatically by what happened later. On the twelfth day the conditions were changed, beginning with B1 (see Figure 5.1). First, the usual token exchange was structured to reinforce cooperative behavior. This was to

Table 5.3. Percent Positive Scores in the Hyperactive and Control Groups for Symptoms Scored Positive in One Third or More of the Hyperactive Group.

Symptom	Group	
	Hyperactive	Control
Overactive	100	33
Can't sit still	81	8
Restless in M.D.'s waiting room	38	3
Talks too much	68	20
Wears out toys, furniture, etc.	68	8
Fidgets	84	30
Gets into things	54	11
Unpredictable	59	3
Leaves class without permission	35	0
Unpredictable show of affection	38	3
Constant demand for candy, etc.	41	6
Can't tolerate delay	46	8
Can't accept correction	35	0
Temper tantrums	51	0
Irritable	49	3
Fights	59	3
Teases	59	22
Destructive	41	0
Unresponsive to discipline	57	0
Defiant	49	0
Doesn't complete projects	84	0
Doesn't stay with games	78	3
Doesn't listen to whole story	49	0
Moves from one activity to another in class	46	6
Doesn't follow directions	62	3
Hard to get to bed	49	3
Enuresis	43	28
Lies	43	3
Accident prone	43	11
Reckless	49	3
Unpopular with peers	46	0

Source: Stewart et al. (1966).

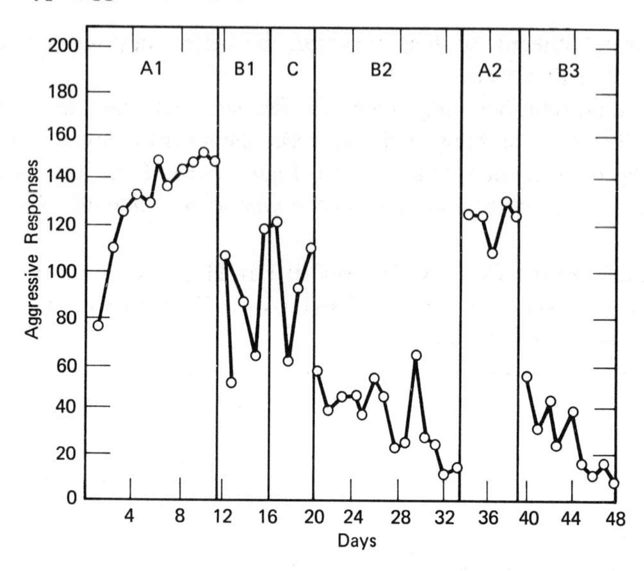

Figure 5.1. Frequency of aggressive sequences by days for five four-year-old boys for six experimental conditions. In A, C, and A2 the teacher attempted to punish aggression but inadvertently reinforced it; in B1, B2 and B3 she turned her back or otherwise ignored aggression and thus did not reinforce the pattern.

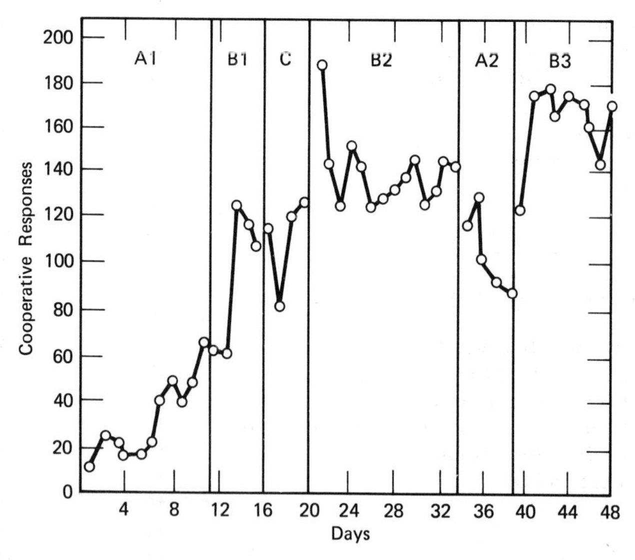

Figure 5.2. Frequency of cooperative sequences for six experimental conditions. In A1 and A2, the teacher structured a weak approval exchange for cooperation and a disapproval exchange for non-cooperation. In B1, B2, B3 and C, she structured a token exchange for cooperation.

develop or strengthen behavior that would replace aggression. Any strong pattern of behavior serves some function for the individual, so the first step in getting rid of a strong, disruptive pattern is substituting another one that is more useful and causes fewer problems. Not only effective remediation of hyperaggression, but simple humanity dictates this.

First, the teacher had to be instructed to avoid reinforcing aggression. Contrary to all her experience, she was asked to turn her back on the aggressor, and at the same time to reinforce the cooperation of others with tokens. Once she was coached and given immediate feedback over a wireless-communication system,[3] she structured the exchanges almost perfectly. The data in Figures 5.1 and 5.2 show the crucial changes: a gradual increase in cooperation—from about 56 to about 115 sequences per day, and a corresponding decrease in aggression from 150 to about 80 sequences![4]

These results should have been satisfactory, but we were new at this kind of experimentation, and nervous. We wanted to reduce the frequency of aggression to a "normal" level, to about 15 sequences a day. So we restructured the exchange system and thus launched C. In C aggression was always punished; the teacher was told to charge tokens for any aggression.

To our surprise, the frequency of cooperation remained stable, about 115 sequences per day; but aggression increased to about 110 sequences per day! Evidently the boys were still playing "Get the Teacher," and the troubled attention and fines were enough reinforcement to continue to increase the aggression. But at this point it became obvious that, for all their

[3] At first we used citizen band transceivers which, because of static and outside transmissions, were not satisfactory. We then moved to a system where the teacher wore a hearing aid with a telephone induction loop and where the experimenter talked into a dispatcher's microphone which was connected with an amplifier which was connected to another induction loop around the perimeter of the experimental classroom.

[4] Data were taken on a 20 channel Esterline Angus Event Recorder. Aggression was defined as an act which produced pain, psychological or physiological, in another. Typical examples for this group: kicking or hitting another, spitting in another's face, choking another, deliberately tearing up the room, throwing chairs or other objects at another, destroying or breaking valuable property, name calling. There were so many aggressive acts that our observers could not keep up, so we invented the aggressive sequence, or series of one or more aggressive acts of the same kind. In other words, if one of the boys kicked the teacher on the shins once or ten times in a row, it was counted as one aggressive sequence. A sequence was considered terminated when the boy switched to another kind of aggression, e.g. throwing chairs at the teacher, or to another activity, e.g. playing with toys. Cooperation was defined as compliance with another's request or spontaneously helping the teacher or another boy. Average interobserver reliability, three different observers over all experimental conditions: 92 percent agreement for aggression totals per child, and 89 percent agreement for cooperation totals per child.

teasing and even abuse of her, the boys—particularly Mike, John and Dan—had grown fond of Miss Sally. They tried to sit by her, jockeyed for the closest position, and sometimes fought for it. This fondness for the teacher, therefore, actually led to greater trouble.

> *Time for reading.* Miss Sally is sitting on the floor with all the boys except Mike. The boys are quite attentive, all listening raptly. Mike decides to join the reading circle, tries to edge in between Miss Sally and John. In an instant, John has his left arm locked around Mike's neck from the back and is choking him. Mike loudly cries and coughs for air. Miss Sally says to John, "If you do that, it will cost you five tokens." John has tokens in the locking hand, he lets go a moment and throws the tokens at Miss Sally; and before Mike or Miss Sally could react, the arm is again locked. Mike again is coughing and screaming. Miss Sally breaks the lock. John draws back, Mike stops crying. Miss Sally starts reading again.

This incident was so outlandish that the experimenters decided to correct the error. Instead of fining the children, the teacher was again told to ignore aggression by turning her back and giving attention and tokens only for cooperation. The frequency of aggression went down to a near "normal" level, to about 16 sequences per day (B2), and cooperation increased to about 140 sequences.

Then, as originally planned, the conditions were again reversed. The boys were given enough tokens at the beginning of the morning to buy their usual supply of movies, toys, and snacks, so these were not used as reinforcers. The teacher was again told to do the best she could. She was not instructed to return to her old pattern, but without the tokens and without our coaching she did—and with the same results. Note A2 in Figures 5.1 and 5.2. Aggression increased to about 130 sequences per day, and cooperation decreased to about 85. While this was an improvement over A1, before the boys had ever been exposed to the token exchange, it was not good.

When the token exchange was restructured (B3) and the aggression no longer reinforced, the expected changes recurred—with a bang! Aggression decreased to 7 sequences on the last day, and cooperation rose to about 175 sequences. In "normal" nursery schools, observations have shown that five boys can be expected to have 15 aggressive sequences and 60 sequences of cooperation per 2.5 hour day. Thus, from being extremely aggressive and uncooperative, our boys had become less aggressive and far more cooperative than "normal" boys.

Here is an example of their new behavior patterns, taken from a rest period—precisely the time when the most aggressive sequences had occurred in the past:

All of the children are sitting around the table drinking their milk. John, as usual, had finished first. Takes his plastic mug and returns it to the table. Miss Martha, the assistant teacher, gives him a token. Goes to cupboard, takes out his mat, spreads it out by the blackboard and lies down. Miss Martha gives him a token. Meanwhile, Mike, Barry and Jack have spread their mats on the carpet. Dan is lying on the carpet itself since he hasn't a mat. Each of them get a token. Mike asks if he can sleep by the wall. Miss Sally says yes. John asks if he can put out the light. Miss Sally says to wait until Barry has his mat spread properly. Dan asks Mike if he can share with him. Mike says no. Dan then asks Jack if he can share with him. Jack says yes, but before he can move over, Mike says yes. Dan joins Mike. Both Jack and Mike get a token. Miss Sally asks John to put out the light; John does so. Miss Martha gives him a token. All quiet now. Four minutes later—all quiet. Quiet still, three minutes later. Time: 10:23 a.m. Rest period ends.

Two or three incidents similar to the following occurred during A1 and A2, and in one of them Mike terminated the episode by punching Dan in the nose, causing it to bleed. But in B3 his response was quite different, suggesting again the depth of the transformation of these boys' behavior patterns:

The children are in the classroom, ushered there by the driver. Mike has some money, which he is showing others. Dan snatches a dime from Mike's outstretched hand, evidently wanting to use the money in the candy machine upstairs. Mike moves toward Dan while asking for his money back. John asks Dan to give Mike's money back. Mike continues to ask Dan for his money. Now he warns Dan that he will not share money with him in the future. (On previous occasions Mike had stolen money from his mother—about $1.75—and had in fact distributed it among the boys.) Time: 9:04 a.m. Miss Sally arrives. Mike tells Miss Sally that Dan has taken his money. Miss Sally asks Dan, who nods and gives the dime back to Mike.

Mike was manifestly frustrated by Dan's snatching; but instead of anger and then direct aggression, he responded several times with a substitute pattern—asking. When this did not work, he came up with a mild threat—he would not share with Dan in the future. Finally, he did what civilized people are supposed to do, though many—including adults—do not: he took the matter to authority for adjudication. *His habitual response pattern had changed!*

These boys actually were double problems; they were not only extremely disruptive, but also washouts as students. Before the token system (A1), they paid attention to their teacher only about 8 percent of the lesson time (see Figure 5.3). The teacher's system of scolding the youngsters for inattention and taking their attention for granted with faint approval, if any, did not work at all. To the pupils, the "Get the Teacher" game was much more satisfying.

After the token exchange was started, in B1, C and B2, it took about twenty days before there was any appreciable effect. The teacher was being trained from scratch, and our training methods were, then, not very good. However, after we set up a wireless-communication system that allowed us to coach the teacher from behind a one-way mirror and to give her immediate feedback, the children's attention began to increase. Toward the end of B2, it leveled off at about 75 percent—from 8 percent! After the token exchange was taken out during A2, attention went down to 15 percent; put back in during B3, it shot back up to a plateau of about 93 percent. Like a roller coaster: 8 percent without, to 75 with, to 15 without, to 93 with. Almost a twelvefold increase.

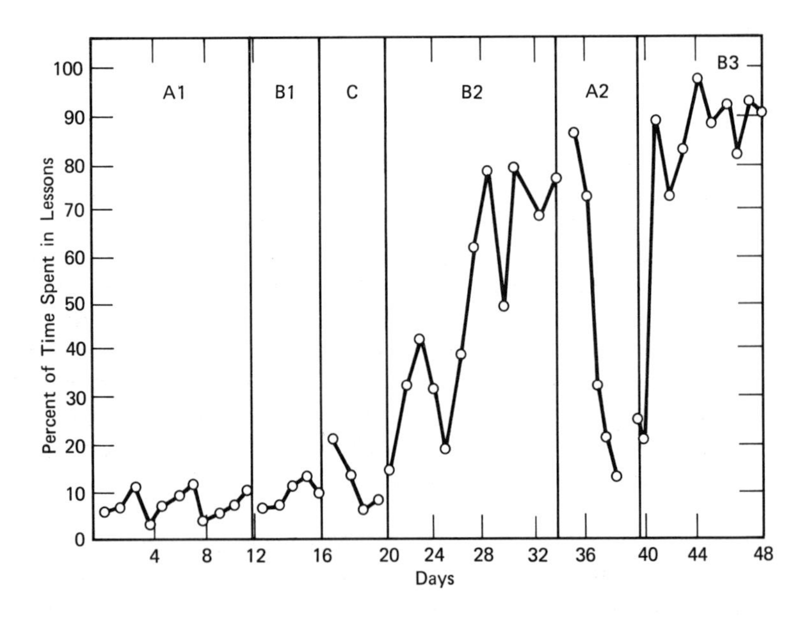

Figure 5.3. Percent of scheduled time spent in lessons by days for six experimental periods for five hyperaggressive boys. In A1 and A2 teacher structured approval exchange for attendance, disapproval for non-attendance. In B1 and C, a token exchange for attendance was structured, but not effectively until B2 and B3.

With more normal children the increase, as might be recalled from Figure 2.1, is at best threefold. Therefore, well-structured exchanges are especially important for working with the disadvantaged—while they do much for normal children, they do more for the purportedly unteachables.

What was the significance of this experiment? It was the first, and by far the most important, acculturation experiment ever done in our laboratories, for it convinced us of the almost miraculous influence that structured exchanges can have in maintaining and modifying the behavior of disturbed children. These were, as noted, tough, barbarous little boys who were so clever at fighting that they always won. Yet, within a few weeks their habitual patterns had changed. Our theories about aggression, about cooperation, and perhaps about behavior in general, seem to have been borne out.

EXPERIMENTS 2 AND 3: DISRUPTIVE PRIMARY & INTERMEDIATE BOYS

We were not the only ones impressed. As word spread that this experiment was going on visitors, interested in young people and education, came to our laboratory to observe. Eventually, our staff received an invitation to run two special classes in one of the local school districts.

We were told the hyperaggressive boys were the most troublesome children, so we requested two classes—a younger and an intermediate group. During the first few months there were four boys, a teacher, and an assistant teacher in each class.

Preliminary Observations

For these two classes the observers changed the coding from simple aggression to disruption (a special case of aggression directed mostly toward the teacher) because the term was more descriptive of what occurred. A "disruption," as we used the term, would in a normal classroom quickly bring a reprimand. Classified as disruptions were: throwing pencils, purposefully tipping over furniture, fighting, yelling, swinging on doors, switching lights off and on, breaking windows, poking holes in the wall. Ordinary conversation, visiting, wandering around or gazing out windows were not considered disruptive in the general pandemonium of these classrooms.

The following is a description of a rather typical few minutes in the primary class during the baseline period when the teachers were allowed to proceed as they thought best. An analysis is interspersed in parentheses.

> John is sitting on a desk kicking his legs, screeching in a high voice, staring at other boys and the two teachers (score several disruptions). Mrs. Linden comes over and tries to drag him off the desk. She pulls at his legs until he is off and sits him in a chair. (Although her inten-

> tions were quite different, she indavertently reinforced his disruption by attending it.) Immediately he climbs back up on the desk (score one disruption). Mrs. Linden ignores this. She goes to the blackboard and completes the stars of the other three boys, giving John an X. Ted, Ralph and Steve are sitting at a table working fairly well. Now John is in his seat, but is still not working. He is sitting with his chin resting on a book staring off into space.
>
> Mrs. Linden stops working with Ted; she is now sitting with Ralph. Ted immediately stops working, turns around, tries to see what Mrs. Linden is doing. He comes back, tries to look in Ralph's desk (disruption). Steve is pounding his desk with his pencil, making a loud noise (disruption). Now Mrs. Snyder leaves John for Steve (reinforces Steve's disruption). With the teacher back at his side, Steve again settles down to his work. With the teacher gone, John stops working. He begins pounding his pencil into the table (disruption). He puts his feet up on the desk (disruption). Ted continues to walk around the room and Mrs. Linden walks to Ted's side, then to his desk, sits down with him. He begins working (she reinforces Ted's disruptive pattern). And so, on and on.

The pattern in this class differs significantly from that of the preschoolers. Mrs. Linden rewarded academic performance, following instructions and kindness to other students. In her class, academic performance was rated from 0 to 100 percent. If deportment was acceptable, she gave stars; if not, X's. All scores could rise or fall during the day. At the end of the day, each child whose ratings were good enough, and who had a completed star, received a candy bar. In addition the teachers consistently reinforced these children, far more importantly, by sitting with them tutoring them on their lessons. And ironically, it was this reinforcement that led to the disruptions. Except for John's, the disruptions were not malicious, designed to tease or upset the teacher, but apparently to finagle an invitation to sit with one of them to be tutored. The strategy usually worked; if it did not at first, the boys would escalate the disruptions until it did. But once a boy had the teacher's attention, he would almost always work well until she was distracted by another boy. When she left for the other boy, the first would usually stop studying in a minute or two and start acting up again.

The following is a description of a few minutes of a typical day (there were worse), in the intermediate class, observed by Buckholdt through the one-way mirror. An analysis is again interspersed in parentheses:

> Miss Tall announces they will be reading for a half hour (an exchange signal), but this doesn't produce any response (they are refusing

> to cooperate in the proposed exchange). The students still sit there, three of them in the classroom and Rudy in the cloakroom. Dave throws his eraser (score a disruption) at Dan who is bothering him (score a disruption for Dan too). Dave and Dan pull faces at one another (score disruptions for Dave and Dan). Miss Tall comes and asks Dan to work (inadvertent reinforcement for Dan—she gave him attention while he was acting up). He says, "Get away from me—get away from me," and refuses to let her talk (disruptions). He keeps this up until she finally leaves (reinforces Dan's disruptions). He jumps up and throws his book (score two disruptions). Now he has his book and seems to be looking for the place where he stopped yesterday. (Note the teacher ignored the last disruptions and Dan stopped disrupting! He is now working.) Dave is making strange noises with paper over his mouth (score a disruption), trying to get Miss Tall's attention, which he does (score one inadvertent reinforcement for disruption). Ned just sits in the corner, thumb in mouth, and watches. He seems to be very bored by the whole classroom situation. Now he slyly shoots Dave with a rubber band (score a disruption).

If we put together and analyze all such episodes in the intermediate class during the first month, the following conclusions would seem logical:

(1) With very few exceptions the teachers ignored the intermediate boys, failed to give them any attention, when they were working well. This was unfortunate because the teacher's attention appeared to be a reinforcer for the boys.

(2) However, the boys found that their disruptive behavior did get the teacher's negative attention, which apparently they also enjoyed. We concluded this from a number of cues; for example, the boys often tipped their hand by smiling behind the teacher's back after putting her through a particularly harassing session. And they would continue to disrupt aggressively as long as the teacher reciprocated with some kind of attention; only when she gave up did they stop. The teacher thought she was punishing the boys, that she was inhibiting their disruptions but she was actually reinforcing them. The sequence, disruption-attention, disruption-attention, continued until she finally walked away.

(3) The boys worked this disruptive interchange whenever the conditions were suitable. (a) They could almost invariably get a reaction from the teacher if, after studying a while, they stopped to act up. (b) Whenever the teacher asked them to work, the boys could always get an upset reaction by being negative, by refusing to do anything.

Looking back it is difficult to avoid the conclusion that the intermediate

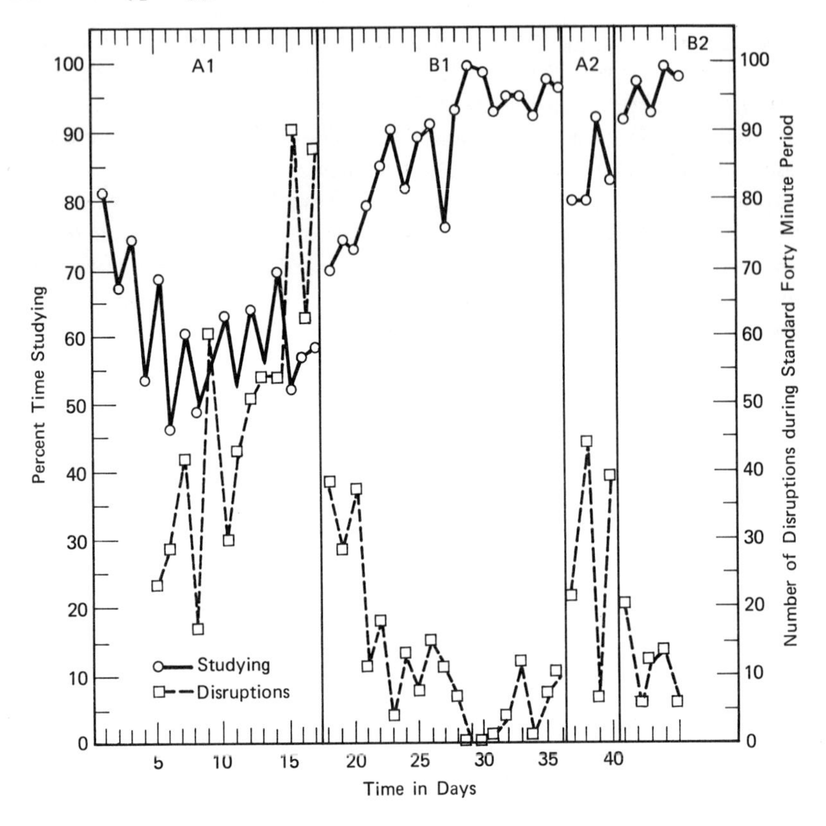

Figure 5.4. The percent time spent studying and the number of disruptions during a standard forty-minute period for four "hyperactive" first and second grade boys through time on a teacher's system (A1 and A2) and on a token exchange system (B1 and B2). The teacher rewarded studying with "stars" which were redeemed in candy at the end of the day, and she scolded disruptive behavior. In the B periods, tokens were continuously exchanged for study and could be traded for recess, swimming, privilege to buy ice cream at lunch, and, at the end of the day, toys. Disruptions were ignored, or if they could not be ignored, the child was timed out.

boys would purposely start studying simply to set up the teacher so she would be sure to retaliate when they began to disrupt, or they would dally on purpose to get her to ask them to do something so they could be negative and thus start a fight.

The Experiments

In these two classes, as before, we had the teachers terminate the exchanges which we thought were repeatedly reinforcing the disruptive patterns and in their place structure attractive token exchanges for studying.

The data for the primary class are given in Figure 5.4.[5] During the baseline period (A1) described earlier, before the token exchange was instituted, the boys, as noted, followed a zigzag course. Even so, in the beginning they spent 80 percent of the available time working at their studies. Their studying then deteriorated until it leveled off at about 55 percent. However disruptions increased, a typical *learning* curve, from 20 per each forty minute period to almost 90. But when the token exchange started in B1, studying quickly increased in a few days to about 95 per cent of the available time; disruptions dropped in a week from almost 90 per experimental period to only about 5, as an average.

When the token exchange was taken out again (A2) studying decreased, if slightly, to about 80 percent, and disruptions increased quickly to as many as 44 per period. With the reinstatement of the token exchange (B2), study went back up to about 96 percent of available time, and disruptions back down to less than 10 per period.

The data for the intermediate class are given in Figure 5.5. The results are essentially similar to those obtained in the two previous experiments with thc younger boys. By the fifteenth, sixteenth and seventeenth days of the A1 period the pattern had become predictable: the boys studied about 28 percent of the time, averaging 66 disruptions for the half hour experimental period.

The change with B1 and tokens was remarkable and rather dramatic. Eventually, the boys studied about 90 percent of the period and made an average of about 5 disruptions.

On the thirty-seventh day we started the reversal—simply by taking the tokens away. Subjectively, to the teachers in the room and to the experimenters watching, everything seemed to fall apart; but the data indicate that much of the improvement was maintained. The teachers were the main problem: without the support of the token exchange they tended to fall back on their old habits—attending to disruptions and failing to reward work. But the boys themselves had changed and all was not lost: in the A2 period they averaged 47 disruptions (compared to 66 in A1) and studied 70 percent of the time, compared to 28 percent in A1.

On the forty-first day we reinstituted the tokens. The boys responded almost immediately, with the usual extra bounce. The disruptions plunged down to less than 10, the studying rose to about 95 percent of total time.

[5] Disruptions were defined earlier in the text. Studying time was defined as time spent reading. Interobserver reliability studies were carried on periodically throughout the experiments with the primary and intermediate classes. The percent agreement on totals for both disruptions and studying time ranged between .81 and .91, the average being .86. Again the data were taken with Esterline-Angus 20-Channel Event Recorders, operated with a bank of press-on-light-on-press-off-light-off buttons.

They were in their new element again and full of fresh appreciation for it. As best we could gauge teacher reactions, they felt at least as much relief as the boys.

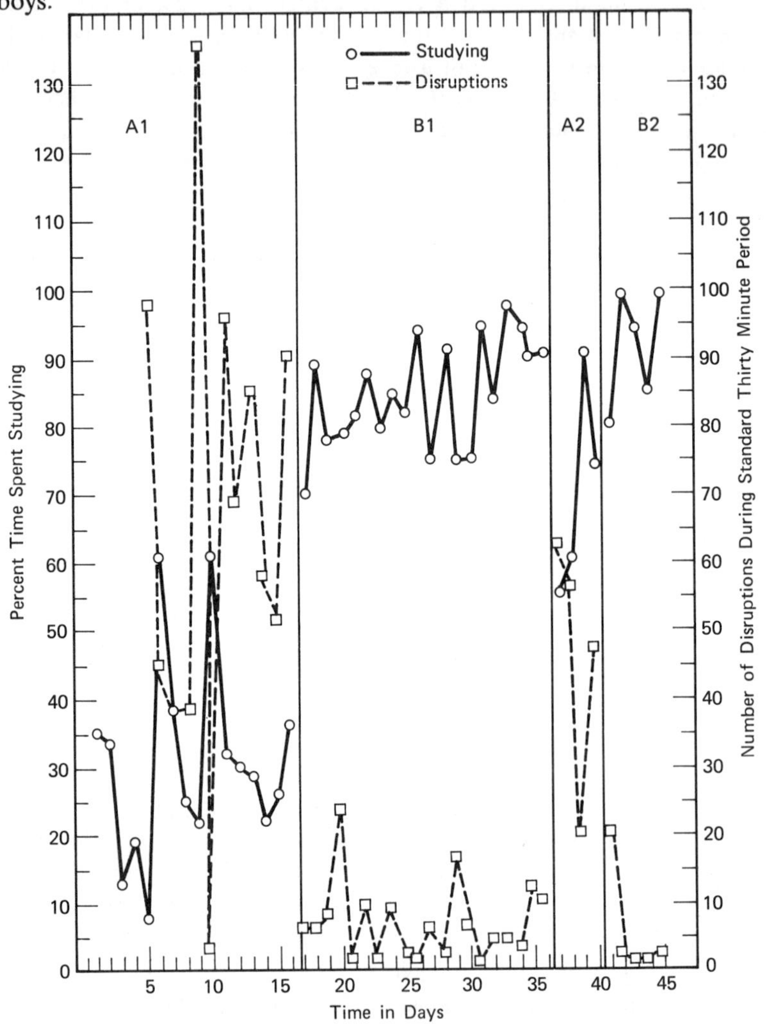

Figure 5.5. The percent time spent studying and the number of disruptions during a standard thirty-minute period for four "hyperactive" fourth and fifth grade boys, through time, on a teacher's system (A1 and A2) and on a token exchange system (B1 and B2). The teacher rewarded studying with help and attention some of the time, and mildly, though consistently, "punished" or scolded the worst forms of disruptive behavior. In the B periods, tokens were continuously exchanged for study and could be traded for recess, swimming, privilege to buy ice cream at lunch, and, at the end of each day, appropriate toys. Disruptions were ignored, or if they could not be ignored, the disruptive child was "timed out" into a small room adjacent to the classroom.

In previous chapters we have seen the equilibria rates of working specific exchanges accelerate or decelerate as the strength of the reinforcers was respectively increased or decreased. In this chapter the illustrations were more complex in that counter exchanges were involved—one behavior was decelerated as another behavior was being accelerated. The counter exchanges were designed to replace aggressive patterns with functional alternatives, that is, cooperative, studious patterns. As expected, increasing the strength of reinforcers for cooperative, studious patterns while simultaneously terminating reinforcers for the aggressive pattern produced rather swift, painless changes in behavior.

The Long Term Experience

By the time the experiment ended in December, the intermediate boys were doing well in the classroom. Like the primary class, they seemed to be working most of the time with only a few serious disruptions. However, with the introduction of two new boys, in December and in February, and with the change of emphasis from maintaining order to obtaining academic productivity and learning, a number of major problems were encountered. While each of the new boys behaved well for the first two or three days while they were learning the token exchange, each then began testing "the system," trying to subvert it. Unfortunately their disruptive patterns were contagious; the other boys joined in. Also these teachers had the problem of trying to manage a continuous exchange for academic achievement. They often ended up reinforcing appearing to work rather than correct work accomplished. Thus, in addition to the periodic disruptions, there was some feigning of work.

A cyclical system developed where the boys would disrupt for a period, causing great turmoil, then as a group would settle down to work or at least to feign work for an hour or so. Then they would agitate again, then settle down again, and so on. When the calm work periods arrived, the teachers were so grateful that they overpaid the boys. Thus during their working periods between the disruptions and agitations, the boys were able to "earn" enough tokens to make the more desirable purchases.

In an attempt to ameliorate this situation, the following exchange was structured: reasoning that these were older, more acculturated boys, it was decided to try a delayed exchange where points were given at the end of each work period. For example, 10 points might be allotted for behavior during each work period and up to 10 points for work correctly done. The delayed exchange, however, did not work. Being hyperactive, they were simply unable to sustain an interest in academic work without periodic reinforcement. Therefore, a periodic token exchange was reintroduced for good behavior during the working period, and a delayed point exchange was continued for work correctly done. This new structure broke the cyclical pattern. Even so, the situation was far from ideal. The boys continued to disrupt at a higher than normal rate, and they were still somewhat lackadaisical about their studies.

Consequently, several attempts were made to increase the power of the classroom exchanges by increasing the value of the backups which could be purchased with tokens. The most successful innovation along this line was a money allowance. Each boy was allowed to exchange tokens for a maximum of 20 cents a day or one dollar a week. Although this allowance seems small, the boys appreciated the opportunity to earn it, and their work did pick up somewhat. Even so, it became obvious that the power of exchange had to be increased further. We essentially faced two choices: spend much more for backups at school or have the parents structure exchanges at home. While we could have enriched the store at school, it seemed more probable that, with the cooperation of the parents, we could structure more meaningful exchanges in the home.

The parents, genuinely worred about their boys, were most cooperative. Hence with them we were able to work out several "cookbook" exchanges which were relatively simple. For John, the most troublesome of all the boys, an exchange was structured so his performance at school each day determined his privileges at home that evening (that is, whether or not he could watch TV, listen to his record player, visit with friends, etc.). In addition his weekend privileges were in exchange for his performance during the week. A second boy, Dave, whose study habits were most unstable, lived to work part time in his father's print shop. Hence an exchange was structured where the privilege of working part time had to be earned. Thus the better Dave did in school, as verified daily by notes to the father from the teacher, the more he could work in the print shop. For other less troublesome boys, a less powerful, more delayed exchange was structured. By behaving well in school and doing their studies, they could earn a special activity with their father each weekend. For example, the father might take the boy for a motorcycle ride, fishing, camping, etc., where the value of the activity was proportional to the boy's verified performance in school.

The combination of the more continuous token and point exchanges at school and the delayed exchanges at home was enough to transform the situation. The boys settled down to work, their behavior was often exemplary and they worked continuously morning and afternoon. In fact, they were so motivated, some of the boys began working right through recess.

It was about this time that the effects of the long term conditioning processes began to be evident. The boys decided among themselves that they wanted to be the very best class in school. Thus, when they attended assemblies, went on outings or participated in gym, they were models of behavior, at least when judged against their past. This pattern was reinforced naturally when the principal, other teachers and other children began to notice what was happening. Every time they participated in public, they began receiving a rash of compliments from surprised outsiders.

Also the parents began to report that the boys were studying at home. A number of the boys started to develop personal libraries. The parents began finding their boys reading in their rooms at night before going to sleep. The parents all noticed a big change in attitudes toward school.

Also, their behavior changed at home. The boys stopped picking so many fights with siblings and neighbor children. And they were finally able to escape the "dum dum" label. For example, Rudy, who had been plagued by the "dum dum" label, talked so ecstatically about school and evidenced so much academic progress that the children who had previously tormented began openly envying him.

At the beginning of the year when this intermediate class settled down so quickly in our initial experiment with them, we dared hope that they would make remarkable academic progress. However, as noted, with the introduction of the new boys, it took us until April to settle the class down into a routine of serious study. Hence, our hopes de-escalated. Even so, these boys did very well as may be noted in Table 5.4. Their median increase in reading was 1.25 levels (four were measured on the California Achievement Test, Upper Primary, two were tested on the Iowa Basic Skills Test) in arithmetic, 1.35 levels.

While this substantial improvement indicates these boys do have the chance of catching up with their peers academically, they still have their problems. Their early classroom experience was so bad that much of it needs to be done over again. While they can now spell third, fourth and fifth grade words, for example, they all too often miss first and second grade words. Put differently, they have curious deficiencies which require remedial work. While this remedial work will slow them down some, many of the boys should reach the normal level during their second year in the program.

The long-term experience with the primary class was not so difficult; the new boys who were introduced after the experiment settled down with little disruption of the normal routine of the classroom. However, as in the intermediate class, it was necessary to structure a periodic token exchange for good behavior, for going through the motions of studying, and a delayed point exchange for correct work.

The data from the before/after levels tests are summarized in Table 5.5. Like the intermediate class, these boys made substantial progress: 1.0 levels in reading and 1.4 levels in arithmetic.

Table 5.4. Grade Level Measures and Changes—Intermediate Class.

Date Enrolled in Tudor School	Child	Subject	Grade Level: At Enrollment	Grade Level: Summer 1968	Change
September, 1967	Rudy	Reading	2.3	3.1	.8
		Arithmetic	2.1	3.2	1.1
February, 1967	Tony	Reading	3.8	4.5	1.4[a]
		Arithmetic	3.6	4.5	1.8[a]
September, 1967	Dan	Reading	5.6	6.8	1.2
		Arithmetic	4.3	4.5	.2
December, 1967	John	Reading	4.8	6.5	1.7
		Arithmetic	4.3	5.8	1.5
September, 1967	Dave	Reading	2.4	3.5	1.1
		Arithmetic	3.8	5.0	1.2
September, 1967	Ned	Reading	1.5	2.8	1.3
		Arithmetic	2.0	3.5	1.5
Median Change in Reading					1.25
Median Change in Arithmetic					1.35

[a] Tony was in the program less than a half year—median change is twice the gains made in 4 months.

These three experiments took two years. Before and during that time, a number of similar experiments have been reported. A brief description of these experiments and their results are given in Table 5.6. While experimental procedures are somewhat variable, the results are usually strong and consistent for social science results. The main variations in outcome appear to be a function of the strength of the reinforcers used in the exchanges instituted by the experimenters; the stronger the reinforcers, the greater the modification in the aggressive pattern. These experiments represent important replications of our experiments and results.

THEORETICAL CONCLUSIONS

(1) The data from these investigations do not bear on the etiology or the original causation of hyperaggression. Rather they bear on its maintenance and modification. Hence, whatever the origins—genetic, biochemical or psychosocial—the hyperaggressive pattern is maintained and modified in ways that are generally characteristic of manipulative or operant behavior patterns. Thus according to the data hyperaggression is maintained because

Table 5.5. Grade Level Measures and Changes—Primary Class.

Date Enrolled in Tudor School	Child	Subject	Grade Level: At Enrollment	Grade Level: Summer, 1968	Change
September, 1967	John	Reading	Knew two letters of alphabet	2.3	1.3
		Arithmetic	Could count to ten	2.9	1.9
September, 1967	Ralph	Reading	1.9	2.9	1.0
		Arithmetic	1.8	3.7	1.9
November, 1967	Bud	Reading	1.5	2.4	.9
		Arithmetic	1.7	3.1	1.4
September, 1967	Steve	Reading	1.1	2.0	.9
		Arithmetic	1.2	2.3	1.1
January, 1968	Randy	Reading	1.4	3.0	1.6
		Arithmetic	1.5	1.5	.0
September, 1967	Ted	Reading	Beginning kindergarten level	1.5[a]	
		Arithmetic		2.0[a]	
Median Change in Reading					1.0
Median Change in Arithmetic					1.4

[a] Teacher's evaluation based on texts used in class; scores not included in median change calculations.

an adult, in the observed cases, is repeatedly and subtly, if inadvertently, reinforcing it. The results also suggest that if the social environment is changed so the hyperaggressive pattern is no longer reinforced but in its place a more adaptive pattern is repeatedly reinforced, then the boys' habit patterns change accordingly. The aggressive pattern extinguishes and the new, more adaptive habit pattern (in our experiments, cooperation and studying) develops in its place. While all hyperaggression may not be so characterized as an operant pattern, at this juncture there have been several approximate replications of our experiments in school situations all yielding essentially similar results. Hence, such a characterization of hyperaggression seems to be generally appropriate, at least among children.

(2) We have found the boys in our experiments variously motivated to be hyperaggressive. They mostly play a teasing game, "Get the Teacher," perhaps to enliven an otherwise deadly dull day, but one class disrupted to get tutoring from the teacher.

More generally, there may be many motives for aggression. It could be quite true that some aggressive exchanges are maintained because one person

Table 5.6. Summary of Research, Remediation of Hyperaggression.

	Subjects	Experimental Treatment	Results
Zimmerman & Zimmerman (1962)	Eleven year old boy who had kicking and screaming tantrums in the classroom.	Teacher began ignoring tantrums. Approached, smiled, talked with him and started him on attractive lesson when he stopped tantrumming, and after he completed assignment.	After several weeks, tantrumming entirely eliminated. (Same system later eliminated baby talk, irrelevant comments and questions.)
Homme & associates (1963)	A class of nursery school children.	With no punishment used to keep order, class disrupted into pandemonium. Homme's group took careful notes of favorite, often chosen activities under these initial conditions. Had teacher signal one of these favorite activities, e.g. running and screaming time, after period of quiet attendance at lesson.[a]	Teacher obtained perfect control after a few days. Class would work at lessons very hard to participate in favorite activities.
Brown & Elliot (1965)	A nursery school class of 27 three and four year olds.	ABAB experimental design: during A periods teachers stopped and punished aggression. During B periods they ignored it stoically and rewarded cooperative peaceful behavior. Rewards: pat on head, saying "That's good," or calling class attention to something good the child had done.	Frequency of observed aggressive acts: A1, 64 per hr.; B1, 43 per hr.; A2, 52 per hr.; B2, 26 per hr.
Becker & associates (1965)	Ten troublesome children, two from each of five classes—six to ten years old.	AB experimental design: A periods teachers attended and punished deviant behaviors. B periods teachers ignored deviant behaviors, attended and praised behaviors which facilitated learning.	Deviant behavior dropped from 62 percent during nine week A period to 29 percent during nine week B period.
O'Leary & Becker	Eight most deviant of 17 nine year old children in a third grade "adjustment" class.	AB experimental design. During A period teacher disciplined aggression or bad behavior. During B period—points redeemable in candy, pennants, comics, perfume, kites, etc., were given for cooperating with the teacher and for school work.	Average of all observed behavior which was "deviant" during A: 76 percent; during B: 10 percent. Same children who had not finished an assignment in two years began to get perfect papers for the first time.

[a] Favorite activities used as reinforcers: running, screaming, chair pushing, puzzle working, plastic cup throwing, wastebasket kicking and giving the experimenter a ride on a plastic chair. Note: treatment and control subjects were not randomly assigned; hence the results could be due to self-selection.

frustrates another, because one person is unjust to another (Homans, 1961) or because one person is trying to protect his territory from the other's invasion (Lorenz, 1966). Certainly there is rather strong experimental evidence that the interference-frustration-aggression hypothesis is true for some people in some situations (cf. Hamblin et al., 1963). And there is anecdotal, if not experimental, evidence for the injustice-aggression and the territorial-aggression hypotheses, at least for some people in some situations.

Perhaps more importantly, most motives for aggression may be served as well if not better by alternative behavior patterns. Talk and reason often substitute for personal fights, trade and commerce for banditry, wages for slavery, law and the judicial process for feuds and so forth.

However, it is apparently essential that these substitute patterns actually serve as well if not better than the aggressive pattern. Our experiments worked because the cooperative-studying patterns were simply much more rewarding than the aggressive patterns, particularly under experimental conditions. The other patterns that supposedly replace the aggressive pattern in larger society apparently work only to the extent they are more feasible than aggression. When they become cumbersome, unwieldy, people generally seem to return to the more primitive aggressive approaches.

(3) Be that as it may, our data suggest the hyperaggressive boys no longer need fail in school; they no longer need to make their own and others' lives miserable. Although they enjoy escalating adults' attempts at punishment into jolly good fights (which they are skilled at winning), hyperaggressive boys do respond typically to rewards. Winning fights takes intelligence, and as we have seen, these boys also do very well academically, if given a chance. Their undesirable behavior does not continue in a nonpunitive, rewarding environment. Is it too much to ask parents and special education teachers to give up punishment and in its place to learn how to reward, that these boys may live productive not wasted, brutalizing, brutalized lives?

CHAPTER 6

Two Aggressive Lives

DAVE REGIA

Dave Regia's reputation at Tudor School had a certain awesome purity in its badness.[1] The boys found him a "bully" and just plain "stupid." The teachers added "disrespectful," "a bad actor" and "anxious and ineffectual." He began to earn that reputation during his primary years in a parochial school, where he had been unwilling to learn, and was very disruptive. Specifically, he was a poor reader and refused to work to get better. He was diagnosed as having perceptual problems, and the teachers could not get him to work to improve them. Instead he caused more and more turmoil in class until he was finally referred to a special education program.

In that first special class, a year before he came to us, he continued to refuse to work. Also, he was disruptive and extremely aggressive, bullying the other pupils. The classroom battles between Dave and the teacher became so frequent that no one was able to work, and the class was in general chaos. He was about to be expelled when we came around asking for the toughest children—and got him, on special assignment.

However, the change of locale did not soften him. He banged pencils on his desk, threw erasers across the room, kicked and pounded the walls and otherwise damaged the floors and desks. In addition, he fought—sometimes in running battles that lasted for days. The teacher would often try to separate him from the others to end the carnage, but later he would be at it again. When fighting, he fought ferociously and unfairly. He lied with heat and without qualm to the teacher about the facts—who started it, what had happened, who was at fault. And, once involved in a fight, he seemed unable to inhibit himself at all, unable to stop.

[1] Buckholdt and Hamblin took the major responsibility for writing this chapter. The case data were gleaned, in part, from social worker and psychiatric reports which were made available to us by the school. Also, Buckholdt interviewed the parents several times during the year.

But fighting, while perhaps his forte, was not his only problem. As suggested earlier, he was a tenuous student at best. His teacher characterized him, in retrospect, this way:

> To Dave, the classroom was a place of anxious trial, of almost certain failure. As he began a day, he would start to make small errors. His small errors would increase his anxiety; his increased anxiety would lead to larger errors; and so on all day long. Consequently, he did not have the confidence to be independent. He showed little self-direction; little initiative. He was so unsure of himself he hesitated to begin his work and once started, his anxiety quickly increased to the point where he would never finish. Thus, he was unable to work for more than fifteen or twenty minutes in any one assignment. Some days he refused to do any assignments at all. These difficulties were compounded because he was unable to tolerate assistance from the teacher for more than a few minutes at a time, perhaps because he felt that help from a teacher was a living demonstration that he was unable to do the work himself.
>
> Thus, Dave was very conscious about his failures in school. He was most ashamed about the discrepancy between his age and the level of work he was doing—"baby work" as he characterized it. As a result he would go into depressive states in which he would sit, drum on his desk top, pick his arm, fidget, look as if he might burst into tears any minute. Also, he had a facial tick which became very severe during these periods; his eyes would blink ten to twenty times faster than normal. In such a state he seemed unable to initiate any satisfying activity. In fact, during these periods, nothing that anybody could do satisfied him. Rather he wallowed in misery, complaining that he felt sick or that he was tired. It was following these periods of depression that he would typically start—or continue—his fights.
>
> Thus, Dave had a poor image of himself. He would often pull his hat over his face or he would try to hide his face in other ways. Several times, for example, he made masks which he placed over his face. Other times, he would lie on the floor with his face down, hidden in his hands, a pathetic figure.

When the token exchange was first introduced in early October, Dave began to improve. His studying increased from about 17 percent to between 80 and 95 percent of the available time. His disruptions decreased from between 8 and 30 per half hour to between 0 and 6. The teachers were very encouraged. However, when the new boys were added to the class in December and then in February, Dave regressed. His studying became very erratic: one day he would be a model student, the next refuse to work altogether.

He was performing at about 50 percent of what we knew his potential to be.

Various explanations were offered: the school clinical psychologist suggested that Dave should be taken off stimulants and given tranquilizers; the principal thought the teachers were too lenient; we felt that the reinforcers were not powerful enough. We tried everything. When Dave was taken off stimulants and given tranquilizers, his behavior did not improve. When the teachers became more demanding, he became worse. Furthermore, we were simply unable to locate any backup reinforcers that would make the token exchange work. These efforts took two and a half months and thus ended in failure.

Finally, one day in late March, Buckholdt simply asked Dave what the matter was. Dave replied easily with the correct diagnosis. His father had opened a small print shop and since January had been paying him $3.00 an hour to work after school. Although technical, the job did not require him to use what he was learning in school. He was making what he considered very good money without knowing how to read or much in the way of arithmetic. Who needed school? His grandfather, a successful printer, had not finished grade school, and his father had dropped out of high school. "Why should I be different?" Dave asked.

Buckholdt promptly conferred with Dave's parents, who were very concerned about his failures and eager to cooperate. The father immediately suggested that Dave not be allowed to work in the shop unless he behaved well and made progress at school. So, as suggested in the last chapter, the teacher began sending home a note each day evaluating Dave's performance. In addition, Dave had to read each print job to his father's satisfaction before he could work on it—and his father was not satisfied unless Dave's reading fluency increased from week to week.

A new zest and interest became evident in Dave's work. He often completed his assigned lessons by noon and spent many recesses and afternoons in free reading or performing mechanical experiments. During reading periods, where the measurements were taken from mid-April until June, Dave studied from 90 to 100 percent of the time and stopped disrupting entirely. At year's end, his teacher's opinion had changed. We give her report in some detail to emphasize the dramatic nature of the change, and the difficulty of ascribing it to any factors other than the working of the new instructional exchanges.

Reading

Before: When he entered the classroom at the beginning of the year, Dave was reading at what I judge to be the middle first grade level. His vocabulary recognition was sporadic, he blocked with a number of words and he was not able to utilize phonics in sounding out new or difficult words. Also, he was subject to reversals, reading "was" as "saw," etc. In addition, his anxiety evidently did not allow him to repeat some words so he repeated the idea instead, for example, substituting pony for horse and fruit for apple. He missed small prepositions and conjunctions. His reading mechanics were poor: he did not read smoothly but stopped and started in a very jerky manner. Also he had difficulty keeping on a sentence line of a page. While he read, Dave would become very nervous, drum on the table, shift his feet or go into rhythmic patterns with his body. He disliked reading; in fact, he seemed to hate it. While reading, he was constantly fighting depression, because he wanted to read at a higher level.

After: The first time I realized the dramatic change in his reading was when he went with Dr. Buckholdt during which time he was rewarded for his reading, not only by the presence of a masculine figure but also with tokens and enthusiasm. This experience gradually changed his basic attitude toward reading, and the change carried over into the classroom. Toward the end of February, I realized his reading was really up to capacity for his phonetic skills, so we began to work with them. His reading continued to improve through March. Beginning in April when I started sending notes home to his father, Dave's progress accelerated. Now two months later, he is able to read independently in middle fourth grade level books. For example, he is able to read well enough in a fourth grade geography book so he is able to answer the questions independently.

In the fall I was told by the school psychologist that because of brain damage, Dave would be unable to learn to read past the middle elementary levels, that at best he might be taught to read enough so he could just get by in his adult years. However, that prognosis seems much too pessimistic in the light of his progress during these last two months. Even his perceptual problems are no longer evident in the classroom. Now when he reads "was" for "saw," he quickly corrects himself. The improvement makes one think that perhaps his reversal problem was just a habit. When Dave is rewarded consistently for *not* making these mistakes, he himself is able to handle the problem.

Dave is now able to read a page from a book without the aid of a marker although he still sometimes relies on one. He does not jump around the page, he does not mix up words from one sentence to another. I would not consider him perceptually handicapped.

Mathematics

Before: When he entered our class, he had been working at the structural arithmetic book and seemed to be working independently at the upper third grade level. However, he was taking cues for his arithmetic answers off the page. He would fuss around giving various answers until he elicited some response from the teacher that would clue him.

He had difficulty thinking abstractly. The first lessons which I gave him were on symbols and symbolism. He had a very difficult time understanding what a symbol is and why we use symbols in arithmetic or in writing.

After: Dave is now able to work independently at an upper sixth grade arithmetic level. He will ask the teacher for different words on a mathematics page which he does not understand, but then he proceeds doing quite well with abstract thinking. He is even now able to work out his own methods for getting an answer to a problem.

Writing

Dave's handwriting has improved. He first wrote a combination of script and printing. Now he is consistent in using one or the other, and his written work is always legible and neat.

Work Habits

Now Dave works during free time, play time, even the noon hour. He is unbelievable. He works during recess in order to get his assigned work finished. And he prefers to stay in the room and eat his sack lunch while doing his work rather than go down to the lunch room to eat with the others. On those days when he does finish an hour or two ahead of the rest of the class, he has enough initiative, enough self-direction, that he keeps himself busy quietly at his seat, reading, doing puzzles or working through programmed learning materials. Now when he hands papers in, they are neat, always stapled together. He is extremely well organized. He knows exactly what he has to do. He starts in the morning by asking for the full day's work assignment, then when he is finished, he wants all of his work checked and graded. He wants his parents to know exactly how well he is doing.

Relations with Teachers

Dave now seems to enjoy getting favorable reactions from his teachers. He likes his teachers to smile at him, and is no longer embarrassed when a teacher returns a look.

Relations with Peers

Dave has gradually become a leader in the class. He often helps the other boys when they have difficulty. He encourages the others to settle down, to read, etc. In public he reacts very well, keeps his presence with adults and wants to be associated with them, identified with them. I would say that Dave has now assumed a position of prestige in the class.

Delinquent Behavior

Dave still lies some and steals some. He is not terribly upset at being caught, nor is he upset if others comment about it. In fact, he is able to talk about his lying and stealing in a way which may or may not be good. Nevertheless, he no longer denies everything.

Taking Tests

Dave has had a history of testing poorly, and he still tests poorly. He blocks and becomes very anxious when taking a test.

Conclusions

As the teacher noted, Dave still has some problems—a mild test phobia and vestiges of his old habits, stealing and lying. Even so, he has just about escaped the behavioral prison into which he had locked himself.

JOHN MUNSEN

Our intermediate class was to be John Munsen's last stop before the state mental hospital. After many suspensions from elementary school, he had been expelled and forbidden entry into any other public school in his community. He had become an increasing source of serious problems in his classes. Social workers and teachers claimed that he stuck pins into his classmates, bullied the smaller children and had injured several boys so badly in fights that they required medical attention. He often left his room without permission, and traveled around the school visiting friends in the gymnasium, the lavatory or in other classes. If a teacher challenged him, he frequently threw books from the window, overturned desks or picked fights. If he felt like it, he left school without permission, and did not arrive home until late in the evening.

The school officials tried patience and understanding, they tried the talking approach—hour after hour of trying to reason with him—but to no avail. He was extremely convincing at feigning penitence, and was clever at lying, until the principal and teachers came to believe nothing he said.

At that point, his mother was asked to spend days at school ready to take John home if he became unmanageable. This, too, was useless; he became more and more disruptive, aggressive, uncontrollable. Finally he was expelled.

John's parents report that for three years before expulsion, he had been seeing a prominent psychiatrist who diagnosed him as having a "character disorder," as being a "sociopath." He told the parents that John very probably had a constitutional or genetic defect and little could be done.

"Essentially, therefore, John was doomed." A residential treatment school in New York might help a little, but a life of constant trouble and turmoil—possibly imprisonment—was almost inevitable for him. The only help the psychiatrist could offer would be to the parents—to help them to live with these facts.

A neurologist came to a similar conclusion. John had a "character disorder" with "excessive involuntary overflow," "myclonic jerk" and uncontrollable aggressive impulses. John could not possibly be contained in a normal classroom; he suggested a "preventative" military or boarding school.

No one had suggested that John's behavior could have been learned; yet his family history was one of turmoil and conflict, the kind that often produces problem children. John was adopted when a few days old by middle class parents who had an older boy. For two and a half years he had a happy family life; but then, according to the father, "all hell broke loose." His mother, for some unexplained reason, became severely punitive with both boys, beating them frequently. Even the smallest mistake or slightest backtalk incurred her wrath. At the same time relations between husband and wife deteriorated rapidly, and they were divorced after twenty-five years of marriage. After the separation, John was shuttled back and forth from father to mother to boarding school. Finally, after three years of bitter fighting between the parents, John's father was awarded custody.

John remembers the time spent alone with his father and brother as very happy. He had escaped his punitive mother, and his father made few demands. This soon changed, however. The father remarried. The new mother, herself divorced after nineteen years, moved in with two daughters.

According to two social worker reports John deeply resented this intrusion and apparently set out to torture his new stepmother. When his father was at home, he behaved well; but when his father was gone, he became a devil. The mother reports that he would mess up one end of the house, then when she came to clean up, he would move to another area and tear that up. This was systematic; it went on for several hours each day. He was also extremely rebellious. If his stepmother asked him to take out the garbage, he would dump it in the back yard. If she asked him to make his bed, he would tear it up.

Mrs. Munsen complained frequently to her husband, but he was not sympathetic. "You just don't know how to handle children." Therefore, with his father's inadvertent support, John felt free to continue to increase the pressure. Finally Mrs. Munsen was driven to the psychiatrist who told her that John's problems were "genetic" and that she would have to learn to live with them. Mrs. Munsen reported that this advice did not help her much.

As John grew older, he broadened his area of attack. He began to have frequent trouble with teachers and students. He had been a shy, withdrawn child in the primary grades but by the fourth grade he was already a developing hell raiser. For a time the school officials punished him in traditional ways—keeping him after school, paddling and temporary suspension. Eventually Mrs. Munsen just waited in the anteroom of the principal's office every day until John was sent home.

This constant turmoil moved Mrs. Munsen to the edge of a "nervous breakdown." She no longer talked to the psychiatrist about John's problems, but about her own. And when John was finally expelled, her days became a living hell. She retreated to her bed. John did not ease up, however. On the contrary, he stepped up his reign of terror at home. He would simply roam the house, taking what he wanted, destroying things and creating havoc.

Since the father felt he could not afford to send John to the residential school in New York as the psychiatrist had recommended, only two options seemed open to him: either the state mental hospital or another divorce. John's father had tentatively decided for the state mental hospital when word came that John was accepted into a special education class. He had been rejected earlier on the basis of the reports of the psychiatrist and the neurologist, but when our laboratory assumed responsibility for the intermediate class, John was admitted. We had asked "for the toughest problems available." And so we got him in December. One condition was that he attend weekly group therapy sessions at a local psychiatric clinic. As it happened, he never did.

John had been out of school about seven months when he came to us, a few days before Christmas recess. His sturdy physique, good grooming and pleasant smile gave no hint of his destructiveness. For the first two days, he sat quietly, almost unnoticed. He caught on quickly to the token exchange, and he worked it well. He completed his work without complaint and cooperated fully. Buckholdt remarked at the time that he could not imagine why such an attractive, well-behaved boy was in a class for disturbed children.

On the third day, however, the first shock came. On a field trip John viciously attacked a classmate. He had to be pulled away and then restrained by two teachers. The next day, the second attack: John jumped on a boy, knocked him to the ground and had his hands around his throat trying to choke him when the teachers were finally able to pull him off. There was no provocation, no warning, apparently no rational explanation. One minute John would be sitting quietly at his desk or standing silently watching the boys play; the next, he would be attacking violently. The teachers privately agreed never to leave anyone alone in the room with him.

Some types of aggressive behavior can be ignored; but not John's. So we outlined a careful strategy. When he attacked another boy in this vicious fashion, his teachers were to avoid entering into aggressive games or contests with him, as had his former teachers; they would restrain him, give the other boy attention, then time John out either in the hall or in the cloakroom. If he left the time-out room to roam through the school, they would not chase him; they would merely inform him that his time-out had to be served before he could rejoin the group. The longer he spent roaming the school, the longer he would have to wait.

John must have found the classroom enjoyable, for he did not like to be timed out. In the time-out room he became sullen, downcast and would frequently inquire if the time were up, if he could come back to the room. Upon return, he would often apologize to the teacher and promise not to misbehave again. The time-out procedure worked very well: John stopped his irrational hostile attacks.

But his other behavior was bad enough. One day he would be a model student; the next, he would tease his classmates, steal items from their desks, throw their coats out the window, drop tacks down their backs and pull their chairs from under them. Then with a smirk, he would return quietly to his seat, leaving the class in complete chaos. Throughout the following day, he was likely to be quiet and industrious. But on the day after that, he would return to the attack.

Despite all this John worked between 60 to 80 percent of the time available to him during the first two months. But he also averaged about nine severe disruptions per week. Although his progress was not as good as most of the other boys, given his history we did not find it too bad. He seemed to enjoy himself in class; he liked the teachers; he even liked the other boys, despite his malicious teasing. He did not like the principal, but that feeling was reciprocated. The psychiatrist, the neurologist and the social workers had predicted that he would not last more than a month in our class; he was doing much better than that.

Even so, about nine weeks after John's arrival, trouble increased again. His study habits did not change much in the morning, but in the afternoon he hardly studied at all. He began, among many other things, to throw paper airplanes and tokens out of the window. He also began to steal tokens from his classmates and to hide their textbooks. At the same time his behavior at home deteriorated. When he started in our class, his attitude toward his stepmother had improved a great deal; now ten weeks later the assault was on again.

The teacher, the principal and the social workers became alarmed; all agreed that his uncontrollable impulses were taking over once more. "He should go on drugs;" "he needs group therapy at the clinic;" "he needs a good licking!"

Our analysis was different. Our exchanges, we felt, were simply not as effective as they should have been. The praise, attention and approval for good work were doing well enough; so was our tactic of simply ignoring (or timing him out) for bad behavior instead of rewarding it with a lot of attention, by chasing, arguing and threatening. John came from a well-to-do family that gave him most of the material things he could possibly want (specifically, pool and ping-pong tables, a personal TV set, a free soda machine, stereo, food or candy any time he wanted them and a rather generous allowance, up to $5 a week). Against this competition, our tokens and the things they would buy at school simply did not turn him on.

Usually, if a positive exchange fails, we increase its power. But what could we possibly offer that his parents were not topping free of charge? So, as with the others, we put him on a different system—we made an arrangement with his parents that they would use these items as backup reinforcers, making them contingent on his progress at school. Each day he brought home a note from the teacher. A total of three points on it indicated a very good day—he had behaved well and had done all assigned work. On three-point days he was allowed all his privileges. On two-point, "fairly good" days (he had done most of the work, but had not quite lived up to expectations), he received all normal pleasures minus an important one such as watching television, playing his stereo or visiting. On one-point days (bad behavior and work, but not so bad that he had to be sent home), he lost most of his regular pleasures, and in addition, he could not leave home or have friends visit him. On zero-point days (sent home early), he was restricted to his bedroom in the evening with no privileges at all.

On Fridays the points were added and the total determined his weekend privileges: twelve to fifteen points, all privileges plus a bonus of one or two extras; nine to twelve points, the usual pleasures minus one important one; on six to nine point weeks, he suffered a species of polite house arrest, some of his in-house pleasures remained intact, but he could have no visitors and he could not leave the yard. Less than six points meant grounding for the weekend—*sans* television, friends, hi-fi.

Results from this more powerful prodding were immediate and dramatic. He began working hard and behaving well. Studying upped abruptly from about 67 percent to about 89 percent of available time; severe aggressions dropped from an average of 9 per week to less than 1. Even in the troublesome afternoons his behavior improved considerably. He abruptly stopped throwing things out the window, teasing and stealing. By the end of the year there were virtually no more problems with John. In fact he formed strong friendships with the boys, charmed the teachers and even made friends with the principal!

The pattern was repeated at home. He started cooperating with his parents, and helped his stepmother with her housework. He became much less rebellious and much more friendly, particularly toward the delighted Mrs. Munsen. "I've decided to be good," he told a social worker. "It's just too hard, too much work to be bad."

Conclusion

It is quite possible that this is merely talk; pious talk comes easy to a "sociopath." John should stay at least another year in our program where our teachers know how to respond to him, working the exchanges both in class and at home. It should take him at least that long until he enjoys behaving more than misbehaving. But allowing these qualifications, his progress to date has exceeded everyone's expectations, including his own.

It is all too easy, when a boy does not seem to respond to the normal sticks and carrots of our culture, to speculate or even assume that the fatal flaw lies deep in him somewhere caused by genetic or organic defect, leaving little hope. But if one analyzes John's history carefully, it becomes obvious that ever since he was quite small, he had been working pathogenic exchanges structured by most of the people around him—parents, teachers, school officials and so on. They did not know they had structured these exchanges, but they had—and their alarmed or resentful reactions reinforced his sociopathic behavior. John's behavior then was in large part what these exchanges molded. As he worked them successfully and repeatedly John developed extreme habit patterns of cruelty, viciousness, rebelliousness and along with them such cleverness in lying and such a charming pattern of verbal penitence that he was seldom punished.

Of course, this is our interpretation. Others may say that a sociopath does not really change his spots. But our interpretation has been borne out by the results of our training. When we terminated the pathogenic exchanges so he could no longer work them, and in their place structured acculturating exchanges for him to work in the classroom and home, John's habitual behavior pattern began to change from those of a sociopath to those of a normal, rather attractive twelve-year-old boy.

John's case has also underlined again a very important principle. When an exchange fails to be effective—that is, when the child refuses to work it —the situation should be restructured with a new, more powerful exchange. During that ninth week when John reverted more and more openly to his earlier disruptive pattern, there was some talk among the staff of giving up, admitting failure. After all, it was said, there are limits to all types of remediating procedures. Why not recognize them and avoid useless work and disappointment? We decided instead to have the parents restructure their exchanges in cooperation with the teachers—with the happy results we have seen. The new exchange made all the difference to John. He was thereby enabled to gain control over himself, to stop the sociopathic pattern of self destruction, to put in its place a more normal pattern that may yet lead him to live usefully with some happiness and fulfillment.

IN RETROSPECT

Although these case studies and the experiments which preceded them appear in the middle of this book, they were actually completed early in the history of our program of research, during the first and second years. While we still have great confidence in the results of the experiments, in the efficacy of the procedures, we have not continued since that time to work with special classes of hyperaggressive children. The reason: we do not think special classes of hyperaggressives are a good idea. Such classes stigmatize a child, damage him socially and psychologically in unnecessary ways. The problems of the hyperaggressive, although they may seem monu-

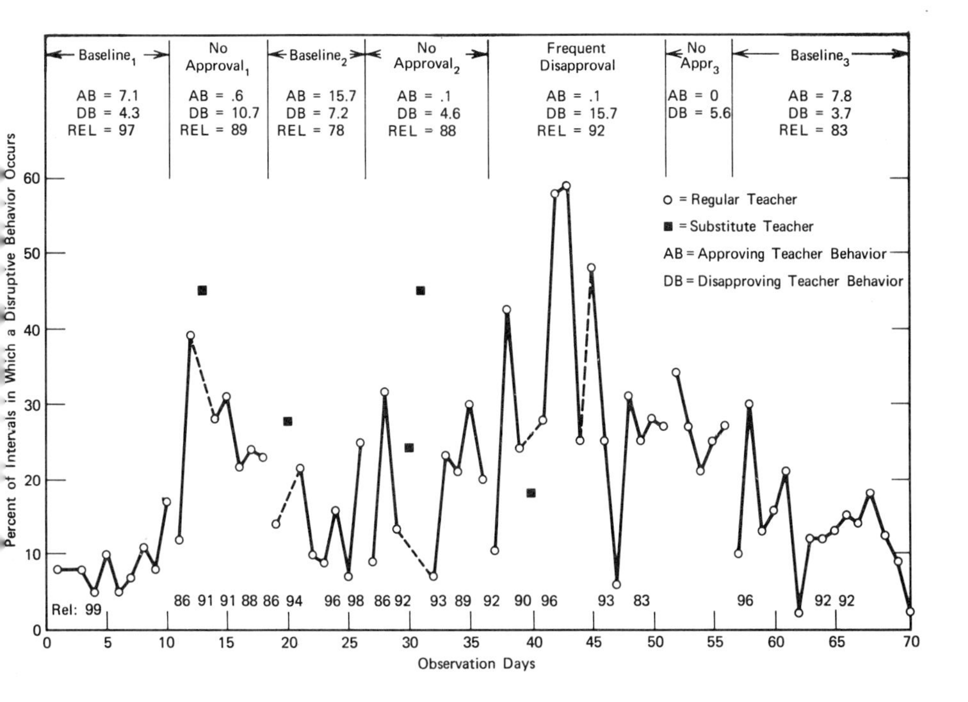

Figure 6.1. Disruptive classroom behaviors as a function of nature of teacher behavior. Data points represent two minute samples on ten children each day. Dotted lines cross observations where the regular teacher was absent due to a recurrent illness, including a ten day hospitalization between days 39 and 41. The dotted line connecting days 44 and 45 represents the Easter vacation break. The data for day 26 were taken with the teacher out of the room. (After Thomas, Becker and Armstrong, 1967.)

mental to teachers and parents who do not know how to handle them, are in actuality relatively easy to remediate. Easy enough for the usual teacher to handle in the typical classroom situation. The essential requirements are simply that she understand, that she be trained properly.

One might object that a teacher in the usual classroom situation is already overburdened, why insist that she handle the load of remediating hyperaggression in addition to all the other problems. We are not suggesting that teachers might not need expert guidance, counsel in handling these problems; it just turns out that the procedures that are effective in handling the extreme cases of hyperaggression are also the best ones for handling the disruptive, aggressive behavior of less bothersome children. There are a number of experiments which show this (cf. Madsen, Becker, Thomas, Koser, and Plager, 1968). The most dramatic, however, is by Thomas, Becker, and Armstrong (1968) who illustrate how a teacher might unintentionally cause previously normal children to engage in a high rate of disruptive behaviors. The data in Figure 6.1 summarize observations of ten children for two minutes each, each day. The children, bright second graders, were observed during a morning reading time when they and most of their classmates were doing seat work.

Under baseline conditions the teacher maintained discipline, using rather frequent approval (7.1 percent of the total responses to the children) and some disapproval (4.3 percent). During those periods the children engaged in some disruptive behaviors, in less than 10 percent of the sample periods. This level may seem high, but it was considered normal for that school. During the next condition, as may be noted in Figure 6.1, the teacher, under instructions from the experimenters, stopped giving approval for appropriate behavior (the percentage dropped from 7.1 to .6 of her total responses). Rather she relied on disapproval for discipline (disapproving behavior increased from 4.3 to 10.7 percent). The result: *the frequency of disruptive behavior increased from under 10 percent to approximately 28 percent.* In other words, when she took away her rewards of social approval, the situation deteriorated, almost immediately.

During the next condition the teacher attempted to reinstitute baseline using approval to reward exemplary behavior and to rely less on disapproval to inhibit disruptive behavior. However, the children apparently found it difficult to settle down. Disruptive behaviors occurred on the average in approximately 15 percent of the sampling periods. During the next three experimental conditions the experimenters instructed the teacher to give no approval, but to vary the frequency in her use of disapproval. Note in Figure 6.1 that when she used disapproval the most (when it comprised 15.7 percent of all her responses to the children), the children behaved their worst, disrupting in over 50 percent of the sampling periods on the extreme days. In the final experimental condition the teacher attempted to return to baseline, relying mostly on approval to encourage good behavior, using some disapproval to inhibit disruptive behavior. The average data show that she never did get the children back to the original condition where they were disrupting less than 10 percent of the time.

The experimenters suggest that this experiment illustrates how to make a bad class out of a good one. The data show rather clearly that whenever this teacher stopped accentuating the positive—that is, using approval to encourage or reinforce good behavior—the rate of disruptive behavior increased. Furthermore, the data show that the increase in disruption was not completely reversible, at least given the manipulations of teacher approval and disapproval. Apparently then, these bright second graders responded much the same way as our hyperaggressive boys did. When the teacher failed to reward them sufficiently for the good behavior, they turned to the more interesting games of getting the teacher.

The above experiments in this and the preceding chapter amply illustrate that teachers who are unaware of what they are doing can create pathogenic learning environments. Hence, we are suggesting that all teachers should learn the behavior management procedures outlined in these chapters and use them routinely in their classes. In our experience in the inner-city school, we find that a teacher, to maintain discipline, has to give some children a few tokens each day for non disruptive behavior. That small concession allows such children to live peaceably in the usual classroom situation and to make normal academic progress.

The few who are not able to progress often need no more than stronger backup reinforcers. It should be possible for the parents to furnish these as they did for Dave and John. It is very simple for a teacher to send home a note each night, if it is needed, or if not, each week and for parents to give privileges at home which are proportional to the noted behavior and progress of the child at school. Even so, such a system may not work with all children. Some may have to be segregated into special classes, some may have to be placed in foster homes where parents are trained in behavior management techniques, as they are in Opportunity Place (an experimental home for delinquent boys established by Montrose Wolf and his associates in Lawrence, Kansas). However, our feeling is that the thrust of remedial work with disruptive children should be in the usual classroom situation by usual teachers trained to spot pathogenic exchanges and to restructure them so their charges may develop in more productive ways.

CHAPTER 7

The Autistic Child: An Introduction

This chapter is an introduction to the laboratory staff's work with a number of autistic children who were severely retarded intellectually and socially when we began to work with them.[1] Autism has been thought by some to be a type of psychosis, the result of physiological defect or damage (cf. Rimland, 1964; Kallmann, 1946; Kety, 1959). Others, such as Bruno Bettelheim (1967), find the cause of the psychosis in extreme emotional disturbance starting very early in life. Both explanations consider the autistic symptoms themselves to be a secondary problem; the "real" disorder is a flaw or sickness within the child himself. In contrast, our research suggests that autism, in some cases at least, may be the natural result of very faulty acculturation and that autistic children have acquired peculiar learning disabilities, the outcome of which are rather severe, insidiously cumulative behavioral problems.

AUTISM

Autism has received considerable attention for research primarily because of its severity as a disorder and its resistance to treatment. Like Mt. Everest, autism is there standing as the ultimate challenge to the scientist interested in early childhood disorders. Even so, until recently the prognosis for autistic children has been poor (Eisenberg, 1956). Almost all are faced with a life of confinement at home or in an institution for the mentally ill. The human costs are enormous: not only do autistic children lead wasted lives but the lives of their parents are full of constant torment from the behavior of the child and feelings of guilt, frustration and hopelessness.

The Characteristics of Autism

In 1943 Leo Kanner, a child psychiatrist, published a description of what he thought was a unique form of schizophrenia which he called infantile

[1] Hamblin, Blackwell, Ferritor and Kozloff took the major responsibility for writing this chapter.

autism. The term autism derives from auto, the Greek word for self. Children with this syndrome are called autistic because to the casual observer they appear to be self contained, essentially uninterested in other human beings in their environment, unreachable in a shell of their own—an empty fortress, to use Bettelheim's phrase. In reading the literature on autism and in observing autistic children interact with their parents or a teacher, one is struck with how many and diverse the symptoms are. Yet, as one analyzes these symptoms, it becomes obvious that many are functional alternatives in that they accomplish the same purposes, but that some are more basic in propagating the disorder than others.

It seemed to us, after study, that autistic children have two cardinal syndromes. If we define these according to their exchange functions, they may be called autistic seclusion and attention-getting behavior.

Autistic Seclusion

"Seclusion," according to Webster, means "the shutting away, or a keeping apart of one's self . . . so that one is either inaccessible to others or is accessible only under very difficult conditions." Thus the autistic child is secluded in the sense of keeping himself apart; he is inaccessible or is accessible only under very difficult conditions and, then, on his own terms. This seclusion, in its extreme form, is manifested in a number of different ways: (1) by gaze aversion—that is, avoiding eye contact with others; (2) by aloof preoccupation in the presence of others; (3) by avoiding the company of other people; (4) by a lack of normal imitation; (5) by a lack of functional speech and (6) by negativism. Of these six the last three are the most pathogenic, for each represents severe learning disabilities.

For a number of possible reasons, which will be discussed, the child does not develop speech to make contact with and thus to learn via instruction from his social world. Rather, he lives mostly in the seclusion of silence or gibberish. Some autistic children are completely mute, that is, they make no sounds whatever; some are near mutes—that is, they have two to fifteen functional words, others engage in gibberish; others echo or parrot sounds and so on.

Speech, as the means people use to negotiate most of the positive exchanges they work in everyday life, is crucial in acculturation. It is essential in the explicit communicating, learning and teaching processes characteristic of human society. It also is man's most normal, most reinforced pattern of attention-getting behavior.

We have found no autistic children who ever imitate the ways their caretakers work the environment for reinforcers. As Bandura and Walters (1963) have documented in great detail, normal human beings ordinarily become acculturated through imitation—that is, they learn to copy behavior they see others using as they successfully work their environments for reinforcers. This is the way cultural patterns of behavior are normally propagated. However, since autistic children do not imitate such behaviors, they do not become acculturated.

Negativism, which characterizes most autistic children, is particularly crippling since it prevents others from relating to them in normal ways. The manifestations of negativism are response refusal (not following instructions, not answering questions), response reversal (doing exactly the opposite of what is requested) and pouting or tantrumming (when something is requested). However it manifests itself, the result of negative behavior is that requests or directions from others are responded to inappropriately, uncooperatively. The result is that negative children gradually thwart attempts by others to treat them normally.

Illicit Attention-Getting Behavior

Autistic children are not unique in repeating behavior and sounds over and over again; all people, even the most civilized, have their repetitious performance rituals. But the autistic children treated in our laboratories—and reportedly all autistic children—seem almost totally preoccupied with bizarre, repetitious performances most of which may be characterized as follows: ritualized hand motions, stereotyped positions, repetitive noise-making, rocking, stereotyped dancing, indiscriminate mouthing of objects, unusual eye movements, bizarre food preferences, drooling, sniffing, dry-eyed crying, creepy touching, lining up objects, spinning objects, irrelevant laughing or smiling, and such self-injurious practices as hand biting and head banging.

As implied earlier, the function of these behavior patterns is to get attention. Most adults will look at such performances, however involuntarily; some even seem compelled to stare. More significant, perhaps, parents have often been observed by the staff hugging and cuddling their children while they were doing these things—in an effort to get them to stop for a while. The usual pattern in such placating exchanges is that the parent ignores the child until his action become so bad they cannot be ignored—then the parent cuddles the child until he stops. Shortly after the child is mollified, the parent will set the child down and once more ignore him. Then generally the whole process begins again: the wild behavior, being picked up and hugged until quiet and so on.

But these bizarre behavior rituals are not the only ways for children to get illicit attention. As the hyperaggressive children demonstrated—disruptions, negativism, malicious teasing, and even violence all serve that function. We consider these bizarre, disruptive attention-getting devices to be alternatives to normal ways of getting attention, easily replaced once the child learns to use normal attention-getting patterns.

Finally, autistic children vary in a number of important ways much the same as other children. Some are hyperactive, some normally active, others underactive. Autistic children vary in intelligence too. Because of our experience in producing massive changes in IQ, we approached this whole problem with caution. At the beginning of their schooling, some autistic children had no measurable intelligence; but afterwards, a number of these youngsters turned out to be quite bright. One was by far, the brightest of all the children we have seen (and this includes the Washington University Preschool children in Chapter 2); he learned to read T.O. and i.t.a. simultaneously, at a faster rate than preschool children learned to read i.t.a.

Table 7.1 illustrates the spread and variety of autistic behavior patterns for the 18 children who have received 8 or more months schooling in our laboratory. All of the children evidence forms of seclusion and attention-getting which are particularly damaging because they also represent severe learning disabilities—that is, lack of normal functional speech, lack of normal imitation, the presence of one or more negative patterns.

Mary and John would probably not be classified as autistic according to what some consider the essential symptom, aloof preoccupation (cf. Rutter, 1968). But both were essentially mute, were extremely negative, and had not developed an imitative pattern when we accepted them for training. As noted earlier, we consider these latter characteristics much more basic to autistic seclusion than the others. Also, of all children accepted, these two were the hardest to live with. Before they came, Mary's mother was considering taking both her own and Mary's life; John's mother had consented, on their pediatrician's advice, to institutionalize him. Their extreme teasing and their violence made life with them hell. Yet they responded to remedial education about as the other children did.

THE ETIOLOGY OF AUTISM

There are many theories about the etiology, the original causation of autism, too many to be reviewed here (cf. Rutter, 1968, for a rather good review). However very little is known about the onset and pre-onset conditions of autism in the home and about any biogenetic aberrations of the autistic child. Furthermore, the etiology of autism has not been the focus of our investigations, rather its maintenance and change.

Regardless of etiology autistic children could respond to instructional exchanges designed to establish normal patterns of behavior and to extinguish autistic patterns.[2] Specifically, to obtain a remedial effect, the child's social

[2] Stroke victims, whose difficulties are obviously physical, respond to physical therapy, to speech therapy which via exercise and learning corrects or compensates for the physical difficulty. Hence even if the original difficulties of the autistic child were physical, they might be corrected by inducing the child to work an appropriate learning environment.

Table 7.1. Inventory of Behavior Patterns—18 Autistic Children.[a]

Behavior Patterns	Mary	Jerry	Larry	Linda	Peter	Joey	John	Jake	Lois	Luke	Kristen	Jeff	Michael	Ross	Sean	Marty
Imitation:																
Motor	—	+	+	+	—	—	+	—	—	—	—	+	—	—	—	—
Verbal	—	—	+	—	—	+	—	—	—	—	+	+	—	+	—	—
Speech:																
Mute	+	+	—	—	+	—	+	+	+	+	—	—	+	—	+	+
Echolalic	—	—	+	—	—	+	—	—	—	—	—	+	—	+	—	—
Gibberish	—	—	—	—	—	+	—	—	—	—	+	+	—	—	—	—
Functional (no. words)	2	2	0	30	0	0	3	0	1	0	30	0	0	0	1	10
Negativism:																
Does not follow requests	+	—	—	—	+	+	—	+	+	+	+	—	+	+	—	+
Response reversal	+	—	+	—	+	+	+	+	—	—	+	+	+	—	—	+
Aggression (offensive):																
Against adults	+	+	+	—	+	+	+	+	—	+	+	—	+	+	—	+
Against peers	+	+	+	+	—	+	—	+	—	—	+	—	+	+	—	+
Malicious teasing	+	+	+	+	+	+	+	+	+	+	+	+	+	+	—	+
Withdrawal:																
Gaze aversion	+	+	—	+	+	+	—	+	+	+	+	—	+	+	—	+
Hands over ears	—	—	—	—	+	—	—	+	+	—	+	—	—	—	—	+
Aloof preoccupation	—	+	+	+	+	+	—	+	+	+	+	+	+	+	+	+
Avoids other presence	—	+	+	+	+	+	—	+	+	—	+	—	—	+	+	—
Blank Facial Expression	+	+	+	+	+	—	—	+	+	+	—	+	+	+	+	—
Tantrumming:																
Whines	+	—	+	—	—	+	+	—	—	—	—	+	+	—	—	+
Screams	+	+	—	+	+	+	+	—	+	—	+	+	—	+	—	+
Destructiveness	+	+	—	—	+	+	+	+	—	—	—	—	—	+	—	+
Self injury	—	—	—	—	+	—	+	—	—	—	+	—	+	+	—	+

[a] "+" equals present; "—" equals absent.

Table 7.1. continued.

Behavior Patterns	Mary	Jerry	Larry	Linda	Peter	Joey	John	Jake	Lois	Luke	Kristen	Jeff	Michael	Ross	Sean	Marty
Clings	+	—	+	—	—	—	—	+	—	—	+	+	+	—	—	+
Cuddles	—	—	+	—	—	—	—	—	—	—	+	+	—	—	—	+
Hyperactivity:																
Overly active	+	—	—	+	+	—	+	—	+	+	—	+	—	+	—	+
Under active	—	—	+	—	—	+	—	+	—	—	+	—	+	—	+	—
Short attention span	+	+	+	+	+	+	—	—	—	+	+	+	+	—	—	—
Bizarre Behavior:																
Ritualized hand motions	—	—	+	—	+	+	—	+	+	—	+	+	+	—	+	+
Hand biting	—	—	—	—	—	—	—	—	—	+	+	—	+	—	—	+
Other self-injury	—	—	—	—	+	+	+	—	+	—	+	+	+	+	—	+
Stereotyped positions	+	+	—	+	+	—	—	+	+	+	+	+	+	—	+	—
Repetitive noise making	+	—	+	—	+	+	—	+	—	+	+	+	+	+	+	+
Spinning objects	—	—	—	—	—	—	—	—	+	+	—	+	+	+	+	+
Rocking and dancing	—	—	—	—	+	+	—	—	+	—	+	—	+	—	+	+
Indiscriminate mouthing	—	—	+	—	+	+	—	—	—	—	+	—	+	+	—	—
Goofy eye movements	+	+	+	—	+	—	—	—	+	+	—	—	+	—	+	+
Unusual food preference	—	—	+	—	+	+	—	+	—	—	—	—	+	—	—	+
Drooling	—	+	—	—	—	—	—	—	—	—	—	—	—	—	+	+
Sniffing	+	—	+	—	+	—	—	+	+	+	+	—	+	—	—	+
Dry-eyed crying	+	+	—	—	+	+	+	+	+	—	+	—	+	+	—	+
Creepy touching	—	—	+	+	—	—	+	—	—	—	+	—	+	—	—	+
Lining up objects	—	—	—	+	+	+	—	—	+	—	—	—	—	+	—	—
Inane laughing, smiling	—	—	+	—	—	+	—	+	—	+	+	+	+	—	—	+

[a] "+" equals present; "—" equals absent.

environment should be modified so he is repeatedly reinforced for babbling and then for progress through the normal development sequences—other successive approximations of normal speech—for imitation, for cooperation and for normal attention-getting patterns. Also, his social environment should no longer reinforce autistic patterns, that is, nonverbal communication and the various bizarre, disruptive attention-getting patterns. In addition, a correctly designed environment should condition the child so he values and responds appropriately to the reinforcers that are used in the usual social exchanges in our culture.

THE BASIC EDUCATIONAL STRATEGIES

Finding Reinforcers

One of the first steps in structuring a remedial exchange is finding a good reinforcer. Autistic children, particularly, must have strong inducements to give up old, fixed patterns. At first we tried token exchanges with them. They worked but they did not work well, at least in the beginning stages of training. We then used food exchanges similar to those that Risley and Wolf (1966) and Lovaas and his associates (1966) had used so effectively. In a food exchange the child is rewarded with a bite of food for following the teacher's instructions—in fitting a piece into a puzzle, looking the teacher in the eye, saying a sound, a word or a sentence. We found that food exchanges increased the rate of criterion behavior of autistic children from three to eight times that sustained by token exchanges. For example, Figure 7.1 shows results typical of verbal changes observed in several experiments in our laboratory.

Figure 7.2 shows how the food exchange worked for Larry. Even though he had been in training over six months, note that he still talked only when necessary to get food. When he was able to get the food without talking, he did not talk, though the teacher tried to carry on a conversation. His is a typical response during the early stages of speech training.

However, through the conditioning processes, the situation changes as working the food exchange has its acculturating effect. Because of this, working the food-talking exchanges after a few weeks becomes quite enjoyable to most autistic children. Larry's case is rather typical. When he had been on a food exchange for talking for about a month, the teacher set two trays containing the same kind and amount of food before him and told him: "You may eat the food on this tray free or you may eat the food on this plate if you ask me for it." We ran the experiment three times—with almost identical results. The first few times Larry ate from the free plate, saying nothing. Then he would turn to the teacher and say, "I want a chip." He would get it, then he would ask for something else and

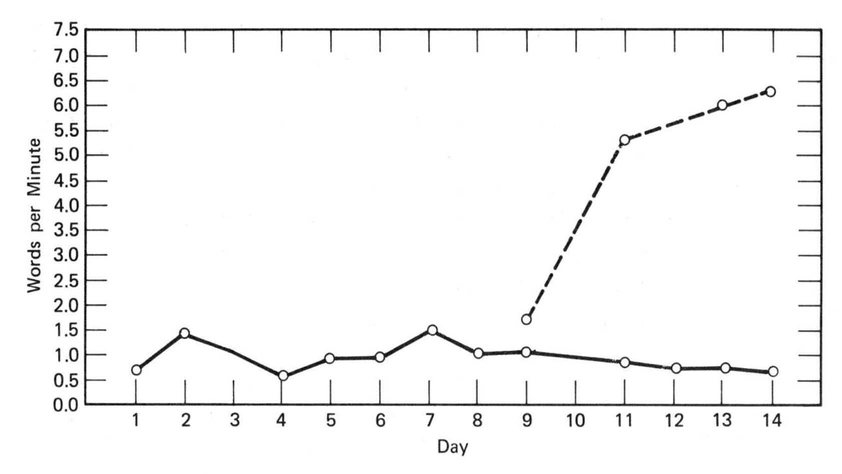

Figure 7.1. Words per minute through time with token-talking exchange (lines) and with a food-talking exchange (dashes). The two exchanges occurred at different times during the last six days of this experimental series. Subject: Jerry is a four year old, non-verbal autistic boy who had been in exchange therapy for four months. Experiment by Ferritor.

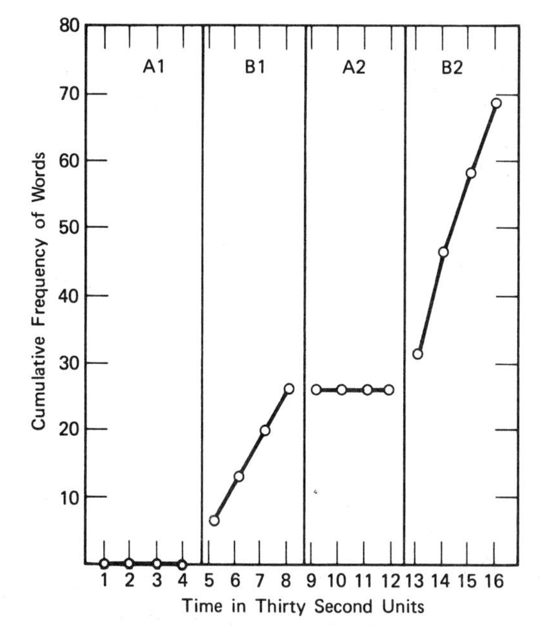

Figure 7.2. Cumulative frequency of functional words by Larry, a four year old echolalic authistic boy who had been in exchange therapy four months, through time. In the A periods, Larry could eat without asking for it; in the B periods, he had to tell the therapist what he wanted. Note: he talked only when the exchange required it. Experiment by Ferritor.

get that, and on and on until he had eaten about two thirds of the food from the teacher's plate. Then he would continue to ask for the food on the teacher's plate, but he did not eat it. He collected it on the napkin in front of him until he had all the teacher's food. Then he would say, "All done." The data in Figure 7.3, from one of these experiments, are rather typical.

The food exchange does have one limitation: children fill up usually in twenty to twenty-five minutes. The food-satiation effect is illustrated with data from an experiment with Sean in Figure 7.4. Note that within each session the response rate increases for a time and then drops rapidly to 0. In contrast, a well-designed token exchange can be run all morning. For those types of behavior that cause autistic children less stress than talking—such as sitting at a table, working puzzles, painting and writing—tokens are adequate. Therefore, with autistic children we shift, as soon as possible, from a food exchange for motor skills to a food exchange for talking; and then supplement that by a token exchange for other activities for one or two additional hours during a normal school day. In this way we are able to add a variety of learning experiences and to work effectively on a number of pro-normal behavior patterns in addition to speech.

Negativism

From the beginning of our research, we noticed that some autistic children were more negative than others and seemed to be more negative with some

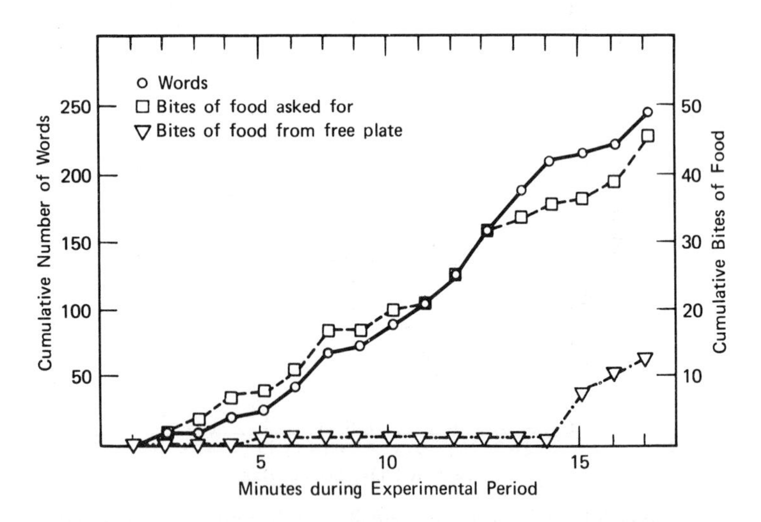

Figure 7.3. Typical experiment with Larry. After six weeks on food exchange for talking, he preferred to ask for food from the experimenter's plate rather than take "free" food from his own plate. (An exception occurred toward the end when Larry decided to eat a favorite food all of which had been consumed from the experimenter's plate. Even then he continued to ask for food.) Experiment by Ferritor.

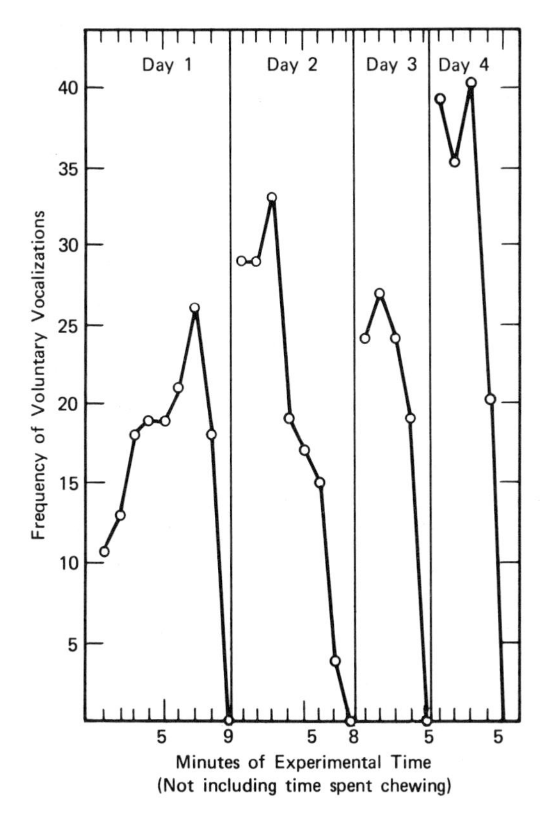

Figure 7.4. Sean was given small bites of food every time he made a voluntary vocalization. Experiment by Kozloff.

teachers than with others. Consequently, we began to observe those situations in which the children were and were not negative in an attempt to pinpoint just what it was that seemed to produce negative behavior patterns. These activities eventuated in a series of experiments by Janet Dehn (1969) for her doctoral dissertation.[3]

Although Dehn's experiments are much too complex to be described in detail here, we will attempt to describe the results of several contrasting procedures on the production and the remediation of negative behavior. While other procedures probably have measurable effects on negative behavior, those she included in her five series of experiments all produced substantial effects with at least some children. There were four types of

[3] The dissertation was done under the direction of Hamblin. Dehn was also counseled and helped at many points in her research by Ferritor who was Associate Director of the Autistic Laboratory when these experiments were conducted.

negative behaviors measured in each of Dehn's experiments: *refusals* measured as the number of requests not responded to within ten seconds; *reversals* measured as the number of incorrect responses accompanied by *smiling* or *laughing* at the mistake; *tantrumming* measured as the time spent shouting, crying, kicking, head-banging, etc; *pouting* measured as the time spent with a sullen facial expression.[4]

Learning with error. Dehn's most fruitful experiments involved a procedure called errorless learning (cf. Terrace, 1963; Hansen, 1959) versus its opposite, trial and error learning. In the errorless learning procedure, the teacher structures the child's environment so that he acquires the criterion behavior almost, if not, without making errors. In each of Dehn's errorless experiments, for example, each child was asked to select a criterion card (with a particular letter on it) from several cards (each with different letters). In the errorless condition the letter on the criterion card asked for by the teacher was outlined in yellow and as the child reached, the teacher moved the board on which the cards lay so that the child's hand fell on the criterion card. Thus on the first trial the situation was rigged so the child picked up the correct card and was, therefore, reinforced with food and approval. In subsequent trials the prompts were gradually faded—that is, the amount of color outlining the letter was gradually reduced and moving the board gradually eliminated—until every time it was requested the child was able to pick the criterion card without prompts. With such procedures then each child learned to make the correct response almost, if not, without making errors. In the B condition the teacher simply asked for the criterion card and reinforced the child when, through trial and error, he happened to pick up the right one. This procedure, then, resulted in the child's making errors on some trials and his not being reinforced on those trials.

While trial and error learning is used with normal children without catastrophic results, Dehn's data indicate that when used with autistic children this procedure instigates great amounts of negative behavior. Note in Figure 7.5 in the trial and error learning conditions Margaret increasingly refused to make responses, ultimately to about 70 percent of the teacher's requests.

[4] Dehn recorded the child's responses during each session on a video tape recorder and then took her measurements one at a time afterwards while playing back the tape. Reliability studies were done in connection with each of the five experiments; inter-observer reliability, calculated as the percentage agreement between different observers, ranged between 98 and 100 percent, the median being 100 percent. Intra-observer reliability, calculated as the percentage agreement between two different scorings of a given session by a single observer, ranged between 98 percent and 100 percent, the median being 100 percent. This high reliability is possible because the observers scored one variable at a time.

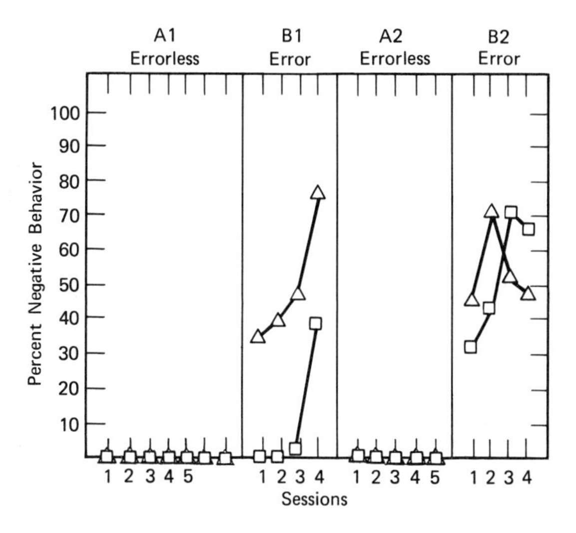

Figure 7.5. Comparison of the negative behavior of Margaret when learning was without and with error: percent response refusals (□— — —□) and percent of time tantrumming (△- - - -△). (After Figure 1, Dehn, 1969.)

In contrast, in errorless learning conditions there were no refusals and no tantrums. While Margaret's negativism was extreme, the other three subjects used in replications of this experiment all showed a similar response: no negativism at all in errorless learning conditions; an average of 31 percent refusals and/or reversals in learning with trial and error conditions.

This experiment is basic, for it suggests that autistic children are aversely affected by trial and error learning. On the other hand, when errorless learning is used negativism is eliminated entirely. Thus these experiments suggest quite clearly that in the early stages of their acculturation instructional exchanges will be successful with autistic children *only if they incorporate errorless learning procedures*. In their early stages of acculturation autistic children are evidently unable to tolerate the frustrations that normally occur with trial and error learning procedures.

Attending incorrect responses. This experiment is an elaboration of our earlier experiments with bizarre, disruptive behavior and, in a different way, the previous one using trial and error learning procedures. It varies from the earlier experiments in two ways. (1) The task was easier. The children were discriminating colors, rather than letters of the alphabet, discriminations they had supposedly acquired at earlier stages of training. (2) In the A conditions if the child's response was incorrect, the teacher responded with negative attention ("No, Anna, that is wrong."); in the B condition with no attention (not looking at the child) but waiting at least ten seconds before making the next request. The same stimulus was used in A1, B1 and A2 and a new stimulus was used in B2. Thus, if any condition should have benefited from more numerous associations between correct responses and reinforcement, it should have been A2.

The data in Figure 7.6 are for Anna. Note that refusals occurred in between 35 and 85 percent of the trials in the A1 and A2 conditions and that the median frequency for reversals during those periods was a little over 10 percent per period. While some refusals and reversals occurred toward the beginning of the B1 and B2 periods, the frequency of these dropped off to 0.

In these experiments, of course, Dehn tested the hypothesis that negative attention was, in fact, a positive reinforcer for these autistic children. The data support that inference and suggest that rates of negativism, like the rates of bizarre and disruptive behaviors, may be accelerated by responding with a "no, that's not right," "stop," etc. and they may be decelerated to 0 by ignoring them altogether.

Multiple requests. Informal observations led several of us to the hypothesis that multiple requests, the tendency to repeat questions that the child does not respond to, results in negative behavior, usually a high rate of refusals. So, in this experiment Dehn used a multiple request procedure in the A conditions and a single request procedure in the B conditions. In

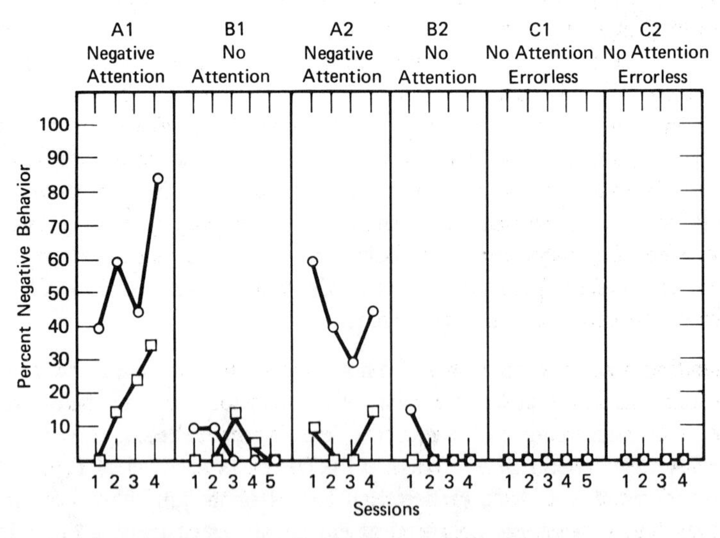

Figure 7.6. Comparison of negative behavior of Anna when negative attention was given to incorrect responses, when no attention was given to incorrect responses, and when discriminations were learned without error: percent response refusals (□— — —□) and percent response reversals (○———○). (After Figure 26, Dehn, 1969.)

the multiple request condition Dehn asked the child to give her a red block, then repeated the question every two or three seconds until the child responded or until ten seconds had lapsed. In the B condition she made the request only once and then proceeded to a different request when the child responded or when ten seconds had elapsed.

The results in Figure 7.7, for Emily, conform rather nicely to the expected pattern: substantial rates of refusals during the multiple request sessions and the decrease of refusals to 0 or near 0 in the single request sessions. However, Emily was an atypical subject. While multiple requests substantially increased the rate of refusals in three out of four subjects, the single requests procedures did not always remediate the refusals. Hence, Dehn used a C condition involving an errorless learning series which did, in fact, remediate the refusals pattern. This may be noted in Figure 7.8 which gives the data for Karl and Anna.

Differential reinforcement. Dehn thought that negativism might occur when children, working on two tasks simultaneously, were reinforced differentially, more for one task than for the other. Thus in Figure 7.9 during the A conditions Margaret responded correctly almost every time on Task #1, even though her correct responses were reinforced intermittently (about 70 percent of the time in A1 and 50 percent in A2). During the B conditions the reinforcement for Task #1 was variable as in the previous A condition, but correct responses for Task #2, interspersed with reinforcement for Task #1, were *always* reinforced. As a result of the lean reinforcement for

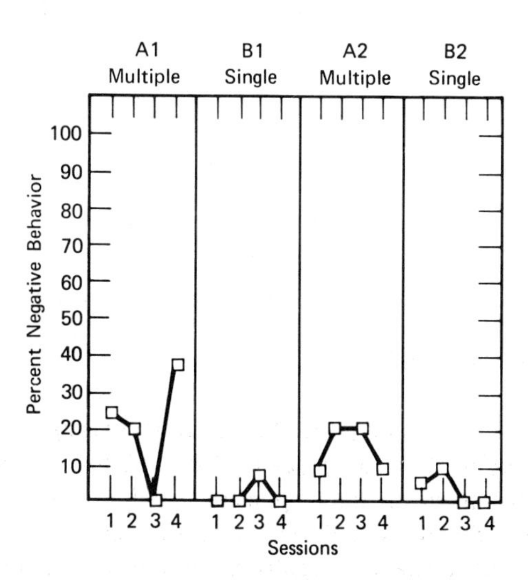

Figure 7.7. Comparison of the negative behavior of Emily during multiple and single request conditions: percent response refusals. (After Figure 28, Dehn, 1969.)

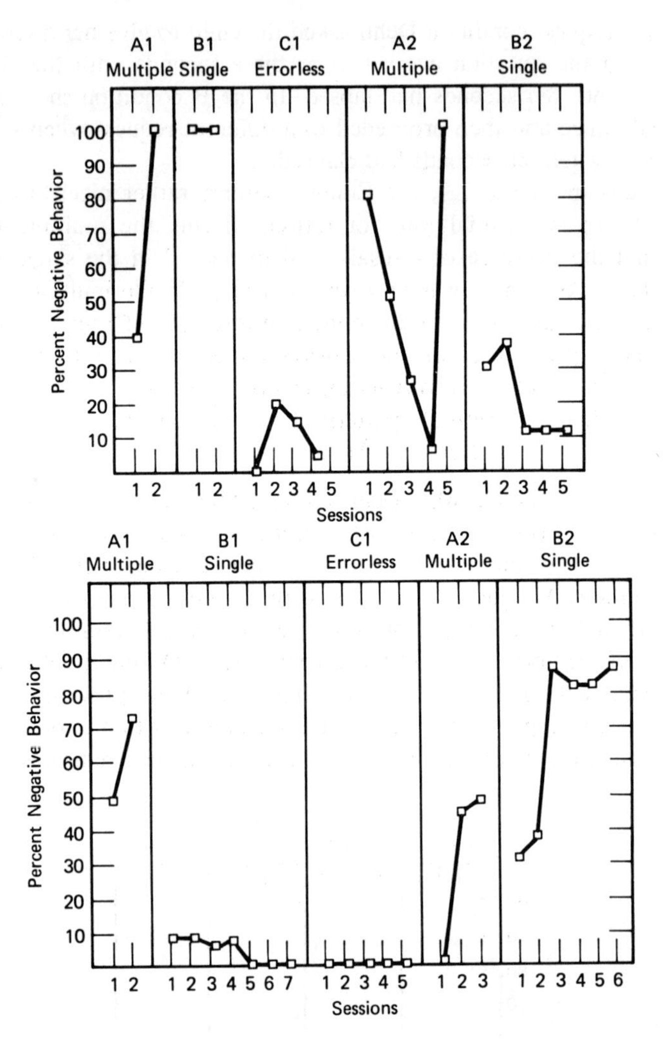

Figure 7.8. Comparison of negative behavior of Karl (top) and Anna (bottom) during multiple and single request conditions and errorless conditions: percent response refusals. (After Figure 29 and 30, Dehn, 1969.)

Task #1 during the B conditions, Margaret increasingly began doing reversals—ultimately to 20 to 30 percent of the teacher's requests. However, reversals were prominent in the responses of only one of Dehn's four subjects (Margaret). So, while differential reinforcement of interspersed responses can produce substantial negativism in some cases, in most it does not.

Abrupt transitions to intermittent reinforcement. This experiment deals with procedures for moving to intermittent reinforcement for the mainte-

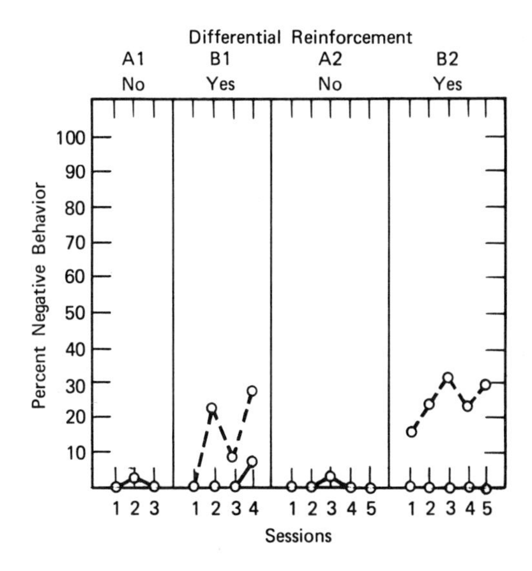

Figure 7.9. Comparison of the negative responses of Margaret when a single response is maintained on a variable ratio schedule (condition A) and when that response is maintained on a variable ratio schedule and a second response is introduced on a continuous schedule. Solid lines indicate behavior on variable ratio schedule; broken lines indicate behavior on continuous schedule; percent response reversals. No refusals. No tantrum behavior. (After Figure 11, Dehn, 1969.)

nance of a response pattern after that pattern has been acquired via continuous reinforcement using errorless learning procedures. In the A conditions the movement to intermittent reinforcement was quite abrupt. In the first period the probability of food reinforcement was .50, of social reinforcement .50 and of no reinforcement .00. In the subsequent periods of the A conditions the probability of food reinforcement was .20, social reinforcement .50 and of no reinforcement .30. The data in Figure 7.10, for Emily whose response is rather typical, indicate an increase in refusals until toward the end of A2 she did not respond to between 20 and 50 percent of the teacher's requests. It may also be noted that the frequency of pouting, a functional equivalent of tantrumming, occurred in as many as 25 percent of the trials toward the end of A1.

In the first part of the B conditions the probability of reinforcement was 1.0 (specifically, the probability of food reinforcement was .50, the probability of social reinforcement .50 and no reinforcement .00). In the second part of the B conditions, the probability of reinforcement was dropped to .9, in the third to .8, and in the fourth and subsequent parts .7, as in the A conditions. However, in the early parts, the bites of food were large enough and the pace fast enough so that the child had food in his mouth most, if not all, of the time. It allowed him or her, without great frustration, to become gradually accustomed to intermittent food reinforcement for correct responses. Note in Figure 7.10 that even this gradual procedure produced some refusals (in 10 percent or so of the trials) toward the beginning of the two B conditions, but the frequency decreased to 0 toward the end of those conditions.

Hence, the data show that negativism occurs during the transition from continuous to intermittent reinforcement and the faster the transition, the greater the amount of negativism.

Summary. The data indicate that the frequency of negative behavior by autistic children may be increased or decreased in an educational setting as a result of certain characteristics of the learning environment.[5] The results of Dehn's experiments indicate the following. (1) In acquisition, errorless learning procedures decelerate negative behavior to zero whereas trial and error learning procedures apparently accelerate negativism in proportion to the difficulty of the learning task. (2) Negativism may be accelerated during acquisition if a teacher tells an autistic child consistently that he is wrong when he is in error and decelerated if errors are ignored. (3) During

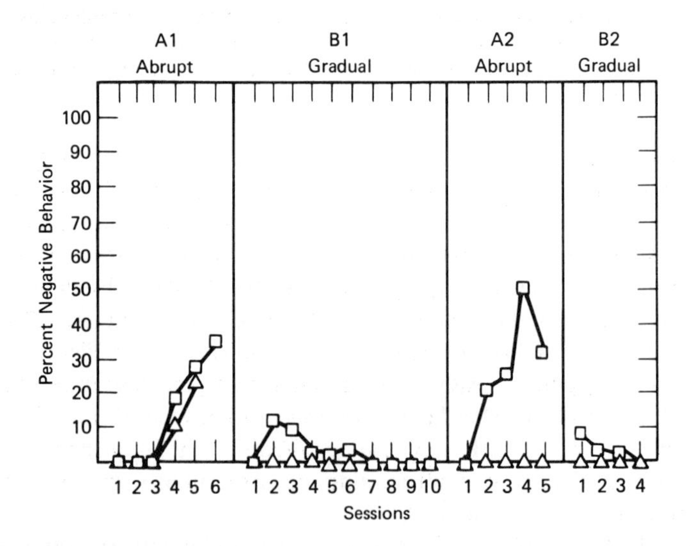

Figure 7.10. Comparison of negative behavior of Emily when reinforcement schedule was changed abruptly and gradually: percent response refusal (□— — —□) and time pouting (△– – – –△). (After Figure 15, Dehn, 1969.)

[5] This is not to be interpreted as a conclusion about etiology or the original causation. Our data do not rule out, for example, the possibility that some patterns of negative behavior are originated or even maintained by genetic or biochemical variables.

acquisition multiple requests accelerate the frequency of negative behavior and single requests decrease the frequency, particularly when combined with errorless learning procedures. (4) After acquisition during the transition from continuous to intermittent reinforcement, negative behavior is increased in proportion to the haste with which the transition is made. (5) In one out of four cases, the differential reinforcement of two interspersed patterns resulted in negativism when the teacher asked for the response where reinforcement was on a less probable reinforcement schedule.

While there are other variables which may well influence the frequency of negativism in its various manifestations at least these experiments give a rather clear indication of what the underlying causal variables are. It seems that any procedure productive of frustration will instigate negative behavior in proportion to the degree of frustration. The errorless learning procedures are so effective in eliminating negativism apparently because they all but eliminate frustration. The gradual transition into intermittent reinforcement is also successful because it, too, almost if not entirely, eliminates frustration. Hence, it appears that the various behaviors we have called negativism are in part, at least, what Maier (1961) has called frustration responses.

But the results also indicate that negativism can be accelerated and decelerated respectively by reinforcement (negative attention to errors) and non reinforcement (no attention to errors). Our inference from the often observed sequence—verbal request, reversal or refusal, parent's or teacher's upset, child's glee—was verified experimentally. Like disruptive-bizarre behavior, negative behavior can become a form of malicious teasing, with the same disconcerting results to those adults who take the bait.

The data in Table 7.2 which summarize all of Dehn's experiments suggest some additional characteristics about negative behavior which are rather interesting. All of the children were engaged in two or more patterns of negative behavior, but some did not have all the patterns. For example, Ann and Max never tantrummed or pouted, Emily never did reversals; the conditions under which the children refused, reversed, tantrummed and/or pouted varied. The data also suggest a modal response pattern to each of the conditions which produce negative behavior in autistic children, particularly if it is assumed that some of the different manifestations—i.e. refusals and reversals, tantrumming and pouting—are functional alternatives.

These experiments are important since they define the general parameters of successful and unsuccessful teaching procedures for autistic children. As we proceed through the next chapter, we will pay particular attention to the errorless learning procedures involved in acquisition and to the gradual transition procedures for maintaining various behaviors once they have been acquired.

Table 7.2. Summary Percentages of Negative Behavior for the Children in Five Series of ABAB Experiments. Note: Most Numbers are Averages for Two Experimental Conditions.

Children	Learning		Teacher's Response to Error		Requests		Transition into Intermittent Reinforcement		Differential Reinforcement of a Second Response	
	With Error	Without Error	Negative Attention	No Attention	Multiple	Single	Abrupt	Gradual	Yes	No
Margaret										
Refusals	32%	0%	0%	0%	0%	0%	43%	0%	0%	0%
Reversals	0	0	6	0	0	5	18	1	19	0
Tantrums	52	0	8	6	0	4	26	0	1	1
Emily										
Refusals	21	0	54	20	18	3	24	3	5	0
Reversals	0	0	0	0	0	0	0	0	0	0
Pouting	29	0	0	0	0	0	16	2	0	0
Anna										
Refusals	7	0[a]	12	2	46	35[a]			2	0
Reversals	26	0	25	0	0	0			0	0
Tantrums & Pouts	0	0	0	0	0	0			0	0
Karl										
Refusals		0[b]	16	5	61	60	12	0		
Reversals		0	20	0	0	0	0	0		
Tantrums		0	0	0	0	0	16	1		
Max										
Refusals	0	0					8	0		
Reversals	29	1					0	0		
Tantrums & Pouts	0	0					0	0		

[a] Averages for four errorless learning series, two in errorless learning experiment, and two in single-request conditions to remediate negativism produced by multiple requests.

[b] One errorless learning series in a single-request condition to remediate negativism produced by multiple requests.

Bizarre, Disruptive Behavior

During the first few months bizarre behavior is generally ignored by the staff, while they help the child acquire pro-normal behavior. Through this very simple counter-exchange process many of the bizarre, disruptive patterns the child brought with him to the laboratory are extinguished, or nearly so. However, an interesting phenomenon occurs. The child typically starts engaging in new bizarre patterns, as though to replace those which he has lost. Sometimes a member of the staff, startled by a new bizarre pattern, will stare at the child and this, of course, reinforces it. Since he is undoubtedly frustrated because the old patterns no longer produce a reinforcer, an autistic child at this stage will persevere on a new pattern that worked once or twice initially. But gradually, if the reinforcement for that pattern is terminated, it too will extinguish. Figures 7.11 and 7.12 show these extinction processes.

This phenomenon strikes a familiar chord: it is similar to symptom substitution often referred to in psychoanalytic literature which claims that unless the deep underlying cause of a bizarre symptom is removed along with the symptom, the symptom will simply reappear in a new guise. But in our experience the bizarre patterns tend to disappear entirely as the child acquires standard cultural patterns which are more effective as functional alternatives. Hence, we spend very little time and effort in eliminating bizarre behavior; only those that cannot be ignored by the teacher are responded to—the child is timed out using procedures described in the previous chapters.

Training Mothers to be Assistant Teachers

In order to observe how Larry and his mother related to each other, we asked his mother to read a story to him. We realized the importance of training mothers to handle their autistic children after observing the following incident:[6]

> Larry is allowed to pick out his favorite book. His mother then attempts to read it to him, but he keeps turning the pages so she cannot. The mother then gets up and goes to the shelf for four more books. Larry gets up and walks away from the table. The mother then *yells* at him to come back. He SMILES!! Mother continues to talk to the child to try to get him back for the story. Finally, he comes over to the table and takes the book away from her. She lets him and goes back

[6] Our staff often does "sport caster" descriptions of sessions in the Autistic Laboratory. The descriptions recorded in a Stenorette are then transcribed by a typist. These observations were recorded by Ferritor.

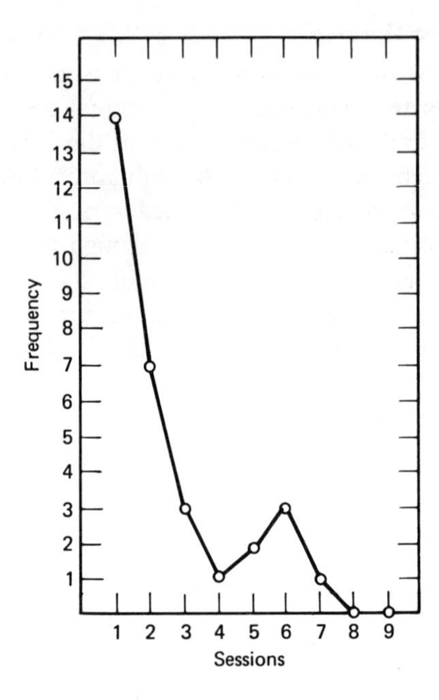

Figure 7.11. Number of random shouting noises from a seven-year-old autistic boy over nine extinction sessions. Experiment by Blackwell.

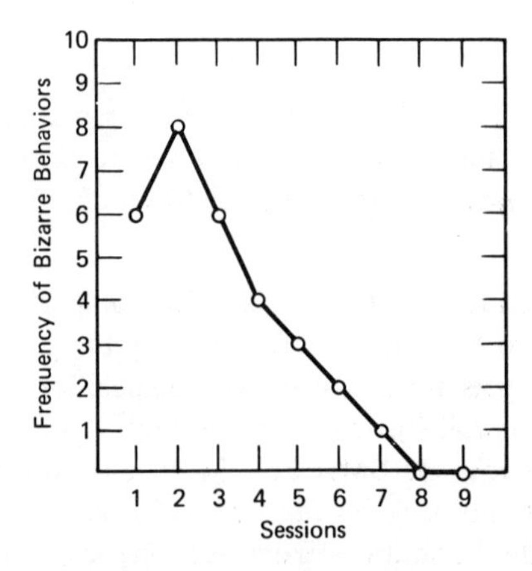

Figure 7.12. Number of bizarre behaviors during nine extinction sessions for a seven-year-old autistic boy. A tally was marked each time the child brushed his hair roughly to the side of his head. Experiment by Blackwell.

to the bookcase for another book. He then sits down and she begins to read. He tries to get up, but his mother pulls him back. Again. Again. She holds him there. He gets away and starts walking around the room. Goes to the toy cabinet. Mother gets up to go over and take a toy away from him. He sits on the floor. The mother comes over and sits down by him. He gets up and goes over by the door, opens it and tries to run out. In an angry voice she tells him he has to stay. He SMILES!! She resumes reading. He gets up and starts walking around the table. She grabs him roughly as he comes by. He SMILES!! He grabs the book away from her and she tries to get it back. She takes the book away from him and pulls him back to the table. Again he grabs the book away from her and she tries to get it back. Now she takes the book away from him and pulls him back to the table. She is very upset. He grabs the book away from her and starts LAUGHING. His mother takes the book back and tries to put him into the hall, on a chair. Now she tries to come back into the room. Larry gets back ahead of her. The mother tries to close the door on him, but he is pushing to keep it open. She cannot or does not close it. Now she pushes him down on the ground and tries to close the door again. He gets his foot in the door and she can't close it again. She picks him up and carries him back to the chair in the hall. Smiling, he races back to the door as she tries to close it.

At this moment the ten-minute period is up and ends with the mother and child at the door. As the experimenter approached, the mother said, "He just does not like to be read to."

When a demand is made of a disturbed child, he will often behave his worst and thus make his disorder most evident. The above incident is typical of Larry's behavior when his mother made demands upon him; it showed his autistic pattern at its worst. Of particular interest here is the record of Larry's smiling. It is rather evident that Larry was pleased, reinforced, every time he could see that he was succeeding in making his mother angry. It is as though Larry enjoyed upsetting his mother and repetitively "pressed a button" to upset her over and over again. Ironically, in her efforts to teach Larry, his mother, typical of all mothers of autistic children observed in our laboratory, had unknowingly involved herself in a pathogenic exchange which was causing Larry to become more and more psychotic.

To make matters worse, Larry's mother had not responded in a way that would reinforce his functional speech, which he had gradually acquired in tutorial with his teacher. His mother reported that Larry was beginning to talk in a meaningful way at home, but in the laboratory she seemed unable to manage a conversation with him, in part because she did not know what to do about his teasing.

Following this analysis, a ten day program was designed by Ferritor and Hamblin to teach Larry's mother to be an assistant teacher, to use the appropriate exchange and non-exchange signals and to use reinforcement meaningfully and effectively (a more advanced version of this program will be described in the next chapter). After that training period her acculturating exchanges with Larry were almost flawless, and Larry's past learning with the teacher then generalized nicely to his interaction with his mother. The exchange analysis interspersed in parentheses at various points in the following episode[7] gives a rather clear picture of a remarkable change—from pathogenic exchange to acculturating exchange in just ten days!

> The mother begins by asking Larry questions (exchange signals). He responds to every question, giving a verbal answer (initiation). She gives approval for every correct response (reciprocation). Then she tries to get him to say, "That is a duck," by asking the appropriate question and pointing to the duck's picture (another exchange signal). He will not say it intelligibly but wants to turn the page. (Refuses to initiate the exchange; instead, he signals another exchange, i.e. turning the page.) The mother says, "As soon as you say 'duck,' you may turn the page" (a more powerful exchange signal). Larry responds, "duck" (correct initiation of the exchange), and the mother turns the page (valued reciprocation). He smiles . . . .
>
> After seven minutes, Larry is still sitting down, they have finished one book, and are beginning a second. The mother turns the page and says, "What is he doing?" (exchange signal). Larry says "Flying a kite" (initiation). Mother says, "What color is the kite?" (exchange signal, she misses reciprocating). Larry replies, "Orange" (an incorrect answer, an unsuccessful attempt to initiate this latest exchange). His mother's typical response once was, "You know that is not orange," but now she just looks away (a non-exchange signal). "Blue," says Larry (an initiation of exchange which his mother had signaled earlier). "That's right," says the mother and smiles at him (reciprocation). By now, ten minutes have passed and Larry is still sitting, responding to the story with his mother.

Note that the mother was able to run this exchange without reciprocating with food. From earlier episodes we had suspected that Larry would value his mother's attention and approval, if he could earn them in a predictable exchange. The autistic teasing pattern seems to occur when the child craves

[7] Again these observations were recorded by Ferritor.

a response from his parents, but does not know how to get it in the usual way, by talking. However, now that the mother had learned how to structure and work an acculturating exchange with Larry, he was able to earn her attention and approval quite regularly when he wished, simply by initiating the exchanges she structured with him.

Larry's mother was trained as an assistant teacher in connection with Ferritor's dissertation (1969) which involved an experiment with a before-training-after-training-follow-up design, measuring various aspects of the child's conversation with his mother in the home during a one hour period on three successive days when the mother and child "were doing what they normally did at home."

The data in Figure 7.13 from Ferritor's dissertation represent the averages for four autistic children and their mothers. Although the training did not bring the mothers up to the teachers' level of competence at once, they showed marked improvement in their ability to reinforce talking, and by

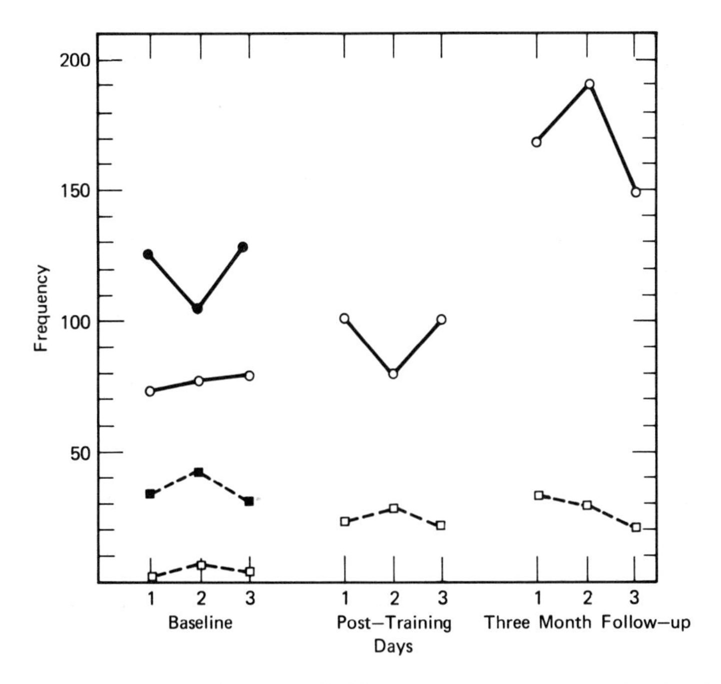

Figure 7.13. Average number of intelligible words (○——○) spoken by the four children in the laboratory with their mothers and the average number of times the children were reinforced (□— — —□) during a story before training, after training, and three months after training. The filled in data points for pretraining represent the average number of intelligible words (●——●) spoken by the four children in the laboratory with their teacher for a comparable period, and the number of times (■— — —■) the teacher reinforced their speech. (After Figures 7.1 and 7.2, Ferritor, 1969.)

follow-up, the children were responding by talking with their mothers about twice as much as they originally had.

More detailed data on the baseline-follow-up comparisons of the children's talking are given in Table 7.3. The follow-up increase over baseline for total number of intelligible words was 239 percent; for number of different words, 232 percent; and for sentences, 183 percent. Hence, training the mothers to run normal language exchanges with their children in the laboratory produced substantial results at home.

Table 7.3. Summary Results of Mothers' Training to Run Normal Language Exchanges With Their Autistic Children.

Child	Baseline	After Training	Three Month Follow-up
Measure: Total number of words used by child in half hour period.			
Mary	199	455	860
Larry	415	781	1331
Jenny	254	326	605
Linda	598	866	695
Average	366	612	873
Percent	100	167	239
Measure: Number of different words.			
Mary	28	103	199
Larry	95	174	243
Jerry	47	65	96
Linda	124	170	151
Average	74	128	172
Percent	100	173	232
Measure: Number of complete sentences.			
Mary	0	1	6
Larry	26	43	70
Jerry	11	33	54
Linda	84	114	89
Average	30	48	55
Percent	100	160	183

SUMMARY

This chapter represents an introduction to the laboratory's work with autistic children. Autism has generally been thought to be a psychosis, the result of a specific physiological deficit or damage or the result of a severe emotional disturbance. Our research suggests, however, it may also be an extremely severe acculturation disorder, a natural result that can begin with grossly inadequate reinforcement for talking in very early childhood. Autism, as was seen, involves two major syndromes: autistic seclusion and bizarre, disruptive behavior. Autistic seclusion is manifested in several ways, but most seriously by the failure to develop functional speech, pro-normal imitative patterns and standard cultural patterns of working the environment for reinforcers. As a result a child develops the second characteristic syndrome of autism—a wide variety of bizarre, disruptive behavior patterns through which he gains attention.

However, regardless of etiology, it was suggested that autism may be remediated, if laboriously, by structuring acculturating exchanges which autistic children are able to work. In the process of working these exchanges, via social learning, they develop behaviors, skills and emotional response patterns which are usual for the culture and, at the same time, eliminate their bizarre, disruptive behavior patterns.

Our research with autistic children has led to several strategies which we have used generally in designing and structuring their remedial learning environments. In the beginning phases of remediation food is used as a reinforcer simply because it sustains a much higher rate of pro-normal behavior than any of the other reinforcers considered. However, food exchanges are designed to condition the child so eventually he is enabled to respond well to a token exchange and then to the conditioned reinforcers typically used in our culture. Secondly, strategies were developed for avoiding and eliminating negative behavior. Thus, errorless learning was found to be extremely effective with autistic children since it almost, if not entirely, eliminates frustration. On the other hand, trial and error learning procedures which work with normal children fail with autistic children, that is, to the extent the procedures are difficult and, hence, frustrating. It was also found that negative behavior can be accelerated in frequency if the teacher routinely told her autistic charges that incorrect answers or responses were, in fact, incorrect. Hence, with autistic children it is generally necessary to reinforce correct responses and to ignore incorrect ones.

Next, our research suggested that the bizarre, disruptive behavior patterns were easily decelerated using counter exchanges, that is, by ignoring the bizarre, disruptive behavior patterns, and thus, not reinforcing them while, at the same time, accelerating culturally prescribed behaviors using food reinforcement and errorless learning procedures. However, we discovered that for a time at least the children will develop new bizarre, disruptive patterns apparently in an attempt to find functional alternatives which would work in their new social environment much as had the old patterns worked in their old social environment. However, these patterns, too, decelerated with no reinforcement. In general, such symptom substitution ceased when the children had acquired culturally prescribed behaviors which, as functional alternatives to the bizarre disruptive patterns, were much more productive of reinforcers and, at the same time, were less costly.

Finally, we found the mothers of autistic children were systematically reinforcing the autistic patterns, and thus were working at variance with our educational program. Hence, as a general strategy we trained the mothers to be assistant teachers, to use procedures at home which would supplement the procedures used at school and, hence, to add to rather than detract from their children's remedial education.

It should be noted before ending this chapter that both Risley and Wolf and Lovaas and his associates have used food exchanges with autistic children. They also spend the major part of their effort in helping the child to acquire language. However, we do not use harsh punishment as they have to inhibit certain very disruptive behavior patterns. Although aversive reinforcers like electric shock may sometimes prevent self-destruction, other less extreme procedures may be as effective. Also, in our view extreme physical punishment makes progress out of autistic seclusion more difficult, particularly in the early stages of remediation.

CHAPTER 8

Autism: Its Remediation

As noted earlier, in educating autistic children we try to focus on establishing culturally prescribed patterns which are functional alternatives to the fundamental autistic habits.[1] In brief outline, here are the eight stages through which we lead the children:

Stage One

Establish eye contact and eliminate gaze aversion through a counter exchange. Almost incidentally, start to eliminate bizarre, disruptive behavior via counter exchange.

Stage Two

Using a food exchange teach the children to imitate movements of teacher. Teach simple discrimination skills via work with puzzles. Begin to teach good work habits, attending to tasks. Continue elimination of bizarre, disruptive behavior through counter exchanges. Train mothers (1) to understand exchange and conditioning theory, (2) to structure simple positive exchanges on the discrimination tasks and (3) to use counter exchanges.

Stage Three

Establish a pattern of vocal response.

Stage Four

Establish verbal imitation: (a) imitation of sounds—b, m, a, e, o; (b) imitation of blends—ba, le, la, lo; (c) imitation of food words—chip, pickle, meat. Continue to eliminate bizarre behavior by counter exchange.

[1] Hamblin, Ferritor, Kozloff and Blackwell took the major responsibility for writing this chapter.

Stage Five

Establish use of functional words in a food exchange, that is, have the child name a food in order to get a bite of it. Develop a vocabulary to identify objects and then pictures of objects. Through imitation establish the use of syntax. Train parents to structure speech exchanges with children at home.

Stage Six

The children's initial group experience, two to three children with one teacher. Establish parallel work patterns. Continue with language development through food-talking exchanges. Establish free play patterns outdoors. Establish the token exchange to supplement the food exchange.

Stage Seven

In intermediate class, establish basic classroom patterns and abilities including the appropriate attentional patterns, the appropriate imitation of competition and cooperatioan with classmates. Work toward an ability to follow complex instructions from teacher. Establish organized play routines indoors. Continue language development. Continue elaboration of token exchange.

Stage Eight

Children are all given developmental tests to locate lacunae in their language, motor, social development. Group curricula designed to remediate common deficits, and individual curricula for particular deficits. The objective is to bring each child's development up to the point where it is normal for his age level.

STAGE ONE: ESTABLISHING EYE CONTACT

Gaze aversion, the avoidance of eye to eye contact, is a general characteristic of autistic children (though not peculiar to them). It is part of the seclusion pattern, an avoidance response. Eye contact in our culture usually precedes all other exchanges; it is a way of signaling another that one wants to initiate or respond to an exchange with him. If one will not meet the other's gaze, then communication and other forms of exchange become strained.

The first step in acculturating an autistic child therefore is to teach him to look other people in the eye. This is essential not only for overall adjustment, but for training itself. Therefore, eye contact is made a precondition for all the exchanges during the first part of training. Parents become very encouraged when their child starts generalizing his training by returning their glances. Such small signs of progress convince parents of our expertise, and thus make them ready to follow our instructions later when we need their help. And, like other children, the autistic child ordinarily has to learn to work normal exchanges. Since eye contact is relatively easy, a food exchange for establishing eye contact is an ideal place to start to learn to work normal exchanges.

The mother brings the child and his lunch to the laboratory for a twenty to thirty minute session each day. On arrival she cuts up the lunch in portions small enough to be tiny bites and arranges the food on a divided paper plate. The teacher takes the child and his lunch into a small room ten feet by twelve feet that is furnished with a low table and two child-size chairs. The teacher seats the child and sits down on the other side with the lunch.

If the child voluntarily looks at the teacher (which he often does, fleetingly), the teacher *immediately* reciprocates with a hearty "Good Boy!" a pat on the back and a bite of lunch. It is important that the reciprocation be immediate and the approval and the body contact precede the bite so they signal that the child will receive food and thus will become conditioned reinforcers.

If the child does not look voluntarily, some method must be devised to entice him into looking. One method used, for example, is to peek at him through a hollow building block. This behavior is bizarre enough that even an autistic child will look in disbelief. As soon as he does, he is immediately reinforced with approval, body contact and a bite of lunch (in that order). As the child continues to work the exchange, the gimmick is faded out, used less and less until it is no longer needed. Or, the spoon can be held in front of the child's eyes and then slowly moved until it is just in front of the teacher's eyes. This, too, often results in the child's meeting the gaze of the teacher; when that happens, he is immediately reinforced.

Immediate reinforcement is extremely important in these early stages. Delays weaken the power of the instructional exchange. It also results in *superstitious learning* (Skinner, 1953), since if other actions occur between the time the child gives the proper response and receives his reinforcer, these other actions will be the ones reinforced. So a good teacher will reciprocate within one to two seconds. With eye contact, the teacher must be very alert because the first glances given by the child may be so fleeting as to be practically unidentifiable.

Once a child makes frequent eye contact, say seventy to eighty times per twenty-minute session, an exchange is structured to modify the child's response until he will look at the teacher's eyes on request. Specifically, the exchange is altered so the child gets his bites of lunch only if he meets the teacher's gaze within five seconds after being asked to do so. If the early training is done properly, the child will voluntarily look at the teacher frequently, so this second step can be easy. Then, once the child will reliably meet the teacher's gaze on request, the length of time he must hold her gaze is gradually increased to ten seconds before he gets his reinforcer.

An exchange analysis of these procedures is given in Table 8.1. Note that both child and teacher are reinforced in these exchanges. Both parties in an exchange must find it rewarding or profitable if the exchange is to be worked repetitively through time at a steady pace. This is true for the party who initiates the exchange and for the party who reciprocates. Also it may be noted that exchange signals (after the child is conditioned to recognize them as signals) become conditioned reinforcers in time because they consistently predict reinforcement.

Typical results are given for eye contact training in Figure 8.1. Note that with consistent food reinforcement the number of eye contacts per session increased gradually, if sporadically, to a median of almost sixty per session (last eight days). The data in this figure also show what happened to this boy's whining—a habitual attention-getting pattern. By ignoring the child every time he whined until he stopped, the teacher extinguished the response pattern by the sixteenth session. It never occurred during subsequent learning sessions. Such extinction results are typical for attention-getting behaviors.

Table 8.1. Exchange Analysis of Eye Contact Training.

Actor	Behavior	Analysis	Reinforcement	
			Teacher	Child
Child	Looks at teacher.	Initiatory response	x	
Teacher	Feeds.	Reciprocatory response		x
Teacher	Holds up toy for child to see.	Exchange signal		
Child	Follows toy with eyes.	Initiatory response	x	
Teacher	Moves toy next to eyes.	Exchange signal		
Child	Eyes follow toy, fleetingly contacting teacher's eyes.	Inadvertent initiatory response	x	
Teacher	Spoons food into child's mouth with haste.	Reciprocatory response		x
Teacher	Says "Look at me."	Exchange signal		
Child	Looks at teacher while teacher counts to five.	Initiatory response	x	
Teacher	Approval, touching, then food.	Reciprocatory response		x

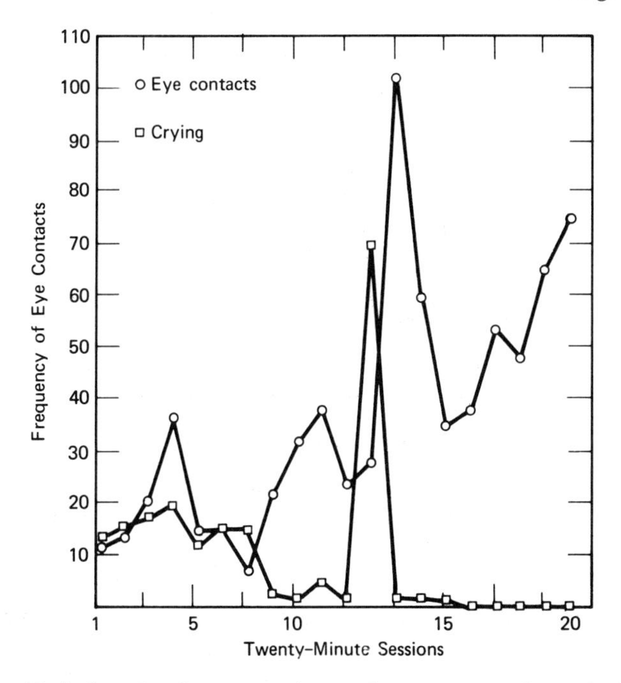

Figure 8.1. Typical results of counter exchange where eye contact is acquired via a food exchange, and bizarre behavior (in this instance whining) is extinguished by totally ignoring it. Experiment by Blackwell.

During eye contact training the autistic child often gets up, wanders from the table. Although other investigators have used restraining techniques of various types (Risley, 1968; Risley and Wolf, 1966), we do not feel these are advisable. But since voluntarily sitting at a table and attending a teacher is essential in all subsequent training, it is important at this juncture to solve this particular problem. Actually the solution is very simple: the initial eye-contact exchange for the child must be structured so he can work it only by sitting at the table *and* by meeting the teacher's gaze. Otherwise, the child is totally ignored. The trouble with this prescription is that no one really believes it works, even teachers in training. Hence, from time to time we run an experiment where a teacher uses the common-sense approach, that is, asks the child to sit down, reasons with him, "As soon as you sit down, you can have some food. . ." In Figure 8.2 are the results of one such experiment with John. This experiment was run during gaze aversion remediation, so John was being reinforced for both sitting and making eye contact. During the first period the teacher purposefully, systematically attended John while he was away from the table, asked him to return, etc. Note that the problem became progressively worse until one session he was

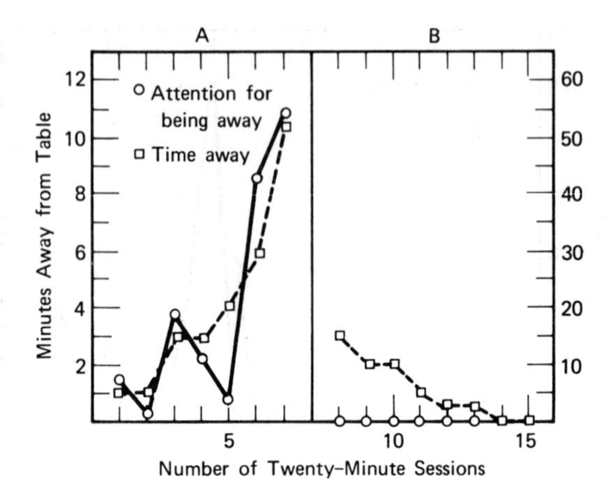

Figure 8.2. During A teacher purposefully looked at John, and repetitively asked him to sit back down until he did. During B, teacher completely ignored John while he was away from the table. Experiment by Blackwell.

away from the table more than 50 percent of the time. Beginning Session Eight, when the teacher began ignoring John's out-of-seat behavior, the problem began rapidly to disappear, until the fourteenth and fifteenth sessions when John was in his seat, attending the teacher throughout the sessions.

We have seen how eye contact, sitting and attending are established, but how are such patterns maintained? As intimated in earlier chapters, there are several strategies for maintaining behavior, but perhaps the best is making the behavior in question into an essential preliminary component of a larger pattern, a chain of behavior, that is reinforced. This strategy is natural for eye contact since, as noted earlier, eye contact is typically used as a signal of interest in starting and maintaining exchanges, particularly those involving verbal communication. Hence the proper approach in training is to use eye contact as a signal, the essential first step in all exchanges. Figure 8.3 illustrates typical results of an experiment in which eye contact is turned into an exchange signal.

STAGE TWO

Motor Imitation of Teacher

During this phase eye contact is established as a generalized signal for the teacher to structure an exchange. Procedurally, the teacher watches the child and as soon as eye contact is made, gives a specific exchange signal, e.g. the teacher puts his hand in the air. This signals the child to put his

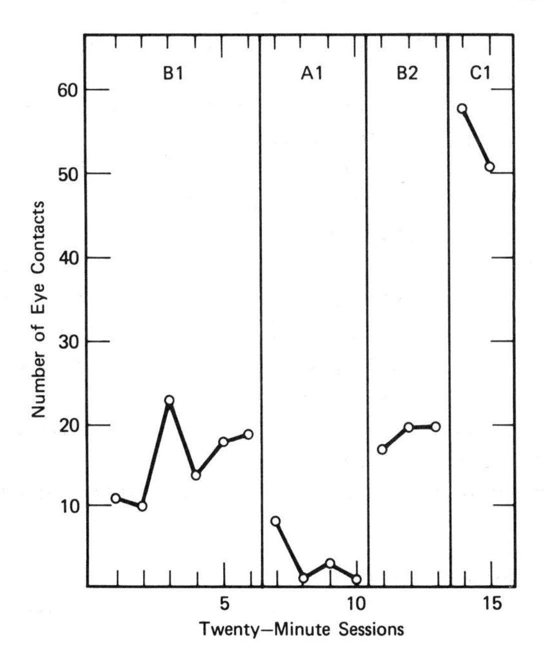

Figure 8.3. Results of a BABC experiment with John. During A, no reinforcement for eye contact, during B, food reinforcement for eye contact and during C, eye contact was a prerequisite. Experiment by Blackwell.

hand up also. Often, after several tries, a child will do it spontaneously. If not, the teacher can *prompt* the child by lifting the child's appropriate hand up with his own free hand. Usually after one or two promptings, backed up with reinforcement, the child will anticipate the reinforcement and thus will spontaneously imitate the teacher. The teacher then does other things—puts his hands down on the table, on his head, to his left, to his right—each time establishing eye contact before signaling the specific behavior the child is to imitate.

At this point it is not always necessary to reciprocate with food. Every second or third exchange may be completed with just approval and a pat. New behaviors, however, must continue to be reinforced as before with approval, a pat, and food every time, for the first few occurrences, at least. New behaviors are costly, and until the child has practiced enough to develop expertise, the conditioned reinforcers, which are still relatively weak, will not maintain an optimal response rate. Also, in successful training, behavior is shaped gradually. At first, the teacher reciprocates only for approximations of the behavior he ultimately wants; everything else is ignored. The next step is to get that approximation closer before completing the exchange by giving the reinforcers; then closer and still closer, as illustrated in Table 8.2, with typical sequences in early imitation training.

Once the child imitates hand positions reliably, the teacher moves on to exchanges involving toys and puzzles. For example, after eye contact is made, the teacher might drop a ball on the table, and after it stops bouncing he puts it in the hand of the child. If the child drops the ball, for whatever reason, the teacher responds with reinforcers. If the child does not drop it, and prompting is necessary, the teacher gently pushes it from the child's hand and completes the exchange. The exchanges are worked over and over again to give the child practice and thereby develop his expertise; then expanded to include more and more tasks, such as putting a three-piece wooden puzzle together, etc.

After a number of imitative response patterns have been established, the teacher begins asking for the behavior as he gives the motor prompts. At first these verbal requests are extra (and redundant) exchange signals.

Table 8.2. Analysis of Imitation Training.

			Reinforcement	
Actor	Behavior	Analysis	Teacher	Child
Child	Meets teacher's gaze.	General exchange signal	x	
Teacher	Holds up one hand.	Specific exchange signal		
Child	Wiggles in chair.	Irrelevant behavior		
Teacher	Ignores child.	No reciprocation		
Child	Looks away.	Non-exchange signal		
Teacher	Puts head down for a second.	Time-out		
Child	Meets teacher's gaze.	General exchange signal	x	
Teacher	Holds up a hand.	Specific exchange signal		
Child	Brushes his forehead.	An approximate initiatory response	x	
Teacher	Approval, a pat and then a bite of food.	Reciprocation		x
Child	Eye contact.	General exchange signal	x	
Teacher	Puts hand up.	Specific exchange signal		
Child	Puts hand up.	Initiatory response	x	
Teacher	Approval, a pat and then a bite of food.	Reciprocation		x

However, they have a subtle function. Because of the conditioning process, the words gradually acquire meaning for the child, and therefore, it is possible after a time to start fading out the behavior to be imitated and to rely solely on the instructions. Hence, the child is taught to respond to the teacher's verbal requests.

In any case, the imitation and request procedures, in combination, are from this point on used to teach the child a large number of motor and discrimination tasks. During this stage of training, the autistic children in our laboratory learn to put together as many as twenty puzzles, to work toys that discriminate for shape or color, and so on.

Training Mothers

As noted in the last chapter, Larry's mother was one of the first to be trained as an assistant teacher in our laboratory. Since then our training program has gradually become more elaborate as we have learned better and better how to help the mothers succeed. It now involves several rather well defined steps.

(1) The mother keeps a daily log describing fully her exchanges with her autistic child. This includes a description of what the child does during the day and what she does in response. She is asked particularly to note when she tries to get the child to do something, what the child does in response to her attempts, and then what she does in response to the child's response. What inevitably emerges from these logs is a description of a placation strategy. Mothers of autistic children generally tend not to ask their children to do anything, rather they placate them by giving in to almost all of their demands. Also, the log usually provides some material which ultimately can be used to sensitize the mother to the teasing pattern which usually typifies the relationships of the autistic child with members of the family. At this time, too, an observer spends several days in the home reporting the flow of the child's behavior including the interaction between the mother and the child. Care is taken to observe different periods of the child's waking hours at least twice. The observer is equipped with a miniature tape recorder and stop watch. He observes from an adjoining room and whispers into the recorder a flat description of events as they unfold in the household. The tape recorder is ordinarily turned up to the point where it picks up any talking which is part of the interaction between the mother and the child. The stop watch is used to get a measure of the duration of the various exchanges which are observed. From this flat description the teacher abstracts the exchange patterns which characterize the interaction between the child and the other members of the family.

(2) After two or three weeks the mother is then asked to read several articles or short books on learning and exchange theory and on reinforce-

ment and exchange training.[2] To help prevent the mother from becoming discouraged, the material is selected to be interesting and is graded easy to difficult. Furthermore, to reinforce her progress, the mother periodically meets with the trainer to discuss the material, particularly its relevance to child rearing practices. This is a crucial step in the training. Without a firm theoretical understanding, mothers find it impossible to be creative later on, and creativity is essential for success.

(3) Once the mother progresses well into the reading, she is allowed to observe her child working exchanges with the teacher. This usually occurs after the child has become accustomed to imitating the teacher's motor responses, particularly after he has gained some skill in working puzzles. We have found it advisable to wait until the child has been acculturated to this extent, if nothing else to continue to establish the teacher's expertise with the mother.

As the mother observes the child and the teacher working the exchanges, the trainer begins to analyze the stream of behavior with the mother, illustrating the various concepts and processes learned about in the reading. This is continued until the mother is facile in analyzing the stream of behavior herself.

(4) Then the mother is allowed to work with a child, taking the role of the teacher, usually running the imitation exchanges on motor tasks. The child that the mother works with in the laboratory is not necessarily her own. If, in the judgment of the trainer, the mother might encounter problems with her own child, she is given a much easier child so her initial experiences will be successful.

(5) Also, to insure the success of these early exchanges, the mother is coached. The experimental rooms in the laboratory are fitted with a one-way wireless communication system.[3] Thus when the mother does not know what to do or when she makes an error, the trainer can make suggestions. With this immediate help and feedback, the average mother is able to do as well as the teacher from the very first day, that is, on exchanges to which the child is accustomed.

It is during this stage that the mother learns how to use exchange signals, how to use questions and direct instructions, to set up the various exchanges. She also learns how to use approval and food to reinforce appropriate responses from the child. She learns how to reinforce quickly within one

[2] Kozloff (1968), Smith and Smith (1966), Risley, Wolf, and Mees (1966), Risley and Wolf (1967), Patterson and Gullion (1968), Williams (1965).

[3] As noted in Chapter 5, we use a one-way communication system involving (1) a regular hearing aid with a telephone induction loop which the mother wears and (2) a dispatcher's microphone hooked to an amplifier and an induction loop which is hidden in the ceiling, around the perimeter of the training room, which the trainer talks into to the mother from behind a one-way mirror from the observation room.

or two seconds of the appropriate response, and how to vary the reinforcement pattern, sometimes using just approval, sometimes using approval as a signal for food reinforcement to strengthen approval as a conditioned reinforcer. The mother also learns how to move from continuous to variable reinforcement.

Also, as mentioned, the mother learns how to use non-exchange signals, that is, how to ignore irrelevant behavior, how to time the child out by dropping her head, looking away or holding her head in her hands when the child is not cooperative or when he engages in moderately disruptive behavior. Also, she learns how to use a time-out room where she puts the child when she simply cannot ignore his behavior. It is always established ahead of time what precise behaviors are to result in a child's being placed in a time-out room and the mother is shown the most effective procedures, that is, not talking while she quickly takes the child by the hand to deposit him in the time-out room. She is instructed in the dangers of wearing out the time-out room; it is effective only if used rarely and then only to the extent the instructional exchange is attractive.

(6) Once she has mastered these basic skills, the mother is then asked to coach one or two other mothers who are also in training. This gives her experience in handling problems which emerge suddenly and further experience in analyzing the flow of exchanges.

(7) Next the mother is trained how to structure new exchanges with the child, how to use prompting procedures, how to use the child's ability to imitate to get new exchanges started. Also, she learns shaping procedures, that is, how to reciprocate for successively better approximations of the desired behavior pattern. She also has to learn how to move back and forth from the accustomed exchanges which are comfortable to the new exchanges which can be frustrating for the child. The goal is to teach her to press ahead until the child begins to evidence the slightest strain and then move back into more comfortable material, pressing ahead again usually a little farther until the child proceeds through the new material and becomes comfortable working the new exchange.

(8) Once the mother has mastered the various instructional procedures in the laboratory, she is given an abstract of the patterns of interaction observed earlier in her home. This abstract, an example of which is given in Table 8.3, is to help her analyze the situation at home. Then the mother is asked to suggest a program for herself and her family to follow in terminating the pathogenic exchanges and structure in their place acculturating exchanges. The trainer coaches the mother through this plan by reinforcing what appear to him to be good ideas with approval and by making suggestions when the mother appears uncertain as to what to do or when she suggests something that obviously will not work. Our experience has been that mothers generally do quite well at this stage. In fact, some become

Table 8.3. Description of Home Interaction Patterns Given to the Mother During Parent Training.

Child's Behavior	Parent's Reaction
(1) Plays in bathroom or kitchen water.	(1) Chases after him, yells at him to stop: "Michael Hare, you get out of that water this very instant." (Usually he stops, then begins again.)
(2) Pulls and pushes for records.	(2) Gives him record—about 50 percent of the time.
(3) Whines and cries if he is not given what he wants.	(3) Cuddles and asks him what is wrong.
(4) Gets into food as it is prepared.	(4) Chases after him, yells at him to stop. (Usually he stops but begins again in a few minutes.)
(5) Gets into pantry or lower cabinets.	(5) Yells at him to stop. (He usually stops, then continues.)
(6) Climbs on top of refrigerator.	(6) Yells at him to come down, or asks him to come down over and over again.
(7) Climbs onto kitchen counter, or pulls a chair up to the counter so as to climb up more easily.	(7) Usually tells him over and over to get down. And sometimes he does, usually not. Eventually, she takes him down bodily.
(8) Plays with his food during a meal (slaps it with spoon, pours it back and forth with spoon).	(8) Repeatedly tells him to stop, sometimes he does, for a minute or so.
(9) Gets into records; pulls them out, creating a mess by the record player.	(9) Goes after him and tells him to stop. Eventually she ends up yelling at him as he continues to get into the records. Then he sometimes stops.
(10) Stands up and rocks back and forth, often with thumb in mouth.	(10) Ignores.
(11) Sits idly fingering silky material.	(11) Ignores—unless it is something she is wearing.
(12) Stands outside and urinates (usually onto sidewalk).	(12) Gives him attention; she usually says, "Why Michael Hare . . . I just don't understand you. . ."
(13) Pours, spills and dumps things onto the floor, right in front of her (looks to see if she is getting upset).	(13) Usually gets upset after he makes a mess. She says, "Michael Hare, you're just doing that to tantalize me." Often hollers at him to clean it up.

extremely creative, often suggesting approaches which turn out to be improvements over early staff procedures. We have the mothers work on just a few problems at a time, the more serious ones first. An example of a plan is given in Table 8.4.

Table 8.4. Prescription Given to Parents to Restructure the Exchange Patterns in the Home.[a]

INSTRUCTIONS:

To Ignore: Do not look at or talk to Michael while he is engaged in inappropriate behavior. Do not tell him to stop, try verbally to divert his attention, scold him, or threaten him with punishment.

To Reward: For the present, give Michael approval in all exchanges. For certain things, food may be given in addition (an afternoon snack for working puzzles for a while, a drink of juice for a household task, etc.) Make sure, of course, that the reward follows the behavior immediately—within a few seconds.

To Time-out: Without speaking, but with some vigor, take Michael to time-out room. Leave him in two minutes for first offense, four minutes for second offense, etc. Do not let him out if he is whining or tantrumming.

Child's Behavior	Your Response
(1) Pulling and/or pushing (a) For records.	(1a) Set aside several periods of the day during which Michael can work for a record (e.g. by picking up toys, clothes, working puzzles). Tell him, "As soon as you . . ., you can have a record." At any other time ignore him. To get it started, ignore him until he asks at an opportune time of the day. (Eventually, working for records was established ten minutes after lunch. It was initiated with Mrs. H. saying, "It's time to work for a record." She would lead Michael to the table and prompt him to work puzzles.)
(b) For bath.	(b) Ignore. Then, when it is proper time, tell him he may take bath.
(2) Crying and/or whining.	(2) Ignore. This will probably occur after he is ignored for pulling.
(3) Playing with stove, getting into food in refrigerator or pantry, climbing on cupboards, getting into food being prepared (assuming that any of these are disturbing to you).	(3) Time-out from the kitchen by removing Michael from kitchen and locking door from inside. Open in approximately three or four minutes and repeat each time he repeats inappropriate behavior. Don't let it escalate; don't wait, letting him do it for a while. Remove him immediately. This will work if he likes being in the kitchen. If he does any of these when you are not in the kitchen with him, remove him and lock the door.

[a] After Kozloff (1969).

Table 8.4. continued.

Child's Behavior	Your Response
(4) Climbing on refrigerator.	(4) Ignore.
(5) Playing with own food (spilling it, slapping it, etc.) or getting up from table to mess around.	(5) Take food away. No food until next meal. Ignore all appeals for food in between.
(6) Water play.	(6) Temporarily, remove him from room and lock door. If he does this during a meal, remove him from the kitchen and take his plate away.
(7) All bizarre behavior.	(7) Ignore.
(8) Self-initiated working at puzzles, looking in magazines, picking up clothing, helping in kitchen, speech (any approximation).	(8) Reward verbally, with strokes and, if convenient, with a bite of food. If he is engaged in such activity for more than a few minutes, reward him several times. Don't just wait until he stops. Reward him during activity if it is longer than ten seconds or so. Be on the lookout for appropriate behavior and consistently reward it.

As may be noted in Table 8.5 from Kozloff's dissertation (1969), the above procedures worked rather well in modifying the mothers' response patterns to their autistic children. It terminated their pathogenic exchanges, their reinforcement of bizarre, disruptive behaviors and accelerated their involvement in acculturating exchanges—constructive play activity, appropriate speech and cooperation.

The data in Figure 8.4 which are typical, depict the through-time changes in behavior of a mother who received the above training and her six-year old autistic boy. The experimental data illustrate rather well the effects of our structuring counter-exchanges to decelerate one pattern, that is, bizarre, disruptive behavior and simultaneously in its place to accelerate another pattern, that is, constructive activity such as chores and play.

In the A1 period, before any training, the child had a very high rate of disruptive behavior and the mother reinforced this at a similar high rate with attention and sometimes even with food. At the same time the child seldom engaged in constructive activity. In the B period after the mother was coached, but only in the Laboratory School, to ignore him, time him out or isolate him for disruptive behavior, the child's disruptive behavior decreased approximately from 50 to 15 per two-hour period. Note, however, that with only the above training, the time spent on constructive activity by the child did not increase significantly in the B period. So for the first six days of the C1 period the trainer coached the mother at home in how

Table 8.5. Patterns of Exchange Reciprocation by Parents for Various Experimental Periods.[a]

Response Class	Percentage of Reinforcement								
	Michael's Parents			Sean's Parents			Peter's Parents		
	Prior to Training	After Training in the Home	Follow-up	Prior to Training	After Training in the Home	Follow-up	Prior to Training	After Training in the Home	Follow-up
Bizarre, Disruptive	73%	0%	0%	72%	0%	0%	54%	0%	0%
Episodes of Constructive Activity	54	100	100	0	100	100	50	None Occurred	100
Appropriate Speech	None Present	100	100	None Present	84	85	64	88	88
Cooperation	60	100	96	0	95	92	69	100	94

[a] After Kozloff (1969).

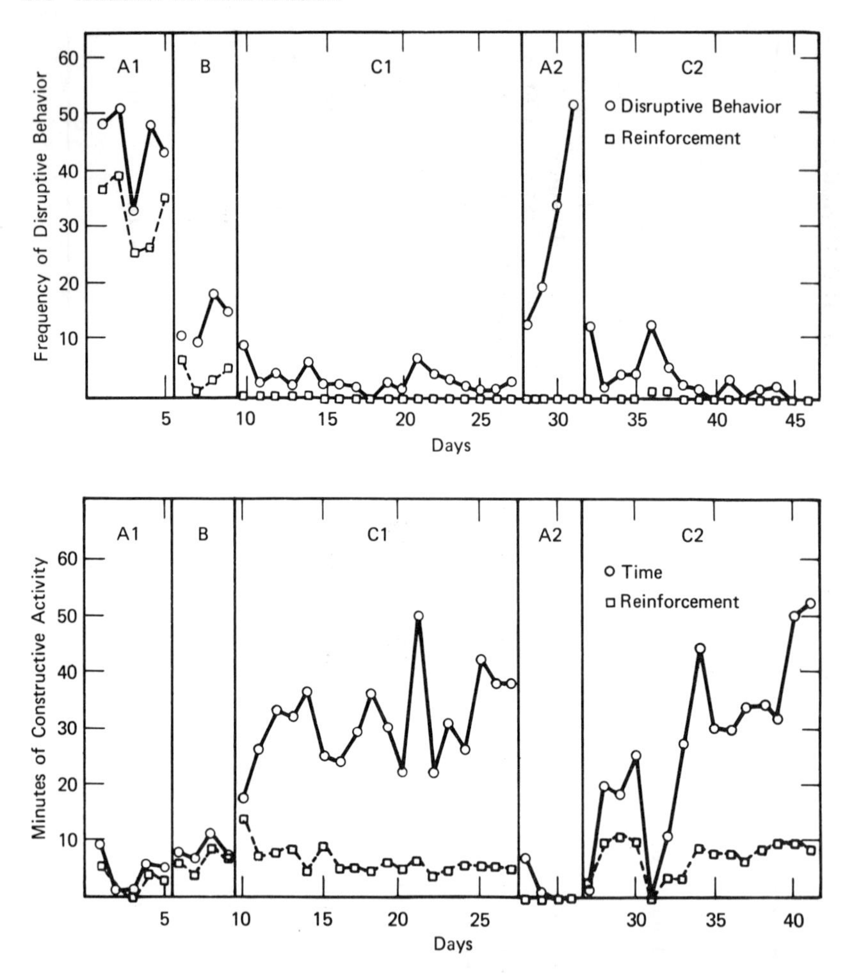

Figure 8.4. Changing the structure of exchanges in the home. The A1 observations of the exchanges between the mother and child were made before the mother was trained. The B observations were made immediately after the mother was trained in the laboratory school. For the first seven days of the C1 period the mother was coached in the home to change the pattern of exchanges observed in the A1 period. In the A2 condition the mother was asked to ignore the disruptive and the constructive exchanges. During the C2 period she was instructed to again reciprocate constructive exchanges and ignore disruptive behavior. (After Kozloff, 1969.)

to structure and maintain exchanges involving constructive activity. During the C1 period the amount of time the child spent at constructive activity increased from about 10 minutes to almost 40 minutes per two-hour home visit. Notice also that the number of disruptive behaviors decreased further as the time spent on constructive activity increased. During the A2 period the mother was instructed to continue ignoring the disruptive behavior and, in addition, to ignore constructive behavior. As Figure 8.4 shows, time spent on constructive activity fell to zero while disruptive behavior rose to its pre-training level. In the C2 period the mother was again asked to reciprocate exchanges for constructive activity. Constructive activity then increased and disruptive activity decreased.

As noted, the mothers work closely with the trainer in designing new programs for their child, and some become quite creative in structuring situations. One good illustration of this was a variation of time-out procedures used on tireless Mary. When she was a baby just home from the hospital, she cried unless her parents rocked her to sleep. This was bad enough, but then she learned to wake up just as they put her down and would cry again until they rocked her back to sleep. This would go on and on, often five or six hours. They could have stopped this interchange abruptly at any time by simply putting her to bed, walking out and letting her cry until she stopped. Eventually she would have given up, extinguished and gone to sleep. Several experiments (cf. Williams, 1965) have obtained such results, and simple extinction would have worked with Mary. But we wanted to see if an alternative strategy could be worked out that would be just as effective but would completely bypass the crying and tantrums, which by now were used routinely by Mary to avoid going to bed.

After discussions with Mary's mother the following procedure, which incorporated a number of her suggestions, was decided upon: About seven o'clock in the evening Mary was bathed, dressed in pajamas and placed with her doll directly into bed under the covers. Her mother sat on a chair at the side of the bed, without looking at Mary, except occasionally out of the corner of her eye. When Mary's eyelids seemed to be closing for the last time, the mother would get up quickly and walk out of the room.

The procedure in the B period was the same except that she placed her chair by the door. In the C period the procedure was again the same except that she sat on a chair just outside the door where Mary could see only her legs. What happened, interestingly enough, was that Mary never did have a tantrum. Furthermore the time required for Mary to go to sleep decreased precipitiously (Figure 8.5) from 2 hours 15 minutes at the beginning to 10 minutes on the sixth night. Eventually a very stable equilibrium was reached; Mary went to sleep about 15 minutes after being put to bed. Her mother chose to sit in the hall every night until Mary fell asleep. During these few minutes she relaxed and read without the other members of the family bothering her. So we left it there!

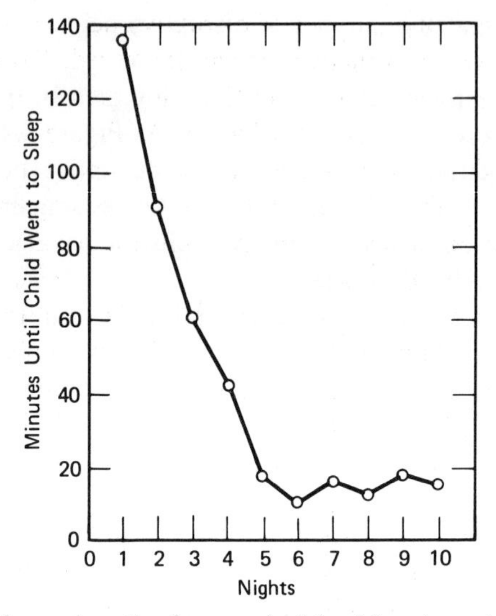

Figure 8.5. Extinction series—the time required for Mary to go to sleep on successive nights, after reinforcement for staying awake was terminated by her mother. (After Ferritor, 1969.)

STAGE THREE: PHONEME EXPANSION FOR MUTE CHILDREN

The procedure used in Stage Three, for mute and near mute children, is omitted for children who use gibberish or parrot sounds, as they already have the skills developed in this stage. A month or so after the mute child begins to follow simple instructions, he will generally begin to babble. That is, he emits spontaneous vocalizations which usually are not recognizable as words or sometimes not even as clear sounds. He does this because the instructions he has been receiving—specifically the sounds of voices—have consistently signaled food reinforcement and have, therefore, come to be conditioned reinforcers for him.

It has been argued (Hurlock, 1964:216) that in the babbling stage the normal child acquires the control over his vocal apparatus necessary for more advanced speech. Be that as it may, the normal child, between the time he begins babbling at three or four months and ceases some time after twelve months, generally voices all the known phonemes. Gradually, however, the babbling pattern is replaced by what Eisenson calls lallation (Vetter, 1969:45), the repetition of the "heard sound complexes and symbols" and the gradual dropping out of the unheard sound complexes. The dropping out of sounds, however, accelerates as a normal child moves into echolalia, begins to imitate without understanding words and phrases which others make. Like babbling, lallation and echolalia are very important processes in normal speech development, for through them the child becomes expert in producing the sound complexes which will become part of the conventional language which he will learn to use in his next two or three years.

In accelerating speech acquisition, it seems to be a mistake, however, to push a child too quickly into lalling and echoing via imitation training where the child is reinforced only for those voiced sounds which approximate the teacher's model. In such training novel verbal responses are defined as incorrect, are not reinforced and, hence, are extinguished. Rather, it is important that the babbling stage continue until the child has developed the capacity to produce most of the pure sounds, the phonemes.

Phoneme expansion involves the acquisition of novel or original behavior. How is a teacher to help a child to produce original utterances? This may seem like an impossible question, but Maltzman (1960:230) suggests that "the way to foster originality is to reinforce such behavior when it occurs." In other words, the suggestion is that originality can be accelerated in much the same manner as other classes of behavior. In fact, Maltzman and his colleagues have trained human subjects to give original responses in free association tests (Maltzman et al., 1960). In one experiment, the most relevant to our problem, an experimental group was given a free association test based upon a list of words. In the process of the experiment, they were presented with this list six times and were instructed to give a different response on each repetition and were reinforced intermittently with approval contingent upon novel responses. The results showed that the experimental group had originality scores significantly higher than those of the control groups which had received neither originality instructions, nor reinforcement for originality. Similarly Pryor (1969:259) successfully trained porpoises to emit original behavior by reinforcing them for novel responses.

However, Maltzman (1960:230) has also suggested "if the baseline rate of novel behavior is too low, conditioning will not be effective, training cannot occur. His human subjects became rather frustrated when the experiment required the repeated production of uncommon responses. Pryor also observed both frustration and stereotypy in some porpoises in the early stages of originality training when their old repertoires no longer produced reinforcement. Hence the procedures used by Maltzman (1960) and Pryor (1969) are potentially treacherous. A teacher who withholds reinforcement from a mute child until original responses are emitted may not generate novel responses but may produce frustration and repetitive, stereotyped behavior.

Therefore, in working out procedures to accelerate the production of novel sounds, to simulate babbling in mute children, we were careful to use successive approximations. The first was suggested by Lovaas (1968), that is, the child is reinforced for all spontaneous vocalizations until his rate of making sounds had been accelerated to a rather high level. Then the teacher moves into the second step, she starts to reinforce the child for making a sound different from that which immediately preceded it. Thus, if the child were to begin a session with "duh," he would be given a bite of food. If his second response were also "duh" he would not be reinforced; if it were "mm," he would be. However, if the response after "mm" were "duh," he would again be reinforced because "duh" is different from the immediately preceding "mm." Notice that this procedure does not require a sound different from any of the preceding sounds. Yet, it was hoped that this less demanding procedure would, in fact, produce phoneme expansion. Data from an experiment by Kozloff, Blackwell and Hamblin suggest that it does.

Bobby, the subject of this experiment, had many autistic patterns when he came to the laboratory. He generally had responded well to the remedial training except in the area of speech. Being mute, he was started on the first step of the Lovaas speech training system where he was reinforced for producing sounds. This initial procedure seemed to work fairly well. After three months the teacher began imitation training which continued for seven months with surprisingly very little success, even though the teacher began with simple utterances and phonemes that the child had used quite frequently in the earlier stage of his training. Hence, it was decided to repeat the Lovaas procedure. Note in Figure 8.6 that when this child was reinforced with food approval and/or for all spontaneous vocalizations that he did respond at a very substantial rate. Although most of the responses were repetitive, he did change his vocal response at a rather substantial frequency. During the B period he was reinforced with approval and, in some instances, food for every spontaneous vocalization which represented a change from the previous vocalization. All repetitions were not reinforced. Notice that it took him a long time, but gradually the frequency of repetitions declined and the frequency of changes in vocal response increased.

More important, however, is what happened to his repertoire of phonemes. During the A period after six months of imitation training, he used a total of nine phonemes. During the B period he used a total of 22. This is a profound increase in phoneme usage from about one fourth to almost two thirds of the phonemes used in standard English. It is also interesting to note that the six months imitation training had actually contracted his usage of phonemes as we suggested earlier that it might. Before imitation training, after three months of being reinforced for spontaneous speech he had a total repertoire of 14 phonemes.

These experimental data then suggest that verbal imitation training may be a trap. Such training should evidently not be rushed. A formerly mute child should be repetitively reinforced for spontaneously emitting sounds

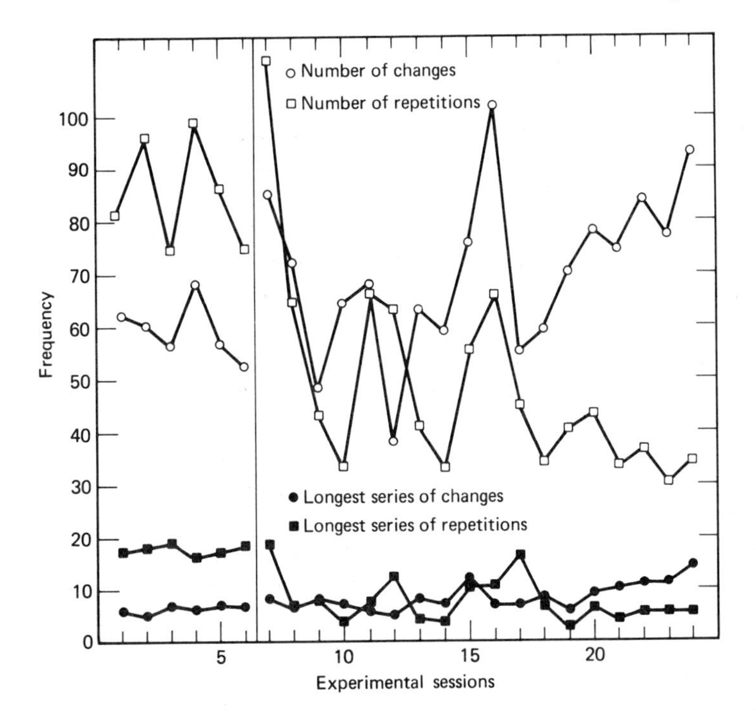

Figure 8.6. Phoneme Expansion in a Non-Verbal Child. In the A period, all spontaneous vocalizations were reinforced with food on a continuous schedule. In the B period, only those spontaneous vocalizations which were changes were reinforced. All repetitions were on extinction. Interobserver reliability averaged 94 percent. Experiment by Kozloff, Blackwell, and Hamblin.

which represent a change from a previous sound emitted until his phonemes are expanded to include at least all those used in standard English. This can be, of course, tedious for the teacher. However, tedium is ameliorated by change and the children seem to benefit from frequent changes in teachers.

STAGE FOUR: VERBAL IMITATION

The goal of Stage Four is to establish verbal imitation response patterns in children who were mute or nearly mute. Almost inevitably, this stage also involves eliminating the negative behavior syndrome. To begin, the teacher makes a sound. If the child responds with any vocalization within 5 seconds, the teacher reinforces. For example, after the child has established eye contact with the teacher, the teacher might make the request, "Say, 'ee.' " If, within 5 seconds, the child says "ee," "ba," "ma," or any other sound, the teacher reinforces him for a first approximation. Now this procedure may seem incongruous to the child for he often knows he has made an incorrect response to the question. This is particularly true of children who are habitually negative—who know very well that they were expected to imitate the exact sound, but deliberately made some other sound instead. Usually such a child will smile after being reinforced, as if to say, "I got you that time."

This procedure has been the subject of lengthy discussions among the staff. Some have felt that it establishes an incorrect response pattern that later has to be undone and that doing it correctly the first time would be easier in the long run. But a number of mute and near mute children have developed talking patterns using this loose approximation method while not even one has succeeded in learning to talk when the more exacting method was used.

Once the child routinely vocalizes within five seconds after the teacher's signal, he is ready to move to the next phase. Then the teacher restructures the exchange so the child must give a fair approximation of the correct answer. For example, if after the child makes eye contact, the teacher asks the child to say "mm" he must make a fair approximation of "mm" before the teacher reinforces him. We find that if a child has not been negative before, he almost certainly will be now. Now he recognizes what is at stake and engages in an all out battle for the survival of the system he has been enjoying.

It is at this point that the teacher must bring up his heavy guns. For a period ranging from one week to a month, the child must eat all of his food in the laboratory. He is brought to the laboratory three times a day for his meals and must earn his food by making on request fair imitations of sounds which he already has in his repertoire. During the first few days the child usually chooses to starve rather than voice the sounds the teacher asks him to repeat, sounds he has already made a number of times a day for a month or two.

These sessions are limited to twenty minutes three times a day. The child has the opportunity to imitate during these periods, and thus earn all of his regular breakfast, lunch or dinner. (The bites at this stage are relatively large.) But if the child will not speak, he is not fed. And some children actually do not eat. They spend their twenty minutes being negative, in some cases tantrumming, for as long as three days (staff sometimes refers to this as the Mahatma Gandhi stage). Eventually, however, the child gives in, sometimes with tears. He starts imitation slowly at first, then at an increasing rate until, after a time, he finally imitates correctly 100 percent of the time. A typical learning curve (for Michael, who had been completely mute, and did not have even one or two functional words when he began training at age 6 years) is plotted in Figure 8.7. When the power

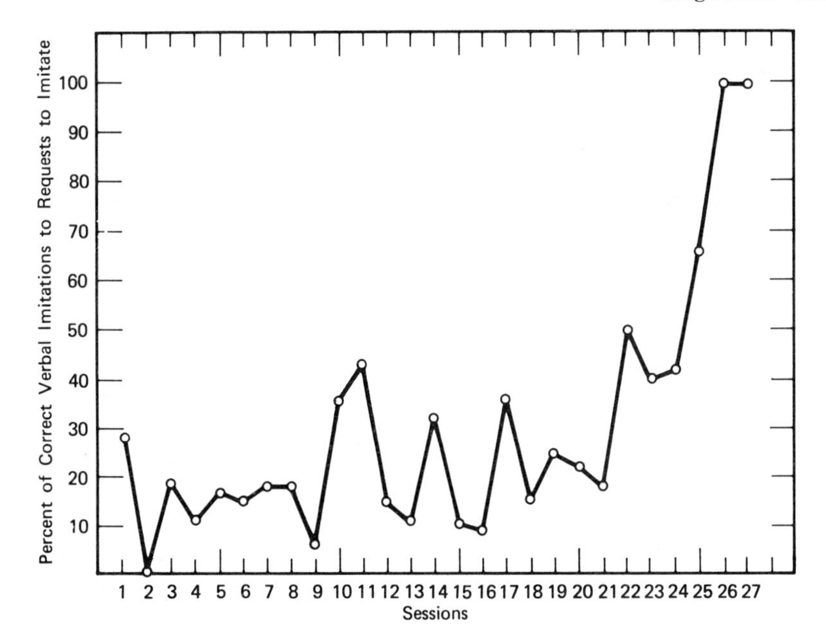

Figure 8.7. Proportion of correct verbal responses to requests during a period when the child received three meals a day in the laboratory. (After Kozloff, 1969.)

struggle is over and the child can imitate simple vocalizations reliably, we return to one session a day. Removing negativism is a taxing procedure for all involved, but it accelerates the child's progress. In fact, if we did not remove it, further acculturation of the child would probably be impossible.

Once the child can reliably imitate sounds that he already knows, the teacher begins to structure exchanges for new sounds until all the vowel sounds are learned. Then new exchanges are structured to teach the child syllables which involve the blending of the vowel sounds with a consonant sound: ba, le, ma, da, etc.

While their speech appears to develop very slowly, actually it does not. Normal children ordinarily take three years to learn how to talk (babbling starts at four to five months, syntax is acquired by forty-two months); an autistic child, who is four years old at the onset of training, on a well-run food-talking exchange will do about as well in two years. But to the teacher, the process seems interminable, so he ordinarily tries to increase the terms of the exchange too fast. At first he might be content to reinforce the child for saying simple sounds such as—ah, ee, o, oo—then simple syllables such as—ba, ma, la, etc. But once he is successful in getting the child to move to a higher level, it is difficult to move back. Yet that is precisely what is necessary in a successful speech training. Like the practitioners of natural childbirth who have to learn to push and then relax, the teacher must learn to increase gradually the the terms of the exchange, thus keeping the child from becoming fixated at a low level, but at the same time he has to be ready to relax to allow the child to regress. Stress comes because the child is being pushed too hard. By allowing the child to slip back to an easier level, the teacher is in effect allowing a natural reversal which a little later will produce an intensification effect when he returns to the more difficult level. The child will thus be more willing to vocalize at the syllabic level when he is allowed at times to slip back to sounding vowels and consonants. Then later he can be pushed to imitate at the word level, being allowed then to slip back to the syllabic level.

The general acquisition process is illustrated nicely in an experiment with Luke with word learning using imitation (pointing to a ball, saying "ball") and gradually fading out the verbal model (just pointing). It is an apt experiment since it also shows how the learning procedures are transferred to the mother. The data are in Figure 8.8.

In condition A a teacher worked with the child while the mother observed. Even under continuous food reinforcement it took the child several days to

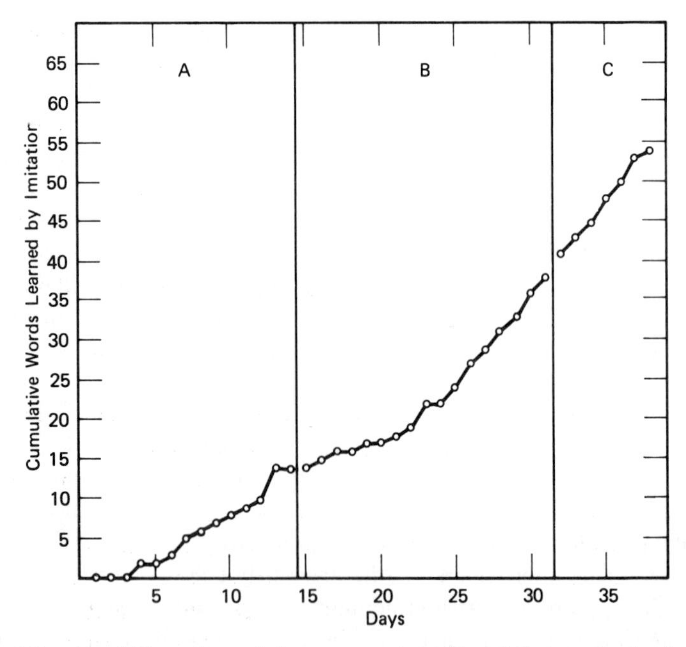

Figure 8.8. Acquisition of speech by a seven year old autistic boy. In the A period a teacher worked with the boy in the laboratory school while his mother observed. In the B period his mother coached by the teacher, worked with him in the laboratory school. In the C period his mother, uncoached, worked with him at home. (After Kozloff, 1969.)

learn his first word, but as the days went by, it took less and less time. The mother's acquisition of the techniques is shown by the fact that in the early days of condition B, in which she worked with Luke, his rate of learning decreased some what. By the middle of condition B, however, his rate of learning new words increased and even exceeded that of condition A. In condition C in which the mother worked uncoached with Luke at home, his learning stabilized at an even higher rate.

At each new stage of development, the behavior has to be practiced until it is habitual, that is, will persevere for long periods without reinforcement. This is illustrated in Figure 8.9 in an intra-session reversal experiment with Luke and his mother. It shows that Luke's speech was indeed controlled by the structure of the food exchange managed by his mother. In the A periods, when his food was on a dole, that is, when he did not have to speak for it, his speech rapidly decreased to 0 in only 2½ minutes. In the B periods when he had to earn his food by speaking, his rate of speech increased immediately and rose to approximately 80 percent correct verbal imitations. This experiment was designed to demonstrate to the mother the importance for Luke's development of the exchanges she and her son worked. Later, after Luke developed considerable expertise and after the pattern had become relatively habitual, it would be possible to maintain Luke's imitating without food reinforcement, as was the case with Larry (Figure 7.3).

At this stage we often encounter the above mentioned multiple-request

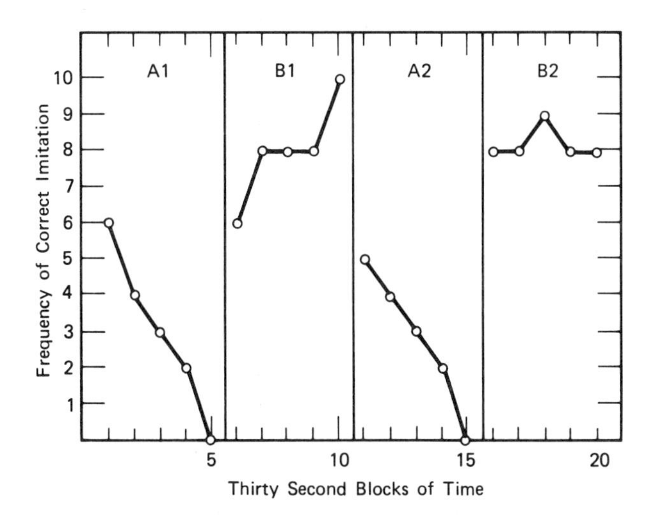

Figure 8.9. Frequency of correct imitative speech responses in the home for thirty second blocks of time. In the A periods the child's food was given to him and his mother attempted to elicit imitative speech. In the B periods she moved his food in front of her and made each bite contingent upon a correct imitative speech response. (After Kozloff, 1969.)

syndrome with our teachers and mothers. When a child or, in fact, anyone does not reply to a request, there is a natural tendency for the person making the request to persevere, to repeat the request until a reply is obtained. When this happens with our teachers and our mothers, the result, as might be predicted from Dehn's experiment in the last chapter, is response refusal and a deceleration of correct responses.

This is nicely illustrated in an experiment with a mother who had fallen into the multiple request pattern with Peter, her autistic son. In Figure 8.10 notice that during baseline when she was using multiple requests and food reinforcement that the child responded verbally only about 4 times per twenty minute period. To correct the situation, in B1 we instructed her to ask each question only one time. If he answered incorrectly or if he did not answer within five seconds, she simply went on to the next question. If he

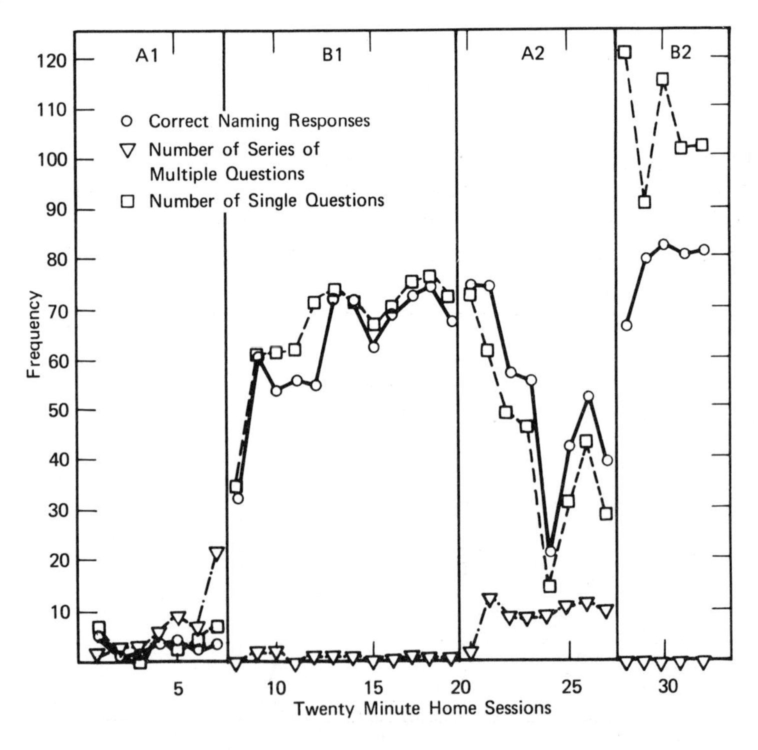

Figure 8.10. Appropriate verbal responses of an autistic boy under various exchanges managed by his mother. In the A1 condition Mrs. Gordon gave Peter bites of food for each correct verbal response to questions about pictures. She was uncoached. In B1 she was coached for two days to ask each question only once. In A2 Mrs. Gordon was instructed to ask multiple questions as in A1. In B2 she was instructed to return to asking each question only once. (After Kozloff, 1969.)

answered correctly, however, she gave him a bite of food. During this condition, the number of correct answers rose to approximately 70 per twenty minute period. In the A2 condition the mother was instructed to repeat the questions as she had done in the A1 condition. The number of correct responses decreased to about 40 per session. In the B2 condition she again asked the question only once. The number of correct responses rose to slightly over 80 per session.

If multiple requests are avoided and if the teacher moves back and forth between easier and harder materials, the child will master a fairly large number of blends in one to four months. The teacher will then start structuring exchanges in which the child is required to say names of the food that he is eating before he is given food. We do this because we have found that mute or near mute children progress much more quickly at the word stage if they are asked to use words which are meaningful to them—if the things the words represent are there for the child to see and experience. Food words are particularly good for mute and near mute children because they already understand these words. When a teacher says "chip," the child already knows that the teacher is referring to a potato chip. Such prior knowledge is a great help. Thus, at this stage the teacher might start the exchange by having the child first imitate a few blends and then proceed by having him repeat the name of each bite of food that he eats. Experimental data with Larry which illustrate these acquisitions were given in the last chapter in Figures 7.2 and 7.3.

After the words relating to food, the children are taught a number of very usable verbs such as move, eat, come, sit. Other researchers who have used talking-food exchanges to teach speech to autistic children have gone from the imitation of sounds directly to the naming of pictures (Risley and Wolf, 1967). But we find that the natural exchanges that one can signal or structure with a vocabulary of nouns is limited, while those made possible by a few verbs is large indeed. Therefore, we try to teach words of maximum use in working natural exchanges both inside and outside the laboratory.

STAGE FIVE: ESTABLISHING FUNCTIONAL SPEECH

Once a child can reliably imitate food words and a few common verbs, the teacher then moves to "speech training" in our laboratories. Toward the middle of the food exchange each day, the teacher asks, "What do you want? A chip or a pickle?" The teacher may have to prompt the child by saying "a chip"; then, later fading by pausing and saying "ch" a few trials, until the child begins to respond without a prompt. As the child works this exchange by saying "chip," the teacher gives him one. If he replies "pickle," he gets that. After a week of these exchanges the child will reliably discriminate among the different types of food and start to ask spontaneously for what he wants. This is ordinarily the first functional speech a mute child has ever used.

Now the mother is instructed to add two or three different foods at each meal without dropping any food that has been used in the past three or four meals. This may result in an unusual diet for a time, but the child quickly enlarges his functional vocabulary. Simultaneously, the teacher might start training the child to use simple verbs. For example, at the end of the training session he might block a doorway the child wants to pass through. As the child tries to push his way through, the teacher resists, while saying, "Say move," or "As soon as you say move I will let you through." With such procedures the child learns in a short time to use as many as one to two dozen common verbs in a functional way. The next step is to enlarge the child's naming vocabulary. The child may be shown concrete objects, particularly toys or pictures of objects. At first we used the procedures worked out by Risley and Wolf which relied on pictures. These worked reasonably well for echolalic children, but were just too much of a jump for mute or near mute children at this stage.

The data in Figure 8.11 show the responses of Peter, a near mute child who had just turned seven when he began therapy. In the A periods, a

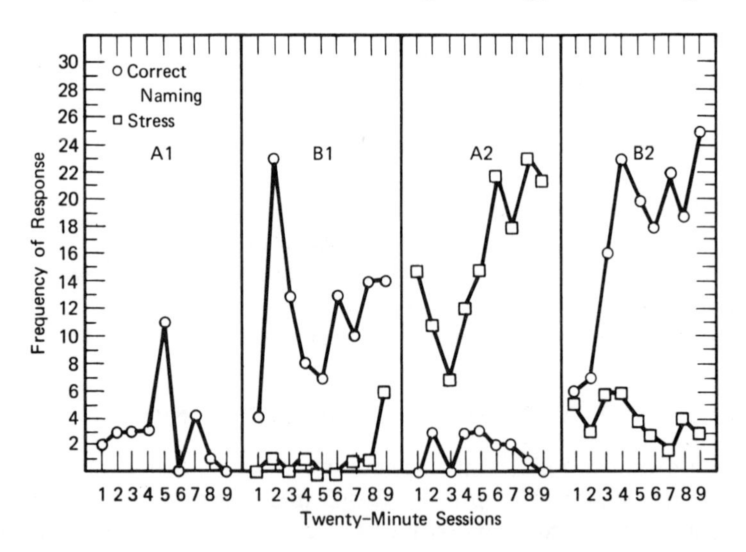

Figure 8.11. Number of correct naming responses and stress behaviors for two conditions. In the A periods, the Risley-Wolf method of picture-naming was employed where the child received a bite of food for each picture correctly named. In the B periods, the child was asked to name a toy. If he named it correctly, he was rewarded with a bite of food and was also allowed to play with the toy while he ate the food. Experiment by Ferritor and Hamblin.

number of pictures were used, including three that Peter could recognize: an apple, a table and a bell. Two additional pictures which he did not know were also included—a picture of a dog and a picture of a bunny. When the experiment started, the teacher asked, "What is this, Peter? This is a . . ." Peter was then to respond with "table," or the experimenter might make the "t" sound. Peter would then often look from the picture to the experimenter's face and repeat the prompt. However, during both A periods, Peter made very few correct, unprompted responses.

During the B period, the child was asked a similar question, "What is this, Peter?" But this time the question was about toys which Peter liked—a ball, a number "1" made out of sandpaper mounted on cardboard, a set of pocket beads, a bubble blower, a wheel, a caster that could be spun in a child's hand. Note how precipitously the number of appropriate responses increased during the B periods, leveling off at about 12 during B1 and 21 during B2.

Toward the end of the A1 period, the staff noticed that Peter began to revert to some of his old bizarre behaviors, perhaps indicating stress. Beginning with the B1 period the number of such stress signals were counted, also plotted in Figure 8.11. Note that the stress responses increased until they leveled off at approximately 22 per session in A2; then decreased during B2 to an average of about 3 per training session.

Once a formerly mute child develops a relatively large naming vocabulary with familiar objects such as toys, it is then possible to increase that vocabulary with pictures. At first we use photographs of familiar objects, preferably of members of the family doing familiar tasks. From this stage we proceed to the acquisition of syntax.

Establishing syntax the teacher generally begins by asking the child a familiar question, preferably about food, "What do you want?" Since the child has already been trained to name the desired food, he will say, perhaps, "chip." Then the teacher says, "Say, I want a chip"; and the child is reinforced only for an approximation of that sentence, such as "Want chip." As in the previous steps, the emphasis is on quantity of response rather than precision, and the teacher will accept very rough approximations. This simple exchange is varied and worked over and over again until the child becomes accustomed to reply to questions in primitive or broken sentences.

The best example we have is a variation used by Mary's mother to teach her to use sentences as though they were giant words (Bereiter and Engelmann, 1966). At this point in Mary's training, her mother's attention and approval had become very strong conditioned reinforcers. The following is abstracted from the transcription of a tape recording. (The mother carried a recorder with her which she called "Carol." Periodically she and Mary would listen to Carol "talk.")

First Day

MOTHER: Good morning Mary. (Slight pause.) Good morning, Mommy.
MARY: Mommy.
MOTHER: Say, good morning, Mommy. (Waits for response.)
MARY: Mommy.
MOTHER: Good morning, Mary. (Pause.) Now you say, Good morning, Mommy. (Note: First day all I was able to get was "Mommy" and a big smile, so I hugged and kissed her and again repeated, "Good morning, Mary.")

Second Day

MOTHER: As soon as we dress, we will eat breakfast. Are you hungry, Mary? (Pause.) I am hungry.
MARY: (Slight reply.) I hungry.
MOTHER: Are you hungry, Mary? (Pause.) Say, "I am hungry." (Note: With slight changes I followed this same pattern throughout each day. Always starting with the above. After the third or fourth day she followed beautifully. Gradually she started initiating conversation. But I still repeated everything she said to me, to let her know I understood.)

After Two Weeks

MOTHER: Mary, are you tired?
MARY: Mary tired, my bedtime.
MOTHER: Yes, Mary is tired and it is her bedtime. As soon as you get into your pajamas, it will be bedtime.
MARY: My bedtime.
MOTHER: Yes, it is Mary's bedtime.
MARY: Daddy, Daddy.
MOTHER: He's outside.
MARY: Daddy.
DADDY: What?
MOTHER: Ask if he wants some ice cream.
MARY: Wanna ma ice cream? Dad, wamma ice cream?
DADDY: No, I don't want any ice cream.
MARY: Me gum me gum me ice cream een ne may.
MOTHER: Daddy doesn't want any ice cream right now? Okay, well, do you want some ice cream, Mary?
MARY: Please.
MOTHER: Okay, just a minute and we'll fix you some ice cream. Where's your bowl?
MARY: He mah bol.

MOTHER: Okay. Hop up to the table now, and we'll have some ice cream.
MOTHER: What do you say to mother for giving you the ice cream?
MARY: Ice cream.
MOTHER: Yes, you're supposed to say thank you.
MARY: Kank you. Kank you.
MOTHER: Very good, Mary. You're welcome.

Last Day of Six Week Syntax Training

MOTHER: What's daddy watching on the TV?
MARY: TV.
MOTHER: Is it a ball game?
MARY: Mah ball game.
MOTHER: He watches ball games, doesn't he?
MARY: May daddy home.
MOTHER: Your daddy's home. He's watching the ball game. Kenny will be home in a minute.
MARY: Mah Ken home in minit?
MOTHER: Uh huh. He's out playing with the kids.
MARY: Play games?
MOTHER: They're playing games. He's playing games with the kids.

A year after this syntax training Mary spoke almost exclusively in sentences. Her speech does not have a parrot-like quality; she is over the giant-word syndrome. She is able to use appropriate sentences to ask for almost anything she wants. She is almost as creative in language as a normal child. She still has a relatively limited vocabulary, but no more so than any normal three year old. (She is actually five, but did not start language training until three and a half.) She still garbles some words, particularly new ones, and has some pronunciation difficulties. She probably will always have some pronunciation difficulties because the palate of her mouth is badly misshapen. Hence, Mary in this sense is not typical. Formerly mute children with normal vocal apparatus have no particular pronunciation problems.

An Alternative Procedure for Establishing Syntax.

The above procedure has worked quite well with younger mute children, but not with the older ones. Hence, we have evolved an alternative procedure which furnishes the child with visual as well as audio prompts via Rebus Reading (Woodcock and Davies, 1969). Rebus is a Latin word meaning, "by things" and each Rebus symbol is a pictured image, the referent of a spoken word, including the more common verbs, articles and conjunctions.

This alternative procedure for teaching syntax via Rebus reading was developed with Luke, an eight year old male who had attended the Laboratory School for two years. He was mute upon his acceptance into the program. After one year he had developed a strong pattern of motor imitation, an ability to attend and to work simple manipulative tasks, and most of his patterns of bizarre, disruptive behavior including severe hyperactivity were almost eliminated. During the second year a strong pattern of verbal imitation and a naming vocabulary of approximately one hundred words and a repertoire of twelve three and four-word sentences were acquired. However, progress was painfully slow. So we decided to try the alternative procedure involving Rebus reading.

Rebus reading. The first step in teaching Luke to read cards involved his learning to associate the appropriate name with ten Rebus cards, all nouns already in his naming vocabulary—table, chair, cat, dog, bird, ball, house, book, tree, car, box. The goal was to have Luke say the name of the object represented on the card when Kozloff, the experimenter-teacher said, "Read this." To accomplish this he held the card up and when Luke looked at it, asked, "What is this?" If Luke did not answer within three seconds, the teacher prompted him with the correct answer; when the child imitated the prompt, which he invariably did since his pattern of imitative speech was quite strong, the teacher reinforced him with a bite of food (the twenty-minute session each day was scheduled in the evening during which time the child took his dinner). The teacher repeated this procedure over and over, gradually fading out the word prompt until the child could name the object on the card ten times in succession when asked, "What is this?" All ten cards were learned to this criterion within the first two sessions.

During this time, after the first two cards had been learned to criterion, discrimination trials were introduced before a new card was presented for learning. In the discrimination trials the cards were placed in front of the child and the teacher would hold out his hand with the request, "Give me the one that says, 'table'." If the child made a correct response, he was given a bite of food; if he did not, the teacher prompted the child by pointing to the correct card. If the child then picked it up and gave it to the teacher, he was rewarded with the words, "Good boy." If, however, the child picked up the wrong card, the teacher closed his hand into a fist and would not accept the card. In other words, the child was reinforced with a bite of food and with praise only if he made the correct discrimination on the first trial. Once a child could reliably discriminate between the cards in this manner he was taught the name of the symbol on another card; once this was learned a new set of discrimination trials was introduced. It only took a few minutes for the child to reach criterion in learning the name of a card and it also took only several minutes to run through a set of discrimination trials. All ten cards were also learned according to discrimination criteria within the first two sessions.

To teach the reading response to Luke, a card was placed in front of him on the table about one foot in front of his face. The teacher then waited for Luke to look at the card. If he did not look at the card within three seconds, the teacher pointed to the card which generally caused him to look. Once the child was looking at the card, the teacher said, "Read this." If the child did not answer within three seconds, he was prompted, and if he imitated the prompt, he was given a bite of food. If the child gave the wrong answer, the teacher replied, "No," and went back to the earlier procedure asking, What does this say?" prompting and reinforcing him for the correct imitated answer, and so forth.

Teaching the child to identify correctly each of the ten cards rotated at random, ten out of ten times, upon a "Read this" request required only one twenty-minute session. On the fourth day, the above procedures were repeated for the ten nouns in a review, and the child learned to read four color cards—black, red, blue and yellow.

Next, Luke was taught to read two-word phrases involving a color card and a noun card. To develop this pattern the teacher placed two cards on the table, a color card on the left and a noun card immediately adjacent on the right. Then the teacher, with the request, "Read this," pointed to the color card, rewarding him with a bite of food when he read it correctly, then pointing to the noun card and, again, rewarding him with food for its correct reading. When errors were made on any card, the teacher, as before, dropped back to earlier procedures, selected the card from among the two, asked the child to name it, prompted him, if necessary, etc. until the child could again respond to criterion. Once the child could read each of the two cards in succession, the teacher began gradually, intermittently omitting reinforcement on the first card, until the child was rewarded only when he read both cards in succession correctly. Then the teacher faded out the pointing prompts for the first card. It took several days until the child could consistently read both cards correctly in succession with less than a two-second pause between the two cards and without requiring any prompts, verbal or pointing from the teacher. By the end of the ninth day, however, the child was reading random color noun combinations from among the four color cards and the ten noun cards, and his rate of correct response was over ninety percent.

On the tenth day the definite article "the" was introduced. The exact same procedures, as in the above steps, were used in teaching the child to read "the ball" or "the house." Learning the card "the" required only a few trials. By the end of this session the child could reliably read all ten combinations of the definite article and the nouns.

During the next two sessions, using the above procedures, the teacher taught the child to read three-word phrases involving the definite article, a color and a noun. As before, the three cards were placed on the table adjacent to one another in the proper order and the child was asked "Read this." The teacher prompted the child, at first by pointing to the first, then to the second, then to the third card and when the child read correctly, he gave the child a bite of food for each word correctly read. Then gradually reinforcement for reading the first and second cards was eliminated until the child received food only for reading all three cards. Similarly, the pointing and verbal prompts were gradually faded. By the end of the second day on this procedure, Luke could consistently and correctly read the three card phrases presented to him.

In the final stage the verb card "is" was added. Using the above procedures Luke was simply taught to name the card correctly, and once he could do this ten times in a row, the used card was placed in its proper sequence among the three other cards, to form sentences of the order: "The ball is blue." The teacher started by simply asking Luke to read the cards which he would do, except he tended to skip over the "is" card. To correct this, the teacher prompted him by pointing to the cards, especially the "is" card. Surprisingly, it took only one day for the child to learn to read the four card sentences. By the end of that session he virtually made no mistakes; he read each of the cards in rapid succession.

The progress in this experiment is pictured in Figure 8.12. Note the inordinate amount of time spent in the early stages when Luke was learning single words and, then, two-word phrases (ten sessions altogether). However, once the basics were mastered, learning to read three-word phrases and four-word sentences occurred rapidly (in just three sessions). This is because of the cumulative transfer of the earlier learning and because the reading system is productive, that is, it involves a series of rules which when mastered allows for certain creative combinations.

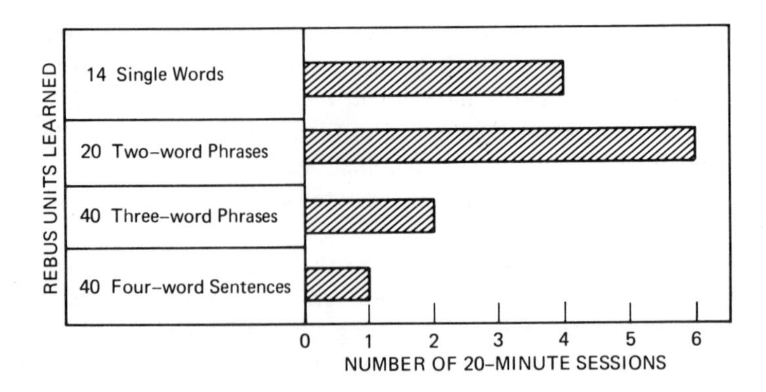

Figure 8.12. Time required to teach Luke to read to criterion Rebus units of increasing length.

Recall. It might be remembered that this series of experiments was initiated with Luke because we simply could not teach him to imitate sentences spoken by the teacher. The strategy, then, was to devise a near errorless learning procedure which allowed him to learn to use words in meaningful units. Thus Rebus reading was the first approximation to establishing a generalized ability to imitate sentences. For the second approximation it was decided to have Luke recall Rebus sentences that he had just read.

Thus on the first day of this experiment the teacher placed a color and a noun card in front of Luke and asked him to read them. As soon as Luke read them, the teacher immediately covered the two cards with a heavy strip of white paper and asked Luke, "What does that say?" It was felt that prompts were needed to help him answer the question. First, the teacher pointed to the first covered card and at the same time said the Rebus word that was on that card. When the child repeated the word, the teacher moved his finger to the next covered card and, if necessary, prompted him. When the child had repeated both prompts, he was reinforced with approval and food. The procedure was then repeated while the teacher gradually faded the prompts. On the second day stronger prompts were used. If Luke did not give the correct name within three seconds, instead of telling him the name of the covered card as he pointed to it, the teacher lifted the paper covering the card for an instant. The teacher then immediately covered the cards again and repeated the question, "What did it say?" In the beginning the child's typical response was to say only the name of that card which he had forgotten. For example, he remembered to say the word "blue," but not the word, "ball," on the first round; then when he was tested on the second round he was likely to say the word "ball" instead of the whole phrase "blue ball." To handle this problem the teacher began to tell Luke to "Say the whole thing" and, if Luke did not respond appropriately within three seconds, to point to the card on the left. It was found that if, after these prompts, Luke was able to recall the first card he was likely to say the second card in sequence. If, however, he did not say both words in sequence, the teacher would uncover the cards completely and repeat the entire procedure, beginning with having the child read the cards. This cycling procedure was repeated until Luke could recall both cards in sequence with no prompts of any kind.

Note in Figure 8.13 that the experiment was continued with Luke recalling three-word phrases or sentences in B and four-word sentences in C and D. Note within each condition a rather smooth acquisition curve obtains. However, as Rebus units were increased from two to three to four words discontinuities appeared, the rate of recall dropped significantly only to recover in subsequent sessions to exceed previous highs.

Also during D a test was run to see if Luke's behavior was actually

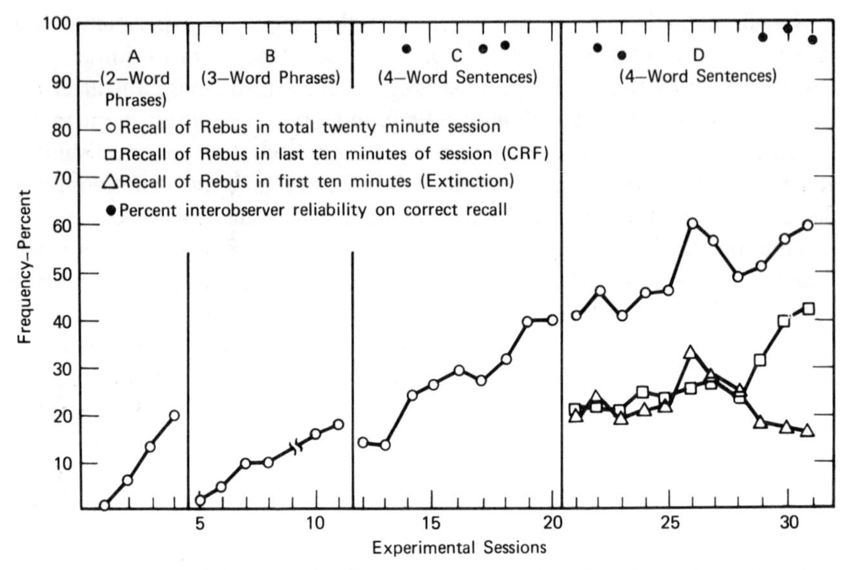

Figure 8.13. Acquisition of Rebus Units of Increasing Length under Various Conditions.

under the control of the food reinforcers. Each session was divided into two segments. In the first ten minutes, no food was given for correct recall (i.e. the child was on extinction), but in the second ten minutes his recall was, as before, reinforced with food on a continuous schedule.[4]

As can be seen from Figure 8.13 the inter-session reversals during D did not produce a contrast between the reinforcement and non reinforcement segments for about eight days. Then the contrast became quite marked. For the last few days of the experiment during the extinction segment Luke would stare at the ceiling for ten to fifteen seconds before responding, and he began to make errors at a much higher rate than he had before. With his first bite of food during the reinforcement segment, however, he began to work intently and quickly, which accounts for the increase in rate.

Spontaneous Speech—Before and After. Note in Figure 8.14, data on spontaneous speech—complete and incomplete sentences—before and after the Rebus reading and Rebus recall experiments. Before those experiments during A1 and B1, Luke did not respond to the differential reinforcement for complete sentences, afterwards during A2 and B2 he did. Also, his mother, subsequent to this series of experiments, reported that Luke was talking at a very high rate at home.

[4] The same cards were used throughout the experiment. Sentences were generated randomly so as to not bias either period, and as might be noted in Figure 8.13 inter-observer reliability was checked almost every day.

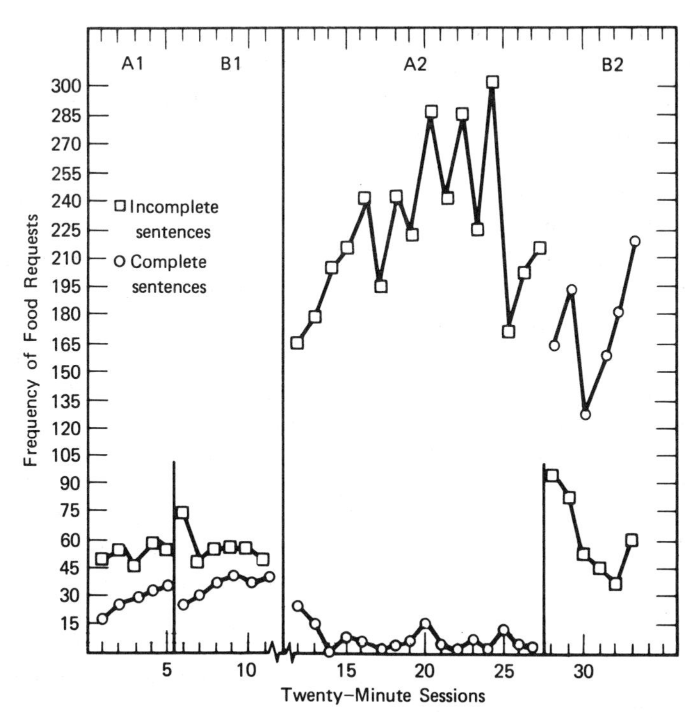

Figure 8.14. Spontaneous Use of Complete Sentences Before and After Rebus Reading and Recall Procedure.

The A1 and B1 periods occurred before the introduction of the Rebus Reading and Recall procedures. The A2 and B2 periods occurred about five months later. In the A conditions, food was given for any request for food, whether or not it was a complete sentence. In the B conditions, the child was on differential reinforcement for complete sentences; all incomplete sentences were ignored. In the A1 and B1 periods, the teacher used prompting and fading procedures to teach the child to use complete and spontaneous sentences. In the A2 and B2 periods, no prompts were used. (Interobserver reliability averaged 93 percent; intraobserver, 94 percent.)

The Remediation of Echolalia

At this juncture echolalic children are put through procedures which are described fully in the following chapter in the case study of Ross Grey. These procedures result in the painless elimination of echolalia, usually within a few weeks. Also, both the echolalic and the formerly mute children are trained to use pronouns properly. Again, the procedure is detailed in the following chapter.

STAGE SIX: THE INITIAL GROUP EXPERIENCE

The primary purpose of Stage Six is to train the children to work with other children and other teachers in a classroom. This may seem like a simple goal; but the transition from working alone with one teacher to a classroom where two or three children must work with different teachers is very frustrating to some children. An example of the way different children react is given in the following excerpt:

> Before the session began, the table had been set up with tasks for each child. When the children came into the classroom, Kristen, Lois and Peter were shown where to sit. Kristen and Lois sat down quickly and began working the puzzles they had worked and enjoyed before. Peter sat down quietly enough and began to work his puzzle, but then he was distracted by Kristen and Lois and he watched them for the next five minutes or so. Suddenly he got up from the table and started to make loud noises while running around the room. The teacher put him in the time-out room. Before he was let out, he had started to cry and had taken off his top and under shirts. As he came back into the classroom he made more noises and climbed onto the table and jumped off. Then he brought his shirts over to the teacher's chair and threw them on the floor. During this performance, the teacher was making a fuss over Kristen and Lois, giving them approval and tokens as they worked their puzzles. Then Peter came over and climbed onto the table on which Lois and Kristen were working (first very primly moving the puzzle pieces, so he would not step on them). At this point he was timed out again. When he was let out, he seemed angrier than before. He began to climb on the toy shelves, and the teacher again timed him out.
>
> Another five minutes and he was timed out again, crying loudly and unhappily. But he was still not about to sit down to work at the table. Rather, he spent the rest of the session jumping off the furniture, walking across the table on which the girls were working, etc. Toward the end he began to approach Kristen, who smiled at him occasionally, but otherwise both Kristen and Lois ignored him and continued with their work. Beginning on the second day, we decided to ignore Peter as much as possible, to avoid placing him in the time-out room.
>
> Peter approached the teacher and pulled her arm for attention; she ignored him. He frowned and fussed and continued roaming around the room. He began climbing again, first on the toy cabinet, then the tables, but was ignored. He was furious at this. He went to the far corner of the room, took off both his regular and his undershirt. Everyone ignored him. He tried to take off his pants, but the button holes were so small he could not unbutton them. This frustrated him further. He came over and looked at Kristen. She ignored him; he hit her. The teacher gave her a lot of attention, and still ignored him.

And so it went for three days, Peter storming around, hitting, taking off his clothes, etc., and during this time the teachers ignored him. Finally, about halfway through the fourth session, he stopped trying to provoke a response from the teacher. He simply came over to the table, sat down and started working his puzzle. From then on, the "class" progressed.

The second objective in this stage is to train the children to work a token exchange, using procedures that are much more direct than those described in the first chapter. (1) The teacher starts by simply handing the children a number of tokens, then points to them and says, "Give me the tokens." The children usually respond readily. The teacher reciprocates appropriately with approval and food. This step is repeated several times to establish the tokens as conditioned reinforcers. Then the teacher asks the children questions about familiar objects: "What is this, Peter?" "This is a ball." The teacher reciprocates with approval and a token; then asks Peter to give the token back as before, and reciprocates with food when the token is returned. This process is repeated with all of the children until the teacher is asking the children to name as many as ten familiar objects. When the children have accumulated their ten tokens, they are allowed to exchange them for a relatively large portion of food, perhaps as many as four swallows of juice, for example. This procedure is extended until the usual twenty minute speech-training session is increased in length to an hour.

(2) Alternatively, a token "machine" is used. This is a homemade device, a four foot by seven foot door which is hung to swing enclosing a corner in one of the classrooms. Cut in the door are two functional openings: one a slot through which tokens may be passed and the other for a paper cup dispenser which is tilted through the slot at a forty-five degree angle. When the "machine" is in operation, an assistant stands behind the door and receives tokens from the children through the token slot and in exchange passes out cups of food and drinks through the dispenser. An illustration of its use is given in the next chapter.

STAGE SEVEN: THE INTERMEDIATE CLASSROOM

Generally when children have progressed to the point where they have functional speech, can work a token exchange, and in general work productively in the initial group, they enter the intermediate class. Usually, the intermediate class has four regular members. These children could not enter the public school system, not even in a special education class because of their lack of basic classroom skills. They lack the ability to respond reliably when called on by the teacher, the ability to attend while others are responding to the teacher during the lessons, the ability to imitate others appropriately and, often, the ability to ignore others' inappropriate responses.

Therefore, the behavioral objectives in this class are to help the children acquire the basic skills and behavior which are appropriate to learning in a classroom situation. At the same time, since all of the classroom activities are mediated by the spoken word, this step is also a continuation of language training.

Procedurally, the children are given tokens for appropriate academic responses, i.e. the correct verbal answers or the correct motor responses. As in the initial group the tokens are exchanged for backup reinforcers. Generally these backups do not include food, but are mostly activities, free play, spinning or riding on a chair, music, see-saw rides, jumping on a trampoline, roughhousing with the teacher and so forth. Children, of course, are allowed to choose which of these activities they wish to buy, and most often they choose to play with the teacher or an assistant teacher. This is a big step for an autistic child, to work for the opportunity to play with another person.

To help the children develop basic classroom skills, they are reinforced with M&M's (by an assistant teacher) for attending to the teacher, particularly while the teacher is attending to another child, while another child is responding to the teacher or while another child is disrupting. An interesting phenomenon occurs at this stage: without prompting, the children often start imitating the answers given by another child or by the teacher.

Through the procedure of systematic reinforcement of spontaneous attending behavior, in a few weeks the children usually settle down to the point where they attend to the teacher almost all of the time. Without the attention from the other children or the teacher for disrupting and with M&M's for not disrupting, the children's disruptive patterns are decelerated rather quickly. Hence, the children learn very quickly to listen to the teacher while she is talking and to watch other children when they are responding to the teacher. In addition to these attending behaviors, the abilities to attend to another child's correct answer and to model that answer correctly are basic requirements for meaningful participation in a classroom.

Also, at this juncture the curricula are enlarged to include a number of motor activities: rhythm games, marching, being part of a percussion band, and imitations, e.g. Simon Says, Follow-the-Leader. Often at first the children dislike and sometimes object strenuously to participation in these activities. Because of this, extensive physical guidance is used (an assistant teacher stands behind the child, grasps the child's arms or hands and moves him through the appropriate response pattern). As the child allows himself to be guided through the appropriate motions, he is reinforced almost continuously with praise and M&M's. Generally at first the children resist such forceful guidance, but after five to ten trials the resistance tapers off and the child begins to attempt the activity by himself. Over time, many come to enjoy such motor activities enough to choose them as backup reinforcers. For example, in the beginning, Peter strenuously resisted marching, but after he acquired the ability to march through forceful guidance, it became his favorite activity. Physical guidance is another errorless learning procedure and, therefore, is extremely useful, if not indispensable in helping these children to acquire appropriate motor patterns.

STAGE EIGHT: THE GROUP LANGUAGE DEVELOPMENT PROGRAM

The Group Language Development Program was designed by Lois Blackwell as the final stage in the remediation of autism prior to the child's entrance into the public school system. By the time the children are ready to enter this program, they will have mastered the behavior skills necessary for acceptable performance in a public school classroom. They know how to respond when called upon and are willing to do so. They are now able to take turns, to share the attention of the teacher with other children, to pay attention while others are responding, to follow directions, to learn from group instruction and to discriminate between those behaviors of other children which are appropriate to imitate and those which are not. The problem henceforth is to maintain these abilities. Toward this objective, the children are intermittently reinforced with M&M's for appropriate classroom behavior. The intermittent schedule is lean, as might be indicated by the consumption of M&M's: a fifty-nine cent bag for five children every three months.

However, the main focus of the Group Language Development Program is on the remediation of the children's developmental deficits. During the years when most children are avidly curious about everything around them, spending their days in unremitting exploration, these children were tightly encased in their autistic shells, spinning and twirling their days away, often wanting little more than to be left alone in an unchanging environment with precise inviolable routines. Consequently, autistic children are plagued with developmental deficits, not only in language and concepts, but also in motor and social patterns. Consequently, this program begins with a systematic inventory of the child's development. Each child is rated on the PAR (Preschool Attainment Record, Table 8.6, and the Vineland Social Maturity Scale, both from the American Guidance Service).

These tests revealed a number of interesting deficits. For example, four of the five children in the class engaged in no imaginative play, no role playing. In addition, they did not have strong patterns of cooperative play; they did not talk with one another; they rarely talked spontaneously to adults (although they would respond to their direct questions); they had large gaps in their conceptual language. Hence, group curricula were designed to remediate these common problems, and individually tailored

Table 8.6. Developmental Sequence for Normal Children.[a]

Age in Years	0–.5	.5–1.0	1.0–1.5	1.5–2.0	2.0–2.5	2.5–3.0
Age in Months	**0–6**	**6–12**	**12–18**	**18–24**	**24–30**	**30–36**
Ambulation	Sits	Stands	Walks	Runs	Balances	Climbs
Class Recap[b]						
Manipulation	Reaches	Grasps	Marks	Unwraps	Takes Apart	Puts Together
Class Recap[b]						
Rapport	Regards	Attends	Initiates	Discrim- inates	Complies	Plays Beside
Class Recap[b]						
Communication	Babbles	Vocalize	Imitates	Invites	Speaks	Talks
Class Recap[b]						
Responsibility	Nurses	Chews	Rests	Minds	Conserves	Takes Care
Class Recap[b]						
Information	Knows Few	Knows Many	Knows Use	Knows His	Fondles	Knows Sex
Class Recap[b]						
Ideation	Resists	Identifies	Gestures	Matches	Counts 2	Compares Size
Class Recap[b]						
Creativity	Demand	Tests	Transfers	Explores	Tears	Drama- tizes Stories
Class Recap[b]						

curricula were included each day to remediate developmental deficits peculiar to each child.

The daily schedule worked out for the class is given in Table 8.7, although insofar as it is possible the activities are switched to different times from day to day. This is done to provide small surprises, to prevent boredom and the tendency to inattention, the concomitants of invariant routines.

Rebus

The aforementioned Rebus program (Woodcock and Davies, 1969) is used to help the children develop skills prerequisite to reading. Thus, the children learn through Rebus reading that a graphic symbol may represent that which is referred to by a spoken word; they learn to read groups of

Table 8.6. continued.

3.0–3.5	3.5–4.0	4.0–4.5	4.5–5.0	5.0–5.5	5.5–6.0	6.0–6.5	6.5–7.0
36–42	42–48	48–54	54–60	60–66	66–72	72–78	78–84
Jumps (Random)	**Hops**	**Circles**	**Skips**	**Jumps (Pattern)**	**Follows Leader**	**Dances**	**Rides Vehicles**
		III	卌 I	IIII	II	卌	III
Throws	**Catches**	**Draws Square**	**Blows Nose**	**Draws Triangles**	**Fastens Shoes**	**Colors in Lines**	**Cuts and Pastes**
	II	I	IIII	II	卌 I	卌 I	卌 I
Plays With	**Plays Cooperates**	**Concen-trates**	**Sings**	**Helps**	**Plays Pretend**	**Plays Competes**	**Plays Rules**
	II	I	IIII		II	卌 I	卌 I
Converses	**Relates**	**Describes**	**Recites**	**Prints**	**Copies**	**Reads**	**Adds**
	III	IIII	卌 I	卌 I	卌 I	卌 I	卌 I
Gets Drink	**Dresses Self**	**Toilets Self**	**Cleans Up**	**Respects Property**	**Conforms**	**Cooperates**	**Observes Rules**
				I	II	卌	卌
Tells Name	**Names Object**	**Knows Day-Night**	**Names Coins**	**Knows Age**	**Knows AM-PM**	**Knows Rt-Left**	**Knows Address**
			卌 I	卌	卌 I	卌	卌
Counts 3	**Compares Texture**	**Counts 4**	**Compares Weight**	**Names Colors**	**Beats Rhythm**	**Counts 13**	**Tells Hour**
I	卌	II	卌 I	II	IIII	卌	卌 I
Builds	**Draws**	**Moulds**	**Drama-tizes Music**	**Paints**	**Invents Stories**	**Solos**	**Experi-ments**
	III	II	卌	III	卌 I	卌	IIII

[a] Based on American Guidance Service, Preschool Attainment Record (Summary and Profile).
[b] The tally is shown beneath the dotted line in each box; "1" for each child who did not pass particular item. There were six children in the class.

symbols as sentences and to answer questions in workbooks based on material they read. These are programmed workbooks; the child answers yes-no questions by wetting the area underneath the yes symbol or the no symbol with a damp eraser. If he has answered correctly, the area turns green; if incorrectly, red.

Also the Rebus orthography, like traditional orthography, helps the child to learn to generalize on the basis of essential similarities and to discriminate on the basis of essential differences. For example, the symbol for house is a little square box with a rectangle representing a door and a triangle representing a roof. In the workbook this symbol must be matched

Table 8.7. Daily Schedule.

Time	Activity	Materials	Behavioral Objectives
9:00–9:10	Set ups.	Puzzles, games, Playdoh.	Keeping the children busy until everyone arrives and settles down.
9:10–9:25	Reading readiness—graphic language.	Rebus Prereading Program, Book 1.	Acquisition of all prereading skills via picture reading. The ability to work independently in a programmed workbook. Development of ability to discriminate and to generalize broadly.
9:25–9:45	Verbal language training.	Peabody Language Kit, Activity I.	Systematic acquisition of listening skills, systematic development of language in expressive, cognitive and associative areas.
9:45–10:00	Experience, e.g. making jello, choc. pudding, popping corn, etc. Taking new roles, e.g. going to dentist, to barber, to store, to farm, etc. Sensory experiences: tasting, touching, smelling, seeing new things. Field trips.	The fixings and equipment for food preparation. Dental and other types of role-playing equipment. Collapsible pegboard.	Acquisition of the ability to tolerate and ultimately enjoy new experiences.
10:00–10:05	Toilet.		
10:05–10:25	Gym, rhythm and rhymes.	Record player with rhythm record, rhythm band equipment, various kinds of gymnastic equipment, e.g. various size balls, bat, gym mats.	Acquisition of coordination, competitive and cooperative play patterns and skills, rhythm, metric language patterning.

Table 8.7. continued.

Time	Activity	Materials	Behavioral Objectives
10:25–10:35	Juices and cookies.	Cookies of various geometric shapes and colors.	Spontaneous use of syntax in a natural situation; learning conventional usage of shape and color discriminations.
10:35–10:45	Experience story, i.e. children describe new experience of the day.	Teacher prints on blackboard the story as it is told. Illustrates with pictures.	Acquisition of the ability to recall and to recount past activities.
10:45–11:05	Verbal language training.	Peabody Activity II materials.	Development of ability to translate verbal concepts into appropriate action.
11:10–11:25	Free play.	Various toys, play equipment.	Designed to test generalization of spontaneous speech and cooperative play patterns.
11:25–11:45	Individual activity; each teacher works with one or two children on the remediation of individual motor, language or conceptual deficits.	Individually tailored curricula.	Acquisition of behavior patterns and skills which are undeveloped in the one or two children being worked with.
11:45–12:00	Stories, fairy tales, nursery rhymes, sometimes read or told, sometimes recited in unison, sometimes acted out.	Books, flannel board materials, costumes and props for dramatization.	Strengthening the ability to role play, to imitate models and to translate words or ideas into action. The ability to recite in unison.

with a number of different pictures of actual houses: some colonial style, some ranch style, some big, some small, some tall and some wide. Also the Rebus symbol for cat is two circles, one on top of the other with a tail and two small triangles for ears. In the workbooks the children learn to generalize this symbol by matching it with pictures of many different species of cats, of different sizes and in different positions, etc. This aspect of the program is beneficial for these formerly autistic children, for they are quite literal minded. It teaches them to be less so in steps that are small enough that they learn to generalize essentially without error.

Verbal Language Training

To insure that no area of language (associate, cognitive and expressive) is slighted, two lessons a day are given from the Peabody Language Development Kit, Level P (American Guidance Service). This language development series was designed specifically to fill in the language gaps which often characterize ethnically disadvantaged children. In addition to being systematic and comprehensive, it remediates the children's language deficits through varied approaches to each of the different areas of language. The first lesson each day (see Table 8.7) is designed to help the children develop their listening skills and to acquire new concepts and words. One of the most effective ways is through their conversations with puppets. The second lesson each day is designed to help the children to translate words or concepts into action. This lesson, then, necessarily involves motor activities and various types of role playing.

Experience

During Experience, the children often make something, such as jello, chocolate pudding or a statue out of modeling clay. Sometimes they preview an experience that they will have outside of school, such as going to the dentist, the barber or the doctor. When the children previewed going to the dentist, the teacher had a set of dental tools at hand; she took the role of the dentist. The children, sitting in a revolving desk chair, played "Open your mouth, let the dentist put the mirror in, let the dentist pick around your teeth, etc." With a little imagination the teacher provides experiences which the children come to enjoy very much and which prepares them to meet real life situations that sometimes are problematical for children.

Experience Story

During Experience Story, the children are asked to describe what they did during that day's new experience. From these descriptions the teacher prints out a story on the blackboard with illustrations. This helps the child to acquire the ability to recall past experiences, to relate them when questioned, and it teaches them that there is another set of graphic symbols (Traditional Orthography) which corresponds to the words he speaks. The experience story, using the children's own words, is then copied on a Ditto Master by an assistant teacher and reproduced. A copy is given to the parents who are asked to spend fifteen minutes with the child at home helping him to recall and to relate what had happened during the experience period. Their copy of the experience story helps them to prompt the child, to ask about those things which the child otherwise might not think to mention. Thus the child has a new experience, he contributes and listens as the experience story is recounted by the group, and then alone at home he has the opportunity of relating the entire story himself. Thus, the experience, the experience story and the talk at home gives the child considerable practice in translating interesting experiences into understandable verbal descriptions. These, of course, are very basic skills in the use of language; they are the foundation of conversation.

Gym

The gymnastic program is also based on developmental levels. The children are put through a program that follows the usual development of ambulatory and manipulative skills. For example, the children are given practice in running, balancing, climbing, jumping, hopping, walking in circles, skipping, following the leader, dancing and riding vehicles. This is the normal developmental sequence as may be noted in Table 8.6 for ambulation. We follow the developmental sequence for two reasons. First, because those skills which develop first are apparently easier, requiring less in the way of physiological development, neural-ripening. Second, they often turn out to be components of the later, more complex patterns and skills.

It is interesting to note how the children were taught to play softball; the successive approximations were rather original. The children's manipulatory skills were so primitive that they were not able to either hit or catch a baseball or softball, so the teacher started with a large beachball. The beachball insured success as the children learned to pitch, to bat and to catch. Then, as they gained experience and developed their skills, the size of the ball was gradually decreased. At this writing they are using a plastic ball just a little smaller than a regulation volleyball. In time, they will be playing with a softball, but meanwhile they are learning to play the game, to cooperate as a team.

Free Play

This activity period is designed less for acquisition than for evaluation. The children are simply allowed to play as they wish with or without toys.

Their choices allow us to gauge their progress. Of interest, is how much of the period each child expends in parallel play versus cooperative or competitive play, how much he talks and to whom. The data in Figure 8.15 shows a through-time comparison in talking for a sample of three of the boys who represent the range of the abilities found among the six students in the Group Language Development Program. Notice that these boys talked as much, if not more, during free play when there were no external material reinforcers from the teacher than they did during the juice and cookie period and during the experience story. Hence, these data suggest that these boys had, at this juncture, finally developed their ability to talk to the point where talking was maintained by the reinforcers available in the natural social environment.

Individual Activity

During Individual Activity the children are tutored; the curricula are designed to remediate deficits that are peculiar to them. On any given dimension these autistic children will have missed some of the simpler behavior patterns and skills, but have developed other later, more complex behaviors

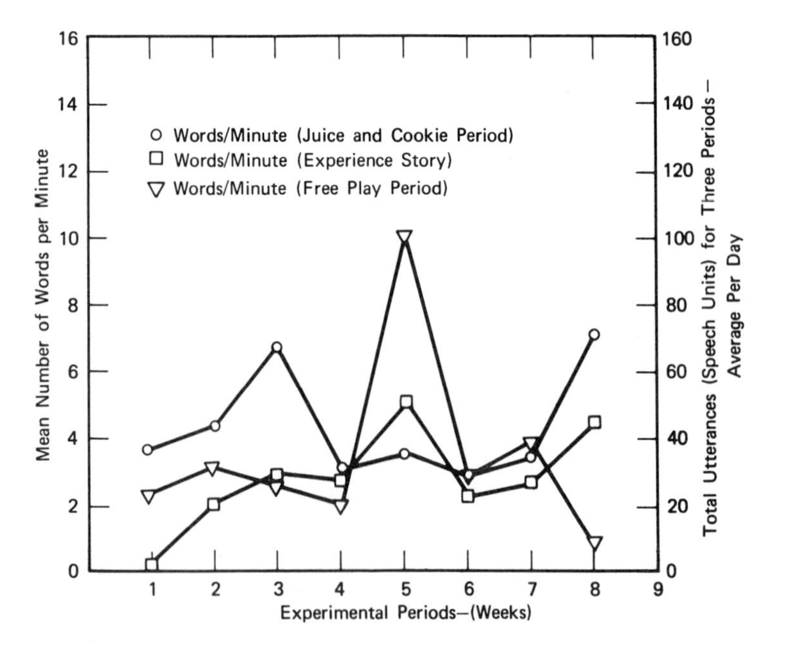

Figure 8.15. Verbal behavior of three representative boys during three periods in the Group Language and Development Program. Material reinforcers for talking were given during juice and cookie periods, M & Ms and teacher approval for talking during Experience Story, natural reinforcers from peers for talking during Free Play.

and skills. (The range of uneven development may cover three to five years.) So this time is used to remediate any of the early deficits, to strengthen behaviors and skills that have been partially developed and to bring the child up to the norm for his age. Some of the children have articulation problems; others, fine motor coordination problems; still others, problems in logical thinking. In addition, if a child is having particular difficulty with some concept that is being taught during the first language period, he will be tutored on that concept. To sum up, the individual activity period is used to remediate individual problems, to bring the individual's development up to a normal level. It allows the child to get extra help where he needs it most.

Imaginative Play and Dramatization

Imaginative role playing is taught by reading the children a nursery rhyme or fairy tale such as Miss Muffet or Goldilocks and, then, carefully outlining the steps on the flannel board. Next, one of the children is handed the flannel board illustration of the last action in the story and is asked to act it out. For example, the last picture showed Goldy running away from the three bears' house; when the child was given the picture, he was to run away from the story area. Alternatively, the child might be walked through the last step of the outlined procedure by being moved through the motions, in imitation of an adult model. In either instance, if the child resisted, he would be reinforced with M&M's as he went through the motions. Once he could reliably perform the last step in a procedure he would be taught the last two steps and so on, adding an earlier part to the later parts until all could be performed reliably. Teaching the last step first and the earlier steps later is a procedure designed to make finishing a task reinforcing. Thus the child is asked to do only that which he has a chance of finishing. Since he almost always has the rewards of finishing, he thereby learns to enjoy finishing tasks.

The main prop in imaginative play is a collapsible toy house made of masonite pegboard. It is large enough for the children to go into, and different props can be quickly and easily attached on the inside or outside, allowing the children to pretend that it is different things at different times—a house, a barn, a store, a postoffice, a barber shop. The children then take the appropriate roles; if the building is a house, they play family; a barber shop, they pretend a haircut; etc.

PRELIMINARY RESULTS

What hope can we bring the parents of autistic children? While it is still too early in our program's history to give an overall evaluation of its effectiveness, preliminary results do give some indication of what we may reasonably hope to achieve. Before/after comparisons are given in Table 8.8 for the autistic children who had been in training at least eight months. The comparisons are on four rather global variables which we feel are the best indexes of the children's progress.

All of our autistic children, except one whose data are excluded from this accounting, were nonverbal before training, that is, were without functional syntax. As noted earlier, such nonverbal autistic children have in the past been least responsive to therapy. After as long as twelve years of therapy, Bettelheim had good to fair success with 92 percent of his verbal sample, as compared with 57 percent of his nonverbal sample. On the basis of Eisenberg's (1956) follow-up study at Johns Hopkins of sixty-three autistic children given mixed kinds of therapy he concluded that nonverbal autistic children (those without functional speech) almost never get better.

Although uneasy about making comparisons at this juncture, we used an adaptation of Eisenberg's and Bettelheim's rating system to estimate the progress of our sample of seventeen nonverbal autistic children in Table 8.9. Our children whose outcomes are rated good are in public schools, in either regular or special classes, and all are functioning quite well. The ones rated fair are progressing at normal rate in speech development and usually are functioning well both in the laboratory and at home. Those whose progress is rated poor are slow in their speech development and/or are subject to behavioral relapses. Note that our results after one to three years of training are approximately equivalent to those of Bettelheim.

Be that as it may, progress in our laboratory varies dramatically with the age at which the child starts training. The malleable age seems to be 5 years or younger. As may be calculated from Table 8.10, 91 percent of the children who started training before they were six years of age have made good or fair progress, whereas only 17 percent of those who started after age six made at most fair progress. The variation in the outcome of training in the younger children seems to depend to a large extent upon the degree to which the mother becomes competent as an assistant teacher. This may be noted in Table 8.11. It is the competent mother of the older children that we feel sorry for. But then their children will probably respond eventually. At least they are making steady if slow progress.

Such problems with mothers as assistant teachers that do occur are: (1) backsliding to their old habits of attending to bizarre, disruptive behaviors, and (2) failing to work out interesting acculturating exchanges which the child can work to fill up his day. One or two of these recalcitrant mothers simply seem to be incompetent people. Another seems to enjoy her child being much less than normal, a baby she can mother, a bizarre toy she can make perform. Even so, the recalcitrants are a minority; most of the mothers are magnificent.

Table 8.8. Presence of Various Classes of Behavior in the Autistic Children in August, 1968.

Child	Age at Starting Training (years)	Duration of Training (years)	Class of Behavior: Friendliness[a]		Speech[b]		Autistic Seclusion[c]		Illicit Attention-Getting Behavior[c]	
			Before	After	Before	After	Before	After	Before	After
Mary	4	2-1/3	1	4	1	4	4	0	4	1
Jerry	4-1/2	2	1	3	1	4	4	0	3	0
Larry	4-3/4	3	2	4	1	4	4	0	4	1
Linda	5-3/4	2	2	4	2	4	3	0	3	0
Peter	7-1/2	2	1	3	1	3	4	3	4	2
Joe	6-1/2	2	1	2	1	4	4	3	3	2
Billy	3-1/4	1	1	2	0	2	4	0	3	1
John	3-1/4	1/2	3	4	0	4	3	0	4	0
Jake	5-1/2	2	1	2	0	2	4	3	3	3
Lois	4-3/4	2	1	3	0	2	4	1	4	2
Luke	6-1/3	2	1	4	0	2	4	0	3	3
Kristen	7	1	1	3	3	4	3	3	3	3
Jeff	5-1/4	1	1	4	2	4	4	1	4	1
Michael	6	1-1/2	1	2	0	2	4	3	4	2
Ross	3-1/2	1-1/2	1	3	2	4	3	0	3	1
Sean	7-1/3	1	1	2	0	1	2	2	3	3
Marty	4-1/2	1	1	3	0	1	3	1	3	2
Barbara	6-1/2	2/3	2	3	0	2	4	2	3	2

[a] 4 = outgoing; 3 = initiate and respond; 2 = reserved but approachable; 1 = unapproachable.

[b] 4 = appropriate speech most of the time; 3 = broken functional syntax; 2 = some functional words; 1 = word and sound imitation; 0 = mute or near mute.

[c] 0 = absent; 1 = present under stress; 2 = only occasionally; 3 = mixed with some positive patterns; 4 = all the time.

Table 8.9. Recovery Rates for Three Samples of Nonverbal Autistic Children.

	Sample		
Recovery	Eisenberg	Bettelheim	Cemrel
Good	0%	57%	35%
Fair	3		30
Poor	97	43	35
Total	100%	100%	100%
N	31	14	17

Table 8.10. Therapeutic Outcome for Autistic Children by Age at Which They Began Training.[a]

Therapeutic Outcome[b]	Beginning Age in Years 3	4	5	6	7
Good	2	2	2		
Fair	1	2	1	1	
Poor	1			3	2

[a] Gamma equals .69.
[b] Rating System:
Good—Has functional syntax, functions well in regular school, excellent in Laboratory School.
Fair —Functions well in lab school and home, making normal progress in speech.
Poor —Slow speech development and/or behavioral relapses in laboratory and home.

Table 8.11. Theraputic Outcomes for Autistic Children by Beginning Age of Training and Competence of the Mother as an Assistant Teacher.

	Beginning Age			
	Younger than 6[a]		Older than 6	
	Mother's Competence as Assistant Teacher			
Therapeutic Outcome	High	Not High	High	Not High
Good	5	1	0	0
Fair	3	1	0	1
Poor	0	1	3	2

[a] Gamma for the younger sample equals .63.

Finally, the third variable that seems to effect the outcome of exchange training is the disruptiveness, the destructiveness, the aggressiveness of the child before training begins. Ironically, it is the disruptive and not the placid autistic child who responds, as may be noted in Table 8.12. Why? There seems to be nothing magic about a disruptive adaptation, *per se*. It just takes considerable energy and intelligence to get away with one. It is not difficult to rechannel both energy and intelligence into a normal adaptation, but without either, progress is tortuous.

The training program outlined here is still in the process of being developed, particularly the later stages. We need better procedures for developing pronunciation, syntax, and in general, speech as a medium for learning and reasoning. We need better procedures for developing peer imitation, cooperation and play. We must work out better programs for mothers to use at home to fill up the child's day in constructive acculturation and for the teachers to use at school to prepare the child for academic work.

There are probably still a number of traps in our procedures which we have not as yet discovered. When and if they are discovered, perhaps we will be more successful with the older children.

As mentioned in the last chapter, very little is known about the onset and pre-onset conditions of autism in the home and about any biogenetic aberrations of the autistic child. These questions, while important to investigate, have not been our concern here. Rather, our investigations have focused on the structure of social conditions in the home while the child is in training in our laboratory and how these conditions relate to the maintenance and remediation of autistic behavior. It seems fair to say that whatever the onset conditions and whether or not we are dealing with a biogenetically sound organism, the behavior of the autistic child, as far as our research indicates, is controlled by the exchanges which are structured in the child's environment. To this extent, at least, autism is an acculturation

Table 8.12. Therapeutic Outcomes for Initially Disruptive vs. Initially Placid Autistic Children.[a]

Therapeutic Outcome	Initial Disruptiveness		
	High	Moderate	Low
Good	5	1	0
Fair	2	2	1
Poor	2	2	2

[a] Gamma equals .61.

disorder. The results further suggest that if this acculturation disorder is caught early enough, the child appears to respond steadily to the remedial training outlined in this and to some extent in the previous chapter. It is now rather obvious that autistic children need not grow up vegetating at home or in the back wards of mental hospitals.

CHAPTER 9

Infantile Autism: A Case Study In Remediation

BEHAVIORAL DEVELOPMENT

Ross Grey, a Caucasian male, was born in July, 1964,[1] the last of five children.[2] His father is an executive in a distribution agency for a nationally prominent manufacturer; his mother lists her occupation as housewife. Mrs. Grey has had some college education and Mr. Grey has received post high school technical training. It should be noted at the outset that pregnancy and delivery were normal. Mrs. Grey had a "natural" childbirth and so received no anesthetic during delivery. Ross was given no oxygen during the first week and was considered to be unusually healthy-looking. His only maladies during the first three months were an eye infection and constipation; during his fifth month he had a respiratory infection which was treated with antibiotics. Ross's early responsiveness to physical stimulation, bright lights, colors and sounds, also appeared to be normal.

Quite early, however, Ross's responsiveness to the people around him indicated substantial autistic aloneness. As an infant he was noticeably stiff and awkward to hold and he did not want to sit on anyone's lap. He often "looked through" others as if they were not there; he rarely met people's eyes when they were talking to him; he rarely saw things out of reach when others attempted to direct his attention to them. Mrs. Grey told us that during his first year of life Ross often had a faraway look in his eyes; he neither smiled nor laughed at others. He seemed to be different. As time passed it became apparent that he did not care to come near other people.

[1] Most of the data in this section were obtained from Rimland's Diagnostic Check List for Behavior-Disturbed Children (Form E-2) which Mrs. Grey filled out when Ross began at the laboratory, also details were filled in during interviews with Mrs. Grey.

[2] Blackwell, Kozloff and Hamblin took the major responsibility for writing this chapter.

In fact, he appeared to be happiest when left alone. He was aloof, neither sensitive to criticism nor responsive to affection. His parents described him as being "in a shell" or so "lost in thought" that he could not be reached. In addition, Ross did not imitate simple models. He was not, however, devoid of all emotion. When pleased, he jumped up and down gleefully, and while tearing out the bars of his playpen he laughed. Also certain objects and noises evoked fear.

Bizarre, Disruptive Behavior

Mrs. Grey reported that Ross sometimes held his hands in strange positions, and he frequently engaged in rhythmic, rocking behaviors for long periods of time. He definitely had odd eating preferences including preferences for certain containers that would be used for his food. Sometimes he whirled himself like a top; he liked to spin objects for long periods of time; he was fascinated by mechanical objects. In addition, he displayed some degree of perseveration of sameness. He sometimes lined things up precisely, insisting that the order not be disturbed. He adopted complicated rituals which, if not followed, made him very upset, and he became slightly upset if changes were made in the house.

Finally, Ross was very destructive. As an infant he repeatedly tore the slats out of his crib; as he grew older he almost totally destroyed his room by slamming his bed against the walls and furniture—his room looked like a battleground. Eventually, as a counter measure his parents bolted his bed to the floor. Although Ross was not aggressive toward others, he was self-destructive, slapping his head with his hands or banging his head against walls, furniture or floors. By the time he was eighteen-months old Ross tantrummed severely whenever demands were made upon him.

Speech

While Ross developed receptive language (as judged from his ability to follow instructions), he never acquired communicative speech. By the age of two, Ross had only one word "buby," and it may not have had any communicative function for him. Between the ages of two and three, Ross began to use a few words: milk, bread, eat, hot, juice, water. However, while his pronunciation was unusually good, these words were not used to communicate. He could name many objects, but he did not make requests, answer questions or talk about his experiences. His speech was echolalic, that is, he randomly echoed or parroted words and phrases of others in a muted, sing-song voice. Rather than answer a question, Ross would repeat the question he had been asked. For example, if someone said, "Do you want to eat, Ross?" he would often respond, "Do you want to eat, Ross?" In addition, Ross did not use the word "I." Like most autistic children, he communicated his wants or feelings using nonverbal gestures. He pulled or pushed his parents to get him the things he wanted; to indicate displeasure or "no" he grunted and waved his arms.

Motor Skill

Despite Ross's speech deficit, his motor skills were highly developed. He learned to walk alone between eight and twelve months with little crawling. He was unusually graceful and rarely hurt himself while climbing, walking and running. He was also exceptionally skillful in manipulating screws, nuts, bolts, etc.; in throwing and catching a ball; in jumping on the trampoline. Mrs. Grey noted that he had perfect musical pitch.

These skills aside, Mrs. Grey described Ross as a child who sat for long periods staring into space or playing repetitively with objects without apparent purpose. He was aloof, indifferent, self-contented and remote.

INITIAL DIAGNOSIS AND TREATMENT

A psychologist observed Ross at the age of two both alone and in interaction with Mrs. Grey. He diagnosed Ross as autistic and provided Mrs. Grey with several methods for teaching Ross to speak. Shortly thereafter, Ross was enrolled in a Montessori school for a short time where he worked part time on a one-to-one basis with a female teacher with whom he seemed to develop some degree of attachment. Concomitant with these two efforts to educate Ross, his labeling vocabulary began to increase in size. He was also placed on the drug Deanol, but we have no information regarding it or its effects other than that it was discontinued. Ross was then taken to New York for diagnosis by a noted child psychiatrist who confirmed the diagnosis of autism and referred the parents to a clinic in St. Louis. From the clinic Ross was referred to a hospital for a complete neurological examination and also to our laboratory for training.

Ross was examined twice at the hospital. The first doctor found Ross to be a well-built youngster showing no obvious deficits in gross or fine motor coordination. The general physical examination was negative. However, based on observations of Ross's behavior, the physician diagnosed him as retarded, particularly in the higher language and communicative spheres. For his second neurological examination, Ross was admitted to the hospital. As a result of his second extensive examination, Ross was diagnosed as having congenital encephalopathy, etiology unknown, severe language retardation, diffuse motor incoordination and autistic social behaviors. His behavior was indeed retarded, but such retardation was not found to be linked to biogenetic pathology.

A final diagnostic indicator is provided by the aforementioned Rimland

Diagnostic Check List.[3] Of the fourteen children whose parents completed the check list, Ross's score was the highest (+25). Rimland states that a score of +20 or more is considered to have a 90 percent likelihood of being "true autism."

In February, 1968 when Ross was three and a half years old, he was enrolled in our laboratory. At that time he had a large echolalic vocabulary. He was extremely aloof and indifferent to others; rather than interacting with others he spent much of his time ritualistically manipulating various objects. He routinely tantrummed to get his own way. During "story reading," a situation which we use to obtain a preliminary picture of the relationship between mother and child, Ross became distracted by objects in the room. His mother's efforts to keep his attention with the story were futile. In fact, the harder she tried by telling him to sit still or to come back to the table, the more disruptive he became, until he tantrummed. In fact, Ross ended by crying hysterically, by climbing onto the table and by hurling himself backwards to the floor. He struck the carpet so hard that his shoes flew off his feet.

EXCHANGE TRAINING

Establishing Exchange Set

Training began with Ross working an exchange where a pat on the shoulder, approval and a bite of breakfast, in that order, were given for his following instructions while putting shapes into a box and working a puzzle, tasks in which he had previously shown some interest. This procedure was used to establish an exchange set and to condition him so approval and physical contact became reinforcers for him, that is, produced pleasurable feelings for him similar to, if weaker than, those produced by food.

Inappropriate Behavior

Both extinction and time out procedures were used to teach Ross to control his inappropriate behavior. Whenever he engaged in repetitive vocalizations such as "airplane, airplane, airplane" he was ignored. In addition, he was put in the time-out room for no more than thirty seconds, whenever he left his chair or began a tantrum. While the echolalia was not markedly affected by the extinction procedure, leaving the table and

[3] Rimland Diagnostic Check List for Behavior-Disturbed Children (Form E-2). Rimland (1964) considers the infantile variety to be the only true autism. The childhood variety induced by trauma, is, according to Rimland, a form of schizophrenia. In our experience the age of onset of the autistic symptoms is not predictive of the outcome of remedial schooling.

tantrumming were eliminated within a week. Consequently, Ross's attention to his tasks soon stabilized at a high level.

As soon as Ross developed an exchange set, that is, understood that he could earn his breakfast by working any exchanges the teacher signaled via her instructions, the training moved on to the second stage.

Eye Contact

Ross almost completely avoided the gaze of others. When asked to look at the teacher, he would repeat some irrelevant phrase like "Turn on the lights, turn on the lights," in his sing-song, odd-toned voice, but he would not look at the teacher. Consequently, a food-eye-contact exchange was structured. Great care was taken to pop a bite of food into Ross's mouth at the moment his glance, however fleeting, met hers. The food was accompanied by a "Good boy for looking at me, Ross," a hug or some other form of caress. After several days of reinforcing spontaneous eye contact, the teacher attempted to bring it under the control of a verbal stimulus, that is, getting him to look at her when she said, "Look at me, Ross." However, Ross did not respond appropriately; he merely echoed the instruction without looking at the teacher. Consequently, the teacher returned to the exchange for spontaneous eye contact. When his spontaneous eye contact reached its previous level, the teacher escalated the terms so that Ross was required to hold her gaze for fifteen seconds, then thirty seconds, before he was given a bite of food.

At this point, then, the teacher again tried the verbal instruction, but made food reinforcement contingent on just a fleeting look. The strategy of increasing and decreasing the terms of the two exchanges apparently worked; Ross started following instructions. At first Ross was reinforced for even a glance if it occurred within five seconds after instruction, but gradually he was required to look at the teacher for longer and longer periods before he received his food. This phase of Ross's training lasted five weeks; by then his spontaneous eye contact and his willingness to hold another's gaze approached normal. Also he willingly and reliably complied when the teacher asked him to look at her.

At this juncture, a procedure was introduced to teach Ross our cultural convention of using eye contact as the first step in initiating exchanges with others. Earlier Ross had evidenced considerable pleasure in working puzzles. So the teacher returned to puzzle working, but this time gave him pieces, one at a time, for spontaneous eye contact. At the same time, the schedules of food and other reinforcement were made increasingly variable. Sometimes food was given for attending the task, sometimes for meeting the teacher's gaze, sometimes for correctly placing a puzzle piece. Also, special approval ("That's the way, Ross!") and an affectionate pat were given on a variable schedule, sometimes in conjunction with and sometimes independent of food. During this period when a number of reinforcers were being used on variable schedules, Ross worked the exchanges at a rapid rate, taking it all in stride. He was seldom distracted from the task at hand for what were now thirty-minute sessions, and he never threw a tantrum.

Tokens and the Token Machine

At the next stage of training Ross and his teacher joined two other children and their teachers; all worked together. This was a minor change which the children took in stride. The token "machine" mentioned in the previous chapter was then used to establish tokens as a conditioned reinforcer. First, Robbie was seated in front of the token machine and given tokens to put in the slot. As soon as the token went through the slot, a paper cup of food came down the chute and in it was a bite or two of Robbie's lunch. Ross and John watched this procedure with great interest. In fact, their attention riveted on Robbie. Ross wanted to get up and put tokens in the machine, so his teacher instructed him to ask to do it. "Ross, say, 'I want to work the token machine.' " Ross replied, "I want to work the token machine." Then he received an enthusiastic, "Good boy!" and some tokens to use in the machine. As his cup of food came shuttling down, Ross, bright-eyed, exclaimed, "Tokens go in, food comes down—tokens go in, cup comes down." Ross repeated this over and over, as though it was the greatest discovery ever.

It should be noted that Ross did not have to be shown how to operate the machine. He had watched Robbie carefully and imitated him. As stated earlier, Ross did not use imitation of models as a learning device. So his modeling of Robbie's working the token machine was a great breakthrough!

At first cups of food were delivered each time a token was placed in the machine. Then to strengthen the pattern and to turn the situation into a game, reinforcement was changed to a variable schedule. Sometimes food would be delivered for one token, and sometimes it would take two or even three before the food cup would rattle down the chute. Also, the "machine" at times held a sponge over the slot so a token could not go in. At first when this happened, the children looked quite indignant. Their teacher then said, "Too bad, I guess you need some more tokens," and *quickly* helped them to earn another token. Then one of the boys put two tokens in and the food cup immediately came down the chute. Eventually when a child attempted to put a token in the machine and it wouldn't go, he would hurry back to his teacher and look directly at her thus signaling his desire to engage in another exchange and earn another token.

During this stage, in addition to the use of the token machine, part of each session was devoted to Ross's speech training. Using pictures cut from magazines and mounted on construction paper, the teacher would ask Ross the names of the objects in the pictures and ask questions about the use of the objects. At the outset Ross's echolalia was very pronounced, illustrated by the following:

TEACHER: What do we do with food, Ross?
ROSS: (No response.)
TEACHER: What do we do with food, Ross? We eat it.
ROSS: What do we do with food, Ross? We eat it.

By emphasizing the answer to the question, by gradually decreasing the volume of the question and by differentially rewarding Ross for repeating the *answer* only, Ross's rate of echolalic responses decreased fifty percent in a month. Also his conversation about the pictures improved as illustrated:

TEACHER: What is this, Ross?
ROSS: It's an airplane.
TEACHER: What do we do with an airplane? *We fly it.*
ROSS: We fly it.
TEACHER: What is this, Ross? *A bed.*
ROSS: What is this, Ross? A bed.
Teacher ignores incorrect echolalic response.
TEACHER: What do we do with a bed? *We sleep in it.*
ROSS: We sleep in it.

The Elimination of Echolalia

We tried another procedure which produced a breakthrough—Ross consciously began to try *not* to echo. That is, he learned to attend to his own responses to see that they were acceptable to the teachers. For a twenty-minute period each day Ross was taken out of the classroom, to a smaller room with both teachers. There his echolalia was treated as if it were functional speech. The following excerpt from a typescript of a session illustrates the procedure:

> Kozloff: "Do you want a cup (of food)?" Ross: "Do you want a cup?" Blackwell: "Yes, I want a cup," and Kozloff gives her the cup Ross was reaching for. She eats the food. Kozloff: "Do you want a pin?" Ross: "Do you want a pin?" Blackwell: "Yes, I want a pin," and she takes it as Ross reaches for it. Blackwell: "Do you want a cup, Ross?" Ross says, "Yes, I want a cup." Blackwell gives it to him and says, "Good boy, Ross." Blackwell, "Do you want a cup?" Ross: "Do you want a cup?" Kozloff: "Yes, I want a cup." Blackwell looks at Kozloff: "Good boy," and hands Kozloff the cup containing a potato chip which Kozloff eats *noisily.*

Blackwell looking at Ross: "Do you want a whistle?" Ross does not respond. Kozloff: "Yes, I want a whistle." Blackwell: "Good asking, Marty," and she gives Kozloff a whistle which he blows. Blackwell: "Do you want a pen?" Kozloff: "Yes, I want a pen." Blackwell gives him a cup with a pen and with a potato chip which he eats. Blackwell: "Do you want a pen, Ross?" Ross: "Do you want a pen?" Kozloff looks at Ross: "Yes, I want a pen." Blackwell gives the pen to Kozloff with a cup and a potato chip. Blackwell and Kozloff ignore Ross and go through this routine several times.

Ross now walks around the room. He plays with a lid. Blackwell to Ross: "Do you want a cracker?" Ross: "Do you want a cracker?" Blackwell: "Yes, I want a cracker," and she eats it. Blackwell: "Do you want a cracker?" Ross repeats, "Do you want a cracker?" Blackwell: "Yes, I want a cracker. Do you want a cracker?" Ross says: "Yes, I want a cracker." She gives him a cracker, a "Good boy," and a hug. Blackwell: "Do you want a cracker?" Ross echoes. Blackwell: "Yes, I want a cracker," and she eats it. Ross says, "Yes, I want a cracker." (But Blackwell has already eaten the cracker.) Blackwell: "Do you want a cracker?" She waits for him to say it after she questioned him again. But Ross walks away smiling to himself.

Blackwell to Kozloff: "Point to the fish." Kozloff: "All right," and he points to the fish. Blackwell gives him a potato chip and he eats it. Ross is sitting on the floor leaning against Kozloff. Blackwell: "Do you want a potato chip?" Ross: "Do you want a potato chip?" Blackwell: "Thank you," and she eats another one. Blackwell: "Do you want a potato chip?" Ross: "Yes," and he eats it. Kozloff: "Do you want a Cheez-it?" Blackwell: "Yes, I want a Cheez-it." Kozloff gives her one and she eats it.

Kozloff: "Lois, do you want the tape?" (Ross has been eyeing the scotch tape and has reached for it a couple of times during the session.) "No." Blackwell: "Do you want the tape?" Ross: "Yes, I want the tape." Blackwell gives it to him. Ross tears some off, spins the wheel around a few times and sticks the tape on the windowsill.

Ross gets up on the table, and then gets down again. Ross: "Do you want to get up?" Blackwell: "Yes, I want to get up," and she stands up. Blackwell: "Do you want to get up, Ross?" Ross: "Yes, I want to get up." So Blackwell lifts Ross up and he looks out the window.

Blackwell: "See the cars." Ross: "See the bump." (He refers to speed bumps painted orange on the street outside the window.) Blackwell: "Yes, I see the bump. Do you see the bump?" Ross: "Do you see the bump?" Blackwell: "I see a bump." Ross: "I see a bump." Blackwell: "Do you want a potato chip?" Kozloff: "Yes," and he eats another chip. Ross is up at the table scooting around backwards. Blackwell: "Do you want a Cheez-it?" Kozloff: "Yes." Ross: "I want to go home." Blackwell: "Oh, do you want to go home, Ross? Say, 'Yes.' " Ross: "Do you want to go?" Blackwell: "No, do you want to go home, Ross?" Ross: "Yes," and he gets down from the table. He went home.

This excerpt shows the tedious repetition required to teach Ross to use his language functionally. For every time that Ross spoke functionally he was reinforced, with food or something else he himself had chosen. Ross attended closely to the interchanges between Kozloff and Blackwell in which sometimes one and then the other initiated and reciprocated. As a result of several weeks of such training, Ross's echolalia gradually decreased and with it the use of the sing-song voice. Both extinguished simultaneously. By February, 1969, the only time Ross echoed was when he was bored with the task he was asked to do or when he was exceptionally tired. In fact, he began having difficulty echoing straight even when he did lapse. For example, one day during a session in February:

TEACHER: What is *your* name?
ROSS: What is *my* name?
TEACHER: Your name is Ross Grey.
And she continued the session without comment or restructuring.

Ross and John

In September, 1968 Ross and John worked together with one teacher.[4] These two children were good models for one another. Ross's speech was

[4] John was within a week of being the same age as Ross and had been diagnosed prior to coming to our laboratory as probably retarded. Although John exhibited some withdrawal behavior—he could not speak up and he refused to answer direct questions—he otherwise appeared to be a normal child. About the time he came to our laboratory John's parents discovered that his vision was extremely poor and had him fitted with glasses. Apparently, for the first time objects farther away than his elbow took on distinct shapes. Instead of seeing moving blurs which took shape only when they loomed directly in front of him, he could now perceive the visual world with clarity. With such little vision, even the brightest of children might be expected to have trouble learning at a normal rate.

loud and clear. On the other hand, John's was low, indistinct, and he did not imitate what was said to him. Ross was more advanced than John in certain areas, as in identifying and naming colors and numbers, while John was more advanced in same-different concepts, in listening to and responding appropriately to what was said.

Each child was reinforced for appropriate behavior the other child evidenced trouble with. When Ross spoke clearly and distinctly, he would be reinforced with a "Good boy for talking so loudly, Ross," and perhaps a pat and an M&M. If John would then speak up audibly, he was similarly reinforced. On the other hand, John would be reinforced for an immediate response to the teacher. If Ross would then attempt an immediate response, he would similarly be reinforced. Also, if one boy answered a question incorrectly, the same question was asked the other. If the other responded correctly, he was reinforced. Then the first boy was asked again, and reinforced if he responded correctly. These procedures facilitated each child's learning many concepts and both developed a general imitative pattern.

"Story time" was effective for John; he began to speak frequently and loudly. Occasionally he anticipated and filled in the proper word in the story, and Ross imitated this behavior. John, in turn, imitated some of Ross's echolalia which was good for him because he had not had the practice in plain articulation that Ross had had. Thus, both boys benefited from working together.

Interestingly enough, the opportunity to respond in itself became reinforcing to both children, as they learned to take turns. The imitation procedure also accelerated the attending behavior of both children to the task at hand, to the teacher and to the other child when he was responding. The exchange structure as outlined above was in effect for about eight months; it was successful in building up functional speech and socially acceptable behavior in both children.

At home Ross began to structure language exchanges with his mother as they were structured with him in the laboratory. If he wanted to know the name of something, he would point to it, or look at it and say, "That's a ______?" He would then wait for his mother to fill in the blank. This was a direct imitation of the picture and object naming procedure used with him at the laboratory. Ross began initiating exchanges with his mother and then in a loud voice giving her the language to use in reply—another example of direct imitation.

ROSS: "Where is Sue?" Then in a loud prompting voice: "She's in her room." Then, "Where is Sue?"

MOTHER: "She's in her room."

His mother was amused at this, and she enjoyed playing along with him for he was talking functionally, correctly.

Use of Pronouns

During October, 1968, Ross learned to use correctly the pronouns I, me, you, your, mine, etc. He would often hesitate when he came to a place in speech where a pronoun would logically be used and appear to be thinking about it. Blackwell structured the exchanges as follows:

TEACHER: "Who does this belong to?"
ROSS: "That is Ross's."
TEACHER: "Yes. Say 'That is mine, Ross's,' or 'That belongs to me, Ross.' "
ROSS: "That belongs to me, Ross."
TEACHER: "Who does this belong to?"
ROSS: "That belongs to me, R. . . "

The teacher would pop the M&M into Ross's mouth before he had a chance to add "Ross." Or she wold interrupt him with, "That's right! Good Ross!"

Then Blackwell began to require Ross to use sentences in reply to questions she would ask him:

TEACHER: "Shall I do it, Ross?"
ROSS: "Ross will do it."
TEACHER: "Say I, Ross, will do it."
ROSS: "I, Ross, will do it."
TEACHER: "That's the way, Ross! Good thinking!"

Or again:

TEACHER: "I, Lois, will give this to you, Ross. What will you, Ross, do with it?"
ROSS: "Ross will put the piece in the puzzle."
TEACHER: "No. *I, Ross,* will put the piece in the puzzle."
ROSS: "I, Ross, will put the piece in the puzzle."
TEACHER: Gives him the puzzle piece. "Good talking, Ross." And gives him a hug.

The purpose of this awkward sentence structuring was to make all concepts in the use of pronouns and their associations explicit and still be communicative. Once Ross had mastered the association between his and others' names and the appropriate pronouns, the teacher faded out the names from the prompts and Ross spontaneously dropped a good many of them. It took Ross about two weeks to establish this firmly. At first he would pause and think about what he was going to say, but with practice, his use of pronouns became more and more facile, spontaneous.

At this point, Ross began to be creative, to say things that he had not been coached to say. Unless one had watched Ross's progress carefully, this might have slipped by unnoticed. For example, one day in October, 1968, the following occurred:

TEACHER: "Thank you, Ross."
ROSS: "You're welcome, Lois."

A small occurrence, but Ross had never been coached to respond that way.

At this point Ross also began to listen to stories and to vocalize his thought associations. One story was illustrated by a picture of a birthday cake. He pointed to it and said, "In the dining room." The teacher asked him if his family had birthday parties in the dining room. Ross replied, "Yes, Michael's birthday was in the dining room." In another story was a picture of a house with a front door. He turned the page and when the house on the back of the first page had no back door, he kept repeating, "Back door, back door," and turning the page back and forth. "Where is the back door?" Finally, the teacher told him that probably the kitchen or back door was on the side of the house and there was no picture in the book of the side of the house where the kitchen door was. The next day, Ross told the teacher that there was a front door on the house in the book, but no back door.

Changes in Routine

At home Ross began to tolerate and then delight in changes in his routine. For instance, he began to enjoy spending the night with his aunt and uncle, and he began to want to go with his father to the store. As long as someone explained to Ross so he knew what to expect, new ventures were not disagreeable to him. Here is an example of how he became prepared for new experiences:

> Ross had not been to a barbershop before he entered our school. In fact, he had never had a regulation haircut even at home. The usual procedure for a haircut involved a patient uncle chasing him, and two or three people holding him down while his uncle cut chunks of hair until he was somewhat trimmed. Unless his uncle, who was the only one who would try to cut his hair, had two or three hours' time to do it, Ross's hair just was not cut. And, of course, the crucial issue was that Ross's extreme behavior made it a very painful experience for everyone involved.
>
> During the winter of 1968 the conversations with the teacher centered around a set of pictures taken from the Peabody Language Development Kit which depicted various occupations: a nurse giving a shot, a carpenter building a house, a barber giving a haircut, etc. Ross was quite interested in the picture of the barber using his clippers. There

followed a detailed discussion about going to the barber—climbing in the seat, the hydraulic properties of barber chairs, having a towel put around one's neck, feeling the clippers, hearing the loud noise the clippers make in one's ears, sitting very still and so on. One day the teacher asked Ross if he went to the barbershop. Ross replied that he did. The teacher asked him who took him and Ross didn't answer. The teacher knew he had never been to a barbershop, but she wanted to see what he would say if he were prompted. So she asked, "Does your Daddy take you to the barbershop?" Ross replied, "Yes, my daddy takes me to the barbershop."

Ross's father happened to be watching that day from behind the one-way mirror. So he decided to "risk" (his own word) taking Ross to the barber. To his father's surprise and relief, Ross climbed up into the chair, let the barber put the towel around his neck and proceed to cut his hair. Ross did not tantrum. In fact, he seemed quite pleased with himself.

Training Lucy

During the fall of 1968 Blackwell made several trips to Ross's home to train the housekeeper to be an assistant teacher. Blackwell began by discussing the principles of exchange training with her, and then by discussing and demonstrating just how to go about implementing these principles. The biggest obstacle encountered was Lucy's fear of losing Ross's love if she were to discipline him. Lucy loved Ross very much and was fiercely defensive of him if someone did not respond to him positively. Alienating Ross constituted a great threat to her. However, once Lucy was convinced that a given procedure was best for Ross, she was willing to go through with it, even to chance losing his affection.

Of interest is that after the first stage of training Lucy told Blackwell that she now felt she was responsible in part for Ross's having had such severe and frequent tantrums. Her analysis showed great insight and, hence, is worth mentioning. Lucy was aware that people commented on Ross's abnormal behavior and that they tried to persuade Ross's mother to place him in an institution for the good of the others in the family. They reasoned that nothing could be done for an autistic child, especially one who had such violent tantrums. As a result Lucy would go to any lengths to placate Ross so he would not tantrum or behave destructively while outsiders were in the house (which was often). Volunteering this information she said she knew now that it made him worse. She intended to do "just exactly" what the teacher told her to do regardless of what people would say if it would help Ross.

The behaviors which were worked on were Ross's nap-taking, his rough treatment of the family dogs, his disruptions at breakfast time and his aggressions toward Lucy.

The nap. When Blackwell set up the procedure for nap-taking, she brought some packages of gum with her and gave one to Sue, Ross's sister. When Ross asked for gum, Blackwell told him: "After your nap you may have some gum, Ross. First, Lucy will fix your lunch. Next you can eat your lunch. Then it is time to take your nap. As soon as you get up from your nap, Lucy will give you the gum." Blackwell repeated this sequence of events several times. Lucy was instructed to repeat the sequence if Ross tried to manipulate her about the nap-time, as he usually did. In addition, Lucy was told to deliver the reinforcement (in this case, gum) immediately upon completion of the task (in this case, taking his nap). No further contingencies were to be placed on him before the reinforcers were given him. Ross was not to be asked to put on his shoes, his pants or anything else before he received the gum on waking up from his nap. If Lucy wanted him to dress before receiving the gum, then that step was to be added to the sequence *beforehand*.

The first time the procedure was tried, Blackwell spent the entire afternoon at Ross's home. Ross tested the system thoroughly, but finally went to sleep about four o'clock in the afternoon. After two or three hours, it was a temptation to allow him to come down without napping because napping so late in the afternoon probably meant a late bedtime. Blackwell suggested that if that happened, Ross was to be awakened early the next morning in order to facilitate that day's nap-taking. However, one afternoon session was all it took; nap-time became a fairly smooth process after that. In the beginning special food reinforcers (such as gum, candy or ice-cream—whatever Ross rarely had and really enjoyed) were used to reinforce nap-taking behavior. These food reinforcers were gradually replaced with privileges; going swimming after his nap, going to the store, etc. After two or three weeks, nap-time became routine and did not always have to be followed by reinforcement.

Rough treatment of the dogs. Ross was very rough with the family's two young dogs. Both had very gentle dispositions and would not snap at Ross to protect themselves, but the problem could not be ignored because Ross was hurting them. So the following procedure was worked out. First, the parents were to praise Ross when they saw him handling the dogs gently. When they saw him handling the dogs too roughly, they were to tell him to stop, that he was being too rough and that he must be gentle with the dogs. As soon as the parents felt that Ross was beginning to understand the meaning of "rough" and "gentle," if he became too rough, they were to terminate his playing privileges. If they were playing in the house the dogs were to be put outside and Ross was to remain inside. If they were playing outside, then Ross was to go into the house and the dogs were to remain outside. He was to be told, "Little boys who play too rough with dogs and hurt them can't play with them."

Within two weeks Ross had stopped playing roughly and hurting the dogs. While Ross's behavior appeared to be just plain meanness, it should be noted that he did not understand the concepts "rough" and "gentle." Terminating his play with the dogs when he was handling them too roughly enabled him to discriminate rough handling from gentle handling of dogs.

Disrupting breakfast. Ross seemed to consider Lucy his own private person and did not like her to be involved with others when he was around. This was especially disturbing in the morning when Lucy prepared breakfast for the other children. Ross would come downstairs, whine and tug at Lucy to help him dress. This annoyed Lucy and occasionally she would stop preparing breakfast and take Ross upstairs to dress him. At other times, he would hit her and in general be so obnoxious that she could not continue working. The following procedures were worked out.

When Ross wanted Lucy to come upstairs to dress him, she was to tell him that first she would fix breakfast for the school kids, next she would dress Ross, and then he could have his breakfast. Or he could go upstairs and put on his clothes himself, then she would fix his breakfast. No deviation from these structured exchanges was to be allowed, regardless of Ross's behavior. If Ross tantrummed he was to be put in the lighted time-out closet for a minute. (He did not trantrum, however.)

After three days of this consistent treatment, Ross went upstairs, put his clothes on, came down and said to Lucy, "Fix my breakfast, please, Lucy."

Hitting Lucy. Frequently when Lucy did not comply with Ross's demands, he hit her. To extinguish this hitting behavior the following procedure was used. Lucy was to simulate the way she would ordinarily attend to Ross when she was talking with someone. She and Blackwell sat at a table near the lighted time-out closet and more or less ignored Ross. When Ross spoke to her, she answered him but her attention was focused on her conversation with Blackwell. After several minutes, Ross began to pull at Lucy. She responded to him briefly but continued talking with Blackwell. Finally, Ross hit her. Lucy (following instructions) held Ross by one arm and matter of factly stated, "We don't hit Lucy, Ross." Before Ross knew what had happened he was in the time-out closet. "I won't hit Lucy any more. Let me out! I won't do it any more, Lucy." After about forty-five seconds Lucy let Ross out. After Lucy saw that this encounter had not made Ross dislike her, she was much more confident and began to use the time-out closet appropriately when Blackwell was not present. During the next two days Lucy timed Ross out four times; that was all that was necessary (until the week when the family was on vacation).

Progress by Spring, 1969

Ross and John were taught to read the words and pictures on lotto cards, to follow dots, to differentiate between "yes" and "no" in relation to questions asked by the teacher. For example:

Teacher: "What do we buy in a toy store?" (No response.) "Do we buy bananas in a toy store?" "No." "Do we buy shoes in a toy store?" "No." "What do we buy in a toy store?" *"We buy toys in a toy store."* "Do we buy toys in a toy store?" *"Yes, we buy toys in a toy store."* Much of the time the conversation centered on a toy farm, a toy circus, and a toy playhouse, all populated with toy animals and people. These were good props because they intrigued the children and at the same time related to their own life experiences. Thus the boys were encouraged to speculate on the activities of the people and animals. For example, when Ross put a cow up on top of the barn, the teacher laughed and said, "Silly boy, cows don't walk on barn roofs. Cows walk in the barnyard." And all three would laugh and Ross would usually put the cow in the barnyard. Later when Ross put the cow in the barnyard, commenting that cows walk in the barnyard, not on roofs, he was reinforced. "That's right, Ross, you know where the cows go!"

All evidences of appropriate thinking, or at least all evidence that Blackwell recognized, were heavily and immediately reinforced with whatever seemed most valuable to the child at the time. During these spring months Ross made remarkable improvement. Not only was his echolalia all but eliminated, but he learned to carry on conversations—asking and answering questions, asking for things, describing past and present situations, speaking of anticipated events, etc.

Language Gaps

Despite Ross's rapid language development, his excellent articulation and his more than adequate conversation, it became apparent to Blackwell that there were substantial, although not obvious, gaps in Ross's grasp of expressive language. Ross would often engage in some activity such as rubbing his hands on a wall, pushing a chair on the floor or pounding a spoon on the table. He repeated simultaneously, "What am I doing? What am I doing?" At first his questions were passed off with, "You know what you are doing, Ross," or something similar. Then one day in class Ross began to pull a chart on the wall up and down. He kept saying, "What am I doing, Lois? What am I doing?" At first, she ignored him; then she realized that Ross was trying to ask the question, "What is the name of the action

I am engaging in?" He wanted to know the language that described his actions. She responded, "You are pulling the chart up and down, Ross, and it's going to fall down!" (At this point it did fall down.) Ross said, "I was pulling on the chart and it fell down."

His parents were instructed to treat as functional all questions that Ross asked, to answer them as fully as possible, to keep in mind that he was not skilled at asking for information. This was a large order, not nearly so simple as it sounds here because Ross's conversation and his expressive language had reached a stage where even those people who knew him well did not recognize that he had difficulty expressing himself. Blackwell was aware that as an autistic child, Ross had not attended to language at the age when certain concepts would normally have been assimilated, and her insightfulness in this instance made it possible to turn apparent meaningless behavior into important learning situations.

The following is an example of another kind of language gap. The session was over and Ross was absorbed in playing. His mother came in to chat with Blackwell for a few minutes. Finally, Blackwell said to Ross, "Do you want to put your coat on, Ross? It's time to go home." Ross did not move from the table, but instead he remained seated and seemed to be consciously screwing up his face to cry. He lifted first one foot and then the other and began to make sounds like crying. It was quite obvious that he did not want to have a tantrum, but that he was extremely frustrated. It was a breakthrough for Blackwell for suddenly she recognized he did not know how to formulate an answer to the question. She quickly intervened, "Ross, if you don't want to put your coat on now, say 'No, I don't want to put my coat on now, Lois.'" Blackwell then posed the question again to Ross, "Do you want to put your coat on now, Ross? It's time to go home." This time Ross replied, "No, I don't want to put my coat on, Lois." Teacher: "All right, Ross, you may play a little longer. Do you want to play a little longer before you go home?" Ross: "Yes." Ross was then allowed to play five minutes longer. Then Blackwell said, "It's time to go home now, Ross. Put on your coat." Ross jumped up from the table, put his coat on and went home quite happily.

After this incident, Blackwell became aware of other times when Ross should have said no, but did not. For example, she asked Ross if he would like to play with crayons. Ross would say yes, but then he would not appear at all interested in the crayons when they were brought out. At the time, Blackwell attributed this to a deficit in Ross's attention span. Later it became clear that he simply did not know *how* to tell her he would rather play with something else.

At the age when a normally developing child usually learns the meaning of "no" and how to say "no," Ross had been autistic and therefore did not acquire this language form. In training, most conversations had been structured so as to elicit "yes" responses. Consequently Ross had no trouble replying affirmatively but simply did not know how to reply negatively. He had to be taught.

One day Blackwell was at Ross's home helping him spell out names with wooden letters. Ross spelled out his own name, and then she spelled out the names of Ross's three brothers and one sister. The teacher asked Ross to show her Ted's name and Ross did. Then she asked for Steve's name, and Ross spelled it out. Then Blackwell asked Ross to give her his sister's name and Ross looked puzzled. Since the answer did not require a verbal response, she suspected that Ross did not know the word, "sister." So she asked Ross to give her Sue's name, and Ross spelled it out correctly at once. Blackwell then explained to Ross that Sue was his sister and that his sister's name was Sue. She also told him that he had three brothers and their names were Steve, Ted, and (she left the blank for Ross to fill in) ________. Ross filled in the last name, Chris. She and Ross then talked about his family, that he had one sister and three brothers and his sister's name was ________. Again, Ross filled in the blank.

During a classroom session in July, 1969, Ross and Mary were sitting next to the same table. They pulled their chairs up to the table at the same time and Ross's fingers were severely pinched between the chairs. He cried very hard and when the teacher asked what had happened, Ross sobbed, "Mary socked me!" No one had observed exactly what had happened, but Mary's behavior did not indicate that she was aware that she had done anything wrong. Mary looked at the teacher and Ross as if to ask, "What happened?" Since Ross's explanation and Mary's behavior were incongruous, Blackwell decided to have the children reconstruct the events. After the reconstruction it became evident what had happened, and Blackwell then explained to Ross that Mary had not socked him. She showed him how his fingers had been pinched between the chairs when he and Mary were pulling their chairs up to the table. The teacher then had Ross tell her that his fingers got pinched when he and Mary pulled their chairs up to the table together.

When Ross played with his brothers he had evidently learned to associate the word "socked" with the feeling of pain. Thus, since Mary was close to him when he was hurt, he concluded she must have socked him. Two weeks later when the children were putting their chairs in a semicircle the incident repeated itself—unfortunately again with Mary's chair. This time, when asked what happened, Ross said, "My fingers got pinched by the chairs." He did not associate the pinching of the fingers with Mary because when he went back in the room, he sat down beside her again. Later, he told his mother that he pinched his fingers at school and that he "cried up" on Lois.

Literally, that is exactly what happened. Blackwell had held him up to her shoulder to comfort him and he had cried on her shoulder.

Vacation with Family, Summer, 1969

It was decided that Ross would go with the family to a Colorado ranch for a vacation for one week and then would fly back with his older brother while the family vacationed for another week. At the ranch Ross enthusiastically participated in everything the family did. While he rode a horse that someone led around the corral, he exclaimed, "Look at me, I'm up on a horse." He also insisted upon taking his nap every day in "the bus (the family camper) that looks like a house. . ." The parents were careful to explain to Ross in great detail what he might expect during his plane flight home with his older brother. Ross apparently enjoyed the trip; he behaved like a veteran traveler.

During the week that Ross was home alone with Lucy (his brother flew back to Colorado), he was under stimulus conditions similar to those in which he had engaged in a great deal of bizarre, disruptive behavior. With his mother, the agent of control, absent Ross reverted to his earlier patterns doing things he had not done for nearly a year. He smeared his food, he refused to take his nap and he had two lovely kicking, screaming tantrums. When Ross's aunt picked him up at school (where his behavior was still exemplary), she informed Blackwell that he had "regressed."

That same afternoon at Ross's home Blackwell had an extended conversation with Lucy. Lucy felt the tantrums and the other bizarre behaviors were designed to test her out rather than a regression to genuine autism. Lucy had been lax in following the prescribed procedures when the family was gone, because she feared that her actions would be misrepresented to Ross's mother by his relatives. It seems they did not approve of his being put in a lighted closet for thirty seconds. However, when Blackwell told Lucy to start following procedures again, she felt the support she needed and she did so quite precisely, with the expected results.

Lucy was instructed to use the lighted time-out closet, as she had done previously and to call to report the results whenever she used it. It was less than an hour after Blackwell left when Lucy called. Ross had hit her, and she had put him in the time-out room. Shortly after that he started on a tantrum, but before he had kicked his legs twice, Lucy put him in the time-out room again. That was the end of his "regression!"

Prognosis

We have now seen in some detail the transformation of Ross Grey from a child who was severely autistic, almost ready for the back ward of a mental hospital, into a child who is essentially normal. So far, his is a remarkable story, but what about his future? Will he continue to progress, or is he destined to regress?

It is possible, perhaps, that the result of Ross's eighteen-months' training could be undone if through some unexpected catastrophy he fell under the care of some incredibly stupid person who happened to do all the wrong things. He, like any other person, is highly dependent upon his social environment and therefore could be shaped into behaving badly, as could anyone. However, his mother and their housekeeper have been trained rather well and at this point are quite competent in providing Ross with a very favorable learning environment. Not that Ross will not have problems. He will; everyone does and will as long as they live. It's just that those who care for him will now know how to respond to those problems to help him work through them.

When a child is given a psychotic label, such as autistic, he is in effect stigmatized so he can be treated differently than everyone else. A psychotic label suggests that the person is not competent to care for himself, that he is physiologically defective. This relieves those around him of the responsibility of acculturating him, rather they can be responsible members of society if they provide him with minimal care and just allow him to vegetate. However, to justify this unusual treatment it is generally necessary for those involved to rehearse over and over again the physiological evidence which justifies the label.

However, via appropriate training it is possible to compensate for some physiological disorders. In this case we do not know of any such disorder: the several physicians who examined Ross very carefully as a young child were unable to find any evidence of a physiological deficit which would produce autism, or autistic-like behavior. This, of course, does not rule out the possibility of an undiagnosed physiological defect.

Be that as it may, when Ross was put into a therapeutic situation he acquired the behaviors, the emotional responses of a normal child at a rather rapid rate. The only exceptional thing about Ross is that he is brighter than average, his Stanford-Binet and WISC IQ's are both 115.

SUMMARY

In conclusion, then, when Ross Grey began at CEMREL's school for autistic children, all of his speech was echolalic, he had extreme autistic aloneness, he tantrummed routinely to get his way and had several severe patterns of destructiveness, of self and of material objects. Within thirty months, using remedial exchanges, designed upon the principles of social learning, Ross became in essence a new child, normally acculturated. Though there are still some conceptual gaps in his language he actively and eagerly engages in conversation with anyone who interests him; he readily responds to the requests and instructions of others; he enjoys playing with other children; his destructiveness and aggressiveness are no longer a problem; he displays a true sense of humor; and he shows affection for others. In fact, he is indistinguishable from "normal" children. He is now enrolled in a regular first grade, and is doing quite adequately. There is simply no reason to believe that Ross will not continue to learn or not continue to develop. In fact, given his caretakers, who are well trained in behavior management, his present prospects for a happy, productive life are good.

CHAPTER 10

Theoretical Conclusions

At the outset we decided to work with several types of children in the hope that each type would be a prism through which we might look at the various facets of the acculturation and the humanization processes.[1] Now, at this juncture, it is time to draw a composite picture of what we have seen, to distill the findings from the separate chapters into a general theoretical statement.

Scientific theories involve a set of definitions, some of them of variables, and a set of interrelated propositions involving the defined variables. The propositions are formulated to describe the underlying cause-and-effect relationships of natural processes. The theories to be developed here involve (1) definitions and propositions about the nature of reinforcers and the conditioning processes which occur as people work exchanges. (2) Other definitions and propositions will involve structured exchanges and the direct learning processes which occur when such exchanges are worked over and over again. (3) There will be a set of definitions and propositions relating to the development of intelligence, perhaps the ultimate of the human abilities. We will now turn to each of these related theories and in doing so, tie together the implications of the experimental work of the previous chapters.

REINFORCER THEORY

A reinforcer, it may be recalled, is a stimulus which, in anticipation and in actuality, produces changes in emotional or feeling states. There are positive reinforcers which men hunger for which produce predominantly pleasant feeling states and there are negative reinforcers which produce painful or aversive feeling states. Since negative reinforcers and the related avoidance and escape learning have largely been beyond the scope of our research interests, we will focus on positive reinforcer theory.

[1] Hamblin took the major responsibility for writing this chapter.

A prime example of a positive reinforcer is food. However, food is only a reinforcer for a person who is hungry. This is true of many positive reinforcers. They are only periodically effective when the related hunger is induced after a period of abstention or deprivation. This periodic activation is often the result of a physiological process which via the hunger stimulates the organism to provide itself with that which sustains its physiological functions.

In learning experiments with animals where food is used as the reinforcer this point is well understood. To insure that the animal has a fierce hunger for food he is (1) put on a forced but gradual diet to eighty percent of his free-feeding weight and (2) starved for twenty-four hours prior to each experimental session. In our food exchanges with autistic children, it was not necessary to go to such extremes. Even so, we found out early that the children would simply not work acculturating exchanges unless they were hungry. Unfortunately most parents had to learn this lesson for themselves via two or three unsuccessful training sessions following their failure to keep the child from eating prior to the session.

Food sustains the organism by providing its nutritional requirements. The organism's nutritional store is ordinarily indicated by the sugar level in the blood which when it reaches a certain low level triggers pangs in the stomach. These stomach pangs, which are mild at first, are the aversive part of the hunger for food. If unheeded, they increase in magnitude until the organism is thereby driven to eat.

At the same time the eating of food produces pleasurable sensations in the taste buds located in the mouth. Possibly due to the operation of the conditioning processes, a psychological component of hunger develops for those foods which produce the most pleasurable sensations during eating. It appears, in fact, that there are conditioned aspects of all physiological hungers—for sleep, exercise and sex, for example. These are usually thought of as "tastes." Other conditioned hungers, however, are apparently purely psychological or social. These involve forms of psychological or social sustenance—for example, attention, love, power, status and the many luxuries that money can buy. Even so, acquired or conditioned hungers seem to dominate people as much if not more than their physiological counterparts.

Some conditioned hungers (for example, the hunger for attention) appear to be rhythmic in nature (at least for some people) and thus are satiable, rather like the hunger for food. However, certain others may be insatiable. For example, Veblen (1968) has suggested that in achieving societies the hunger for status is essentially insatiable. Certainly some people behave as though the Veblen thesis were true; they work for status fourteen, sixteen, eighteen hours a day only stopping when the physiological hungers for food, sleep and sex become so strong that they can no longer be ignored. Also, as we saw first in the chapter on hyperaggressive children, the hunger for negative attention appeared to be insatiable. At least, never once in all our observations did we see these boys terminate an aversive exchange with the teacher because they became satiated or bored, rather it was the teacher who always terminated the exchange by, in effect, giving up, by turning her back and by walking away. Similarly autistic children apparently have an insatiable hunger for the incredulous look in response to their bizarre behavior. Even so, satiability or insatiability of certain conditioned hungers is an interesting empirical problem which will requre much investigation before it is fully understood.

Most of the learning occurring in the everyday acculturation processes apparently involves conditioned reinforcers: a loved one's voice, attention or approval, a favorable comparison, a correct answer and so on. The almost exclusive use of conditioned reinforcers in acculturating children has the advantage of being subtle, unobtrusive, but it has an enormous, if heretofore hidden, cost for a few. Without the experiences which result in the conditioning of these reinforcers a few children never learn, are never acculturated and, therefore, become retarded and otherwise deviant in development. Also, without periodic backup, conditioned reinforcers tend to lose their power and, hence, retard acculturation.

It is difficult for people to realize that learning does not occur without meaningful reinforcers but we have seen very convincing examples. One involves the so-called ethnically disadvantaged children who apparently are not well conditioned to the reinforcers used in traditional classrooms. The results are graphically illustrated by the Coleman data, a cumulative deficit in academic achievement. We have seen repeatedly that such children can learn at a *better* than normal rate if they are allowed to work educational environments for reinforcers which are *meaningful* to them—food and other material reinforcers.

In correcting deviant patterns in children it is, therefore, not enough to work artificially constructed environments to develop normal behavior patterns. It is also crucial, as Lovaas, et al. (1966), has so effectively argued, that their therapeutic environment be so structured that while they are working it to develop normal patterns, they are simultaneously conditioned to respond appropriately to the reinforcers typically used in everyday society so the normal patterns, once learned in therapy, will be maintained, even elaborated in everyday life.

It may be recalled that anything which repeatedly signals reinforcement gradually becomes a conditioned reinforcer. While we have not subjected this principle to experimental test, we have used it over and over in designing our learning environments. It may be recalled that our teachers generally signaled token and other material reinforcement with "thank you," "that's correct," and a pat or a touch to condition these as reinforcers for the children. And it may be recalled that these conditioned reinforcers were then used, preferentially, to maintain established patterns (the more powerful material reinforcers are generally reserved for acquisition).

Also we have been careful in selecting those behaviors which the children must use in working the instructional exchanges. For those behaviors—eye contact, talking, doing puzzles, reading, writing, arithmetic and so on—all become positive reinforcers, that is, intrinsically pleasant for the children, since all repeatedly proceed and thus signal reinforcement in the acculturating exchanges. As a result the children come to require less and less in the way of extrinsic reinforcement to maintain their behavior.

We have repeatedly seen this phenomenon occur in the experiments in prior chapters particularly with talking. In our first experiment with nonverbal inner-city children it took extrinsic material reinforcers to get them to begin talking, but after a three-month training period they talked normally without special extrinsic reinforcers. This also occurred with the autistic children. While it took extrinsic material reinforcers to teach them to talk, after several months of conditioning it was possible to fade out such reinforcers without having their verbal communication patterns deteriorate. This does not mean, however, that all outside reinforcement was withdrawn. Verbal communication is the normal medium used in getting attention, in negotiating exchanges and is, therefore periodically, if indirectly reinforced with attention, material and other reinforcers.

The fact that social life is structured in terms of repetitious social exchanges means that many things do or can become conditioned reinforcers. However, precisely because of this many find learning theory and, by extension, exchange theory a slippery enterprise. Yet this plasticity of reinforcers, for good or for evil, allows man to be the adaptable animal that he is, to be acculturated, humanized. Even so, at any given time, it is useful, if not crucial, to be able to identify that which is reinforcing for any given individual.

It may be recalled that we began by assuming that reinforcers produce anticipatory and then direct changes in the emotional or feeling states. We also assumed with the ethologists that internal feeling states are generally reflected externally via reflexive response patterns and that the magnitude of the internal feeling is generally gauged by the magnitude of the external response which reflects it. It seems to us (1) that the anticipatory emotional response, part of a natural or the essence of a conditioned hunger, is reflected in what might be called fond or wistful looking, (2) that a person will work for a positive reinforcer, (3) that they will show evidence of pleasure such as a smile when experiencing a positive reinforcer. Likewise, people will look at negative reinforcers with discomfort or fear. They will work to avoid or escape a negative reinforcer, and they will show evidences of pain or discomfort when experiencing a negative reinforcer and relief when escaping it.

In our analyses of what reinforces what in ongoing streams of social interaction, we have attempted to use these cues, and we have found a general consistency. People generally will look wistfully at what they will work for, at what will cause them to smile and otherwise evidence pleasure over. Unlike some adults children tend not to disguise their feelings, in their actions and in their words. Even so, learning and exchange theory are at their weakest when used to analyze streams of ongoing interaction. Determining what is and what is not reinforcing in ongoing social interaction is somewhat chancy. Even so, it is possible, as we have seen, to use rather standard reinforcers in the experimental context and routinely obtain rather remarkable learning effects.

The Contrast Effect

Contrast usually magnifies the value of any natural or conditioned reinforcer. The effect occurs, apparently, when something that produces a negative emotional response immediately precedes the occurrence of something else which produces a related positive emotional response, the value of the latter response being heightened by contrast with the former.

The contrast effect has long been used by writers of fiction and dramatists to produce strong, sometimes exquisite emotional responses in their readers and audiences. It apparently makes little difference what the negative emotional response is as long as it precedes the positive response immediately in time. Thus the pleasure of safety is heightened by the prior escape from danger, the pleasure of goodness is heightened by the prior escape from the miseries of evil, the satisfaction of problem solving is increased by the prior anxieties of failure.

Similarly, we have noted earlier that the rate of response is higher, holding the value of the reinforcement constant if the reinforcement schedule is variable rather than constant. This appears to occur because of the contrast effect which is built into variable reinforcement. When on a variable reinforcement schedule the individual is never certain he will or will not receive reinforcement. Hence, a person working an exchange on a variable schedule will necessarily experience some anxiety, some fear of failure every time he attempts to work the exchange. Presumably this fear of failure will be enhanced the more frequently one in fact fails to receive reinforcement. However, the fear of failure as it increases in magnitude should via the contrast effect increase the net strength of the reinforcement when it does in fact finally occur. Hence the general but paradoxical rule, the smaller the ratio of reinforcement (with 1 to 4 being a smaller ratio than 1 to 2) the higher the rate of response. However, all principles have their limits and the limit here is that the ratio of reinforcement to response has to be decreased gradually or the response pattern of the person working the exchange will deteriorate very rapidly to naught.

The contrast effect is also responsible for most of the satisfaction one experiences in games. In winning one derives some pleasure from a favorable comparison of his performance with that of others, but this pleasure of winning is apparently heightened substantially in close contests by the suspense, the fear of failure which precedes and thus contrasts with winning. Some of our more successful experimental teachers used a wide variety of educational games to heighten the effect of material reinforcement.

Finally, in the school situation tests seem to involve substantial contrast effects. Tests, by their very nature, involve exchange contingencies which in turn always involve the possibility of failure. In general, the greater the fear of failure, as Maier (1961) has documented, can increase to the point where people become nonrational, in effect, intellectually crippled. But then any behavior pattern may be carried to the extreme or the grotesque—even talking and studying. Be that as it may, the effects of contrasts which strengthen reinforcers is crucial to understand, both from the point of view of appreciating the old, the existing learning environments but also for designing that which is new, perhaps better.

Intensification by Reversals

In the ABAB experiments with suburban children in Chapter 2, the inner-city children in Chapter 3, and the hyperaggressive children in Chapter 5, we encountered the intensification-by-reversals effect. We found that the experimental reversals designed initially to evaluate causal assumptions in our theory produced what to us then was an unanticipated therapeutic effect. After the reversal in the B2 period, the behavioral equilibrium was higher than it was before in the B1 period. The equilibria data for the ABAB experiments in Chapters 2, 3 and 5 are summarized in Tables 10.1 and 10.2.

The data in Table 10.1 involve behaviors which were supposed to be acquired during the ABAB series. The A period represents baseline where the reinforcers (the usual conditioned reinforcers) were generally weak. During the B periods the exchanges were nearly continuous with tokens and material backups added to the conditioned reinforcers. Note that the equilibria in the B2 periods were consistently higher after the A2 reversals than they were before in the B1 periods. There is not a single exception to this rule in the 10 sets of data reported in Table 10.1. On the average the B1 equilibria are only 84 percent of the B2 equilibria.

The equilibria data for the A1 and A2 periods are also interesting. They,

Table 10.1. Equilibria and ABAB Acquisition Series: A, Weak Reinforcers; B, Strong Reinforcers.

	A1	%	B1	%	A2	%	B2	%
Hyperaggressive Preschoolers								
Studying (percentage, scheduled time)	7	8%	78	87%	13	14%	90	100%
Cooperation (sequences)	50	29	138	80	83	43	172	100
Hyperaggressives, primary class								
Studying (percentage, scheduled time)	58	59	95	97	84	86	98	100
Hyperaggressives, intermediate class								
Studying (percentage, scheduled time)	32	33	87	91	63	66	96	100
W.U. Preschoolers								
Studying (percentage, allotted time)	18	23	68	88	14	18	77	100
Peer tutoring (percentage, allotted time)	10	14	58	78	12.5	17	74	100
Words Learned	1.5	35	3.0	71	2.5	58	4.25	100
Webster Preschoolers								
Studying (minutes)	NA	..	48	92	18	35	52	100
Peer tutoring	3.0	22	13.5	77	9.5	54	17.5	100
Assignments learned to criteria	NA	..	4.0	80	NA	..	5.0	100
Medians		26%		84%		43%		100%

Table 10.2. Equilibria for ABAB Extinction Series: A, Conditional Reinforcers; B, No or Almost No Reinforcers.

	A1	%	B1	%	A2	%	B2	%
Hyperaggressives, preschoolers								
Aggression (sequences)[a]	150	100%	22	15%	124	83%	16	11%
Hyperaggressives, primary class								
Disruptions (sequences)	75	100	9	12	31	41	8	11
Hyperaggressives, intermediate class								
Disruptions (sequences)	71	100	7	10	52	73	2	3
Medians		100%		12%		73%		11%

[a] For purposes of comparison B1 here corresponds to B1-C-B2 in Figure 5.1, A2 to A2 and B2 to B3.

too, show an intensification. On the average they changed from 26 percent to 43 percent of the final B2 equilibrium. According to the data in Table 10.1, holding the level of reinforcement constant, the equilibrium before an increase in the strength of reinforcers is always lower than the equilibrium obtained after the reversal, after the reinforcers are restored to their original strength.

In the second chapter we suggested that the increased levels after change were the result of an increment in expertise learning, the result of the increased reinforced practice obtained during the reversal. While this explanation could fit the data in Table 10.1 which all involve ABAB acquisition series, it does not fit equilibria data for ABAB extinction series, such as those found in Table 10.2. Note that the aggressive and the disruptive behavior which were extinguished in the ABAB series reported in Table 10.2 show a decrease rather than an increase after reversal. The level of the behavioral equilibria in the A2 period averages only 73 percent of the level of equilibria in the A1 periods, and for the B1 and B2 periods, respectively 12 and 11 percent of the initial A1 equilibria. In other words in an extinction series, the second behavioral equilibrium is not heightened by the reversal, or the change in the strength of the reinforcers, rather it is lowered.

It does not seem plausible that children in these extinction experiments became less expert after a reversal and, hence, were less *able* to be aggressive or disruptive. Rather, in both tables, it would seem that they progressively changed their taste for the behavior in question. How could that happen? Possibly, in several ways. However, remember that these extinction series occurred in the context of what we have called a counter exchange. During the B period when the strength of the reinforcers for aggressive and disruptive behaviors was reduced to zero or near zero, the strength of the reinforcers for an alternative behavior—studying, cooperation—was increased substantially by adding tokens and material backups to the conditioned reinforcers used in the A periods. Apparently, this *contrast* in the strength of the extrinsic reinforcers used in the B periods conditioned the children in a way that changed the intrinsic value of the behaviors involved and, thus, changed their strength as conditioned reinforcers. Apparently the cooperation was subjected to a favorable contrast which resulted in the children's being positively conditioned so in subsequent periods these behaviors became stronger as intrinsic conditioned reinforcers. This change was then apparently reflected, as is the increase in the strength of any reinforcer, in increased equilibria levels in A2 and B2. Conversely, the aggressive, disruptive behaviors were subjected to an unfavorable contrast. Therefore, the children were apparently conditioned so the strength of those behaviors as intrinsic reinforcers was decreased. This decrease in the strength of the behavior as an intrinsic, conditioned reinforcer then apparently showed up in the relative decreases in the equilibria levels in A2 and B2.

Of course, the above explanation is offered as a theory, one that needs to be checked out systematically. However, the heightening and lowering of equilibria values after reversals appear to be both consistent and important phenomena. As we have noted, substantial therapeutic effects are involved in the process. The explanation offered here suggests that the therapeutic changes in behavior reflect basic changes in attitudes and values. Such conclusions are not firm, however, without the support of additional research.

STRUCTURED EXCHANGE THEORY

Our work with several types of children has perhaps more than anything else documented the theory that social learning environments are structured as exchanges. It is now time to summarize what we know about such exchanges.

It seems that the fundamental social exchange is always between two parties. We have observed more complex exchanges, but these can usually be analyzed fruitfully in terms of the two party paradigms. Hence, to simplify our analysis, an exchange will be thought of as involving two parties, one taking an initiator role and the other, a reciprocator role.

The initiator always starts the actual exchange by behaving in a way that has reinforcing consequences for the reciprocator. The reinforcing consequences may be pleasureful and thus valued by the other or they may be painful and thus aversive to the other. The reciprocator completes the exchange by behaving in a way that has reinforcing consequences for the first party, the initiator. Again, the reinforcing consequences may be pleasant or painful.

It should be noted that both the initiator and the reciprocator may signal or otherwise arrange the terms of the exchange. The initiator role is not acquired by arranging the terms but by being first in providing a reinforcer to the other. Thus in a typical employee-employer relationship, the employee first does his work and then is paid by the employer. Therefore, the employee, by providing first that which is reinforcing to the other, is the initiator and the employer is the reciprocator.

Social exchanges are structured if they are being worked repetitively and if reciprocation is patterned enough to be reliably characterized by a rule by sensitive observers. Structured exchanges are important because they, not transient exchanges, produce social learning and social conditioning.

Social exchanges become structured in several ways. Although some are negotiated so the terms are set explicitly by verbal contract, the vast majority are structured implicitly as it were, without verbal negotiations. People are generally unaware of the thousands of implicitly structured exchanges in which they are involved every day and, like the mothers of autistic children, they are often oblivious to the learning and conditioning that occurs as a result. For that reason alone it is worth making a distinction between contractually and implicitly structured exchanges. A second reason, however, is that the propositions which describe the cause-effect relationships capitalized on in our experiments involve implicitly structured exchanges.

(1) The central variables in a theory of an implicitly structured exchange have to do with the frequency with which such an exchange is worked. In gauging the frequency with which any exchange is worked, one may count the frequency with which either party to the exchange provides that which is reinforcing to the other. As we have seen, in most instances the frequency comes into an equilibrium, a relatively steady state characterized by a cyclical fluctuation but no long-term upward or downward trend.

(2) The frequency of working an implicitly structured exchange apparently equilibrates at the point where, *for both parties*, the effort and other costs of working the exchange balance value received in reinforcers.

(3) If the strength of the reinforcers, and hence the value received, is for some reason increased by one of the parties, then the frequency with which the other party works the exchange will increase until a new equilibrium is established where again value received balances the costs incurred.

(4) Conversely, if one of the parties, for some reason, decreases the strength of the reinforcers and, hence, decreases the value the other receives for working the exchange, then the frequency with which the other works the exchange will decrease until a new equilibrium obtains where value received again balances costs incurred. As we have seen, these generalizations, (3) and (4), referred to as the acceleration-deceleration principles, have been confirmed in experiment after experiment at least when the reciprocator did the changing.

(5) When the strength of the reinforcers for initiating the exchange is increased, the frequency of initiating may abruptly increase to the new higher equilibrium or gradually increase as pictured in Figure 10.1. In the latter case, what is involved is an acquisition curve. In general, acquisition curves are obtained because two processes occur which progressively reduce response time. As the person repeatedly works the exchange for reinforcers, (1) the contingencies became progressively clarified, so the person better and better understands exactly what behavior produces the reinforcers and (2) he acquires expertise wherein the essential parts of his behavioral pattern (those which actually produce the reinforcers) are gradually strengthened and the

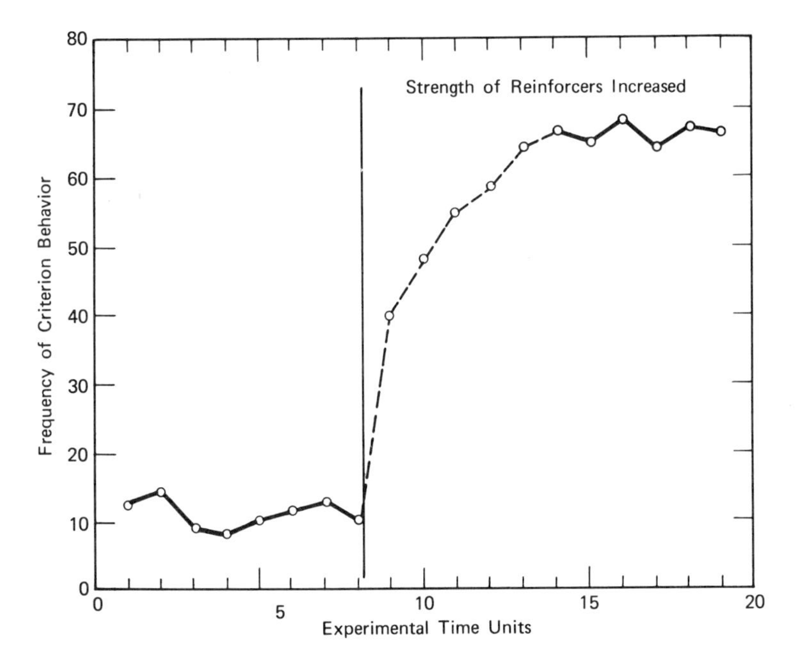

Figure 10.1. Theoretical type 1 learning curve, acquisition series. The black lines indicate initial and final equilibria, and the dotted line, the acquisition phase.

superfluous parts weakened. The strengthening simultaneously increases accuracy and speed and reduces the fatigue generated by the repetitive response pattern. This gives the acquisition curve fixed mathematical properties: when the methodology of an experiment approximates, even roughly, the expected standards, acquisition data consistently approximate a power function (See Appendix A).

(6) The gradual versus the abrupt changes referred to in (5) occur lawfully, as a function of the transfer of prior learning. Thus, as may be noted in Table 10.3 a second acquisition series occurs much more quickly than does the first (a median of 1.5 sessions until equilibrium for second acquisition versus 9 sessions for the first).[2]

(7) The initial transition from a low equilibrium into acquisition occurred in most of our experiments shortly after the exchange contingencies were improved, i.e. after the strength of the reinforcers for the behavior in question was increased. A number of variables apparently influence the

[2] There are other characteristics of transfer which will be introduced later in this chapter. However, transfer is a complex subject which is best understood in the context of the mathematical analysis in Appendix A.

Table 10.3. Transfer-of-Learning Effect: Acquisition—Hyperaggressive Boys.

	First Acquisition		Second Acquisition	
	Experimental Period	Latency, New Equilibrium	Experimental Period	Latency, New Equilibrium
Preschoolers	B1-C-B2			
Studying	B1-C-B2	17 sessions	B3	3 sessions
Cooperation		9 sessions	B3	2 sessions
Aggression	A1	5 sessions	A2	1 session
Primary Class				
Studying	B1	12 sessions	B2	1 session
Disruptions	A1	18 sessions	A2	1 session
Intermediate Class				
Studying	B1	7 sessions	B2	2 sessions
Disruptions	A1	1 session	A2	3 sessions
Median		9 sessions		1.5 sessions

speed of this contingency learning and, hence, influence when the transition into acquisition occurs.

(a) The evidence suggests that children attend the reinforcers in their environment in proportion to the strength of those reinforcers. This occurs because attending reinforcers, it will be recalled, produces pleasant anticipatory emotional reactions similar to those produced by the reinforcers themselves. Apparently the more children attend reinforcers, the more quickly they will be able to spot exchange contingencies between the production of behavior and the reception of reinforcers. Hence, the stronger the reinforcers, the more children will attend them, and consequently will more quickly spot or learn the exchange contingencies, i.e. what it is they have to do to earn the reinforcers.

(b) Immediacy of feedback in an exchange, whether that feedback is reinforcement *per se* or process cues predictive of later reinforcement, is related to the speed of contingency learning. In general, the more immediate the feedback, the more quickly a person will learn new exchange contingenies.[3]

[3] This proposition may not be true in the case of negative reinforcers which seem to have generalized inhibiting effects.

(c) Structured exchanges may also vary in the degree to which the reinforcement and the process cues predictive of later reinforcement are consistent or invariant. In general, the more consistent the feedback, the more quickly a person will learn new exchange contingencies.

In this book, our experimental focus has been more applied than theoretical. So whenever a structured exchange has been inadequate as a social learning environment we have almost always strengthened it by simultaneously manipulating the strength of the reinforcers and, if possible, their immediacy and consistency. The result has been that in almost all of our experiments the transition into acquisition has occurred during the same period in which the contingencies were actually changed by the experimenters. Even so, the theory in this section requires thorough investigation for human subjects.

(8) When the strength of the reinforcers for initiating an exchange is decreased, the frequency with which the children work that exchange may decrease abruptly or gradually as pictured in Figure 10.2. In the latter case, an extinction curve is obtained. Extinction curves apparently result when the pattern of initiating the exchange has become habitual where the response occurs almost, if not automatically, in the presence of accustomed

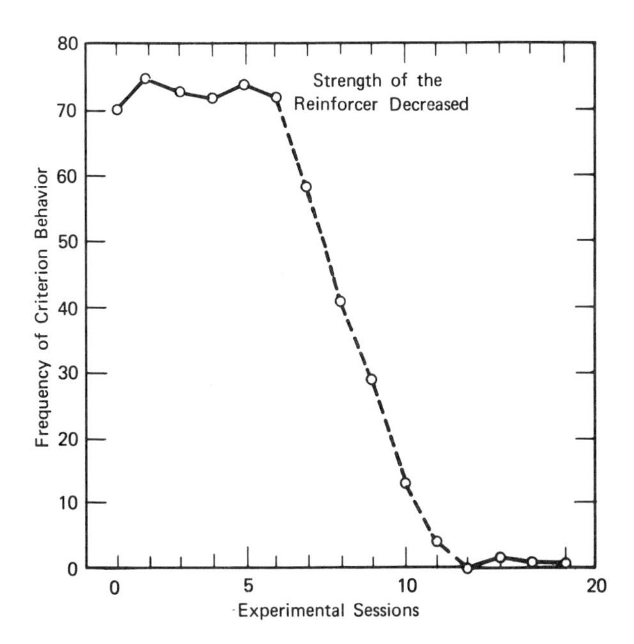

Figure 10.2. Theoretical type 2 learning curve, extinction series. The black lines indicate initial and final equilibria, and the dotted line, the extinction phase.

exchange signals. It is as if the person finds it impossible to believe that his behavior can no longer work the exchange for strong reinforcers. However, just as habits are strengthened through repeated reinforcement, they can be weakened through repeated non reinforcement. Hence, when contingencies are changed to weaker or to no reinforcers as, for example, they sometimes are in an experiment, the frequency of the habitual manipulative pattern deteriorates.

In general, speed of extinction is a function of the transfer of prior learning. The data in Table 10.4, although not entirely uniform, suggest that in a second extinction series the new equilibrium is obtained much sooner (the median is one experimental day) than in a first extinction series (the median equals six days).

(9) Structured exchanges may be classified any number of ways, but the classification that seems to be crucial to children's acculturation problems involves the consequence of the actions of each party to the other party of the exchange. Basically, with respect to their consequences for the other party (the initiator or the reciprocator) there are three types of responses: (1) valued responses which are experienced by the other as predominantly pleasureful; (2) aversive responses which are experienced by the other as predominantly painful; (3) neutral responses which the other experiences are blah, neither pleasureful nor painful. Note that the third type, neutral responses, because they are not reinforcing are excluded from exchange analysis.

Any exchange to be worked through time, as Homans has noted, must provide a short term profit for each party to the exchange—the pleasant

Table 10.4. Transfer-of-Learning Effect: Extinction, Hyperaggressive Boys.

	First Extinction		Second Extinction	
	Experimental Period	Latency, New Equilibrium	Experimental Period	Latency, New Equilibrium
Preschoolers Aggression	B1-C-B2	22 days	B3	9 days
Primary Class Disruptions	B1	6 days	B2	1 day
Intermediate Class Disruptions	B1	1 day	B2	1 day
Median		6 days		1 day

must exceed the aversive consequences. Thus a person's response pattern may have mixed consequences for the other as long as the total pleasure outweighs the total pain. It follows then that there are four basic types of structured exchanges as pictured in Figure 10.3

A structured exchange where both the initiator's and reciprocator's response patterns have predominantly mixed consequences for the other may be called an aggressive exchange or, more simply, a fight. In an aggressive exchange, each party's intended response pattern is aversive or punishing to the other: his unintended pattern, evidencing hurt from the other's punishment apparently gives the other satisfaction or pleasure, at least enough to maintain his part of the fight. In addition, there is an issue at stake in every fight and the ultimate reinforcement is to win, for the other to capitulate. It is the party who is unable to absorb the other's punishment as well as the other absorbs his, who usually capitulates or loses. War is an extreme example of a fight; even so, fights occur perhaps less cataclysmically at all levels of social interaction, every day in numerous situations. Fights are common whenever a person uses punishment in attempting to modify another's offensive behaviors. A fight usually starts when the person being punished decides that he does not want to change, or that the other's punishing behavior should be modified and, so, he punishes back.

Predominant Reinforcing Consequence for the Initiator	Predominant Reinforcing Consequences for the Reciprocator: Mixed–Painful and Pleasant	Predominant Reinforcing Consequences for the Reciprocator: Pleasant
Mixed: Painful and Pleasant	An Aggressive Exchange (A Fight)	An Exploitive Exchange
Pleasant	A Teasing Exchange	A Normal Exchange

Figure 10.3. The Four Types of Structured Exchanges.

In a teasing exchange, the initiator's responses are mixed for the reciprocator, but ironically, the reciprocator's response pattern is predominantly pleasureful to the initiator. We have noted that encounters with hyperaggressive and autistic children typically develop into this kind of exchange. This pattern seems to occur when the reciprocator thinks that his responses are aversive to the other, that he is involved in a fight to persuade the other to modify his offensive patterns. However, in a true teasing exchange, the reciprocator never wins, for his supposedly aversive response patterns are actually pleasant to the other party who will continue to initiate the exchange until he is either satiated and, hence, terminates or until the reciprocator gives up and, hence, terminates. As we have seen with both the hyperaggressive boys and the autistic children, the giving up or placation strategy does not solve anything in the long run, for the children just wait for another opportunity to start teasing. Thus the teasing exchanges seem to get progressively worse from the reciprocator's point of view. In fact, in the long run, the reciprocator typically will adopt a new strategy to modify the teasing or will terminate permanently. Autistic children and the worst of the hyperaggressive boys are frequently sent to a custodial institution of one kind or another.

In an exploitive exchange the initiator's response pattern is predominantly pleasureful to the reciprocator, but the reciprocator's response pattern is mixed to the initiator. Ordinarily the exploitive exchange is maintained by virtue of the reciprocator's superior aversive power and his willingness to use that aversive power to structure the exchange so the other will experience even worse consequences if he fails to provide the reciprocator with that which he wants. An exploitive exchange is unstable for the initiator typically tries to escape the relationship, tries to organize, to force a change in the terms of the exchange or failing these engages in various types of sabotage. In the latter instances, the relationship degenerates into a subtle fight.

The basic conditions for direct social learning are present in these three types of exchanges. Depending upon which role one takes in each type of exchange, one will learn various contingencies (ways of working the exchange) and will become progressively, habitually expert in those ways. Thus if one participates seriously in fights, one will learn different ways to win fights and will become progressively, habitually expert in those ways. If one initiates teasing exchanges enough one will find many ways to tease and will become progressively, habitually expert in those ways of teasing. If one repeatedly reciprocates exploitively then one will learn ways of exploitation, will become progressively, habitually expert in exploiting others. If one is repeatedly teased or exploited, then one learns different ways of escaping teasing and exploitation and becomes habitually expert in working these escape patterns. In other words, men, because they are equipped with biological learning mechanisms, adapt to their environments; it may take some time, but they adapt.

It also follows that working structured exchanges will produce gradual changes in emotional response patterns. This is because the situation is repetitive and because many aspects of the situation are constant enough to signal reinforcement repeatedly. As suggested earlier, any aspect of an exchange which repeatedly signals reinforcement will gradually become a conditioned reinforcer which will produce anticipatory sensations similar to, but slightly weaker than a sensation produced by the original reinforcers. Thus, people who frequently fight with one another and attempt to modify one another's behavior will, at best, be ambivalent about each other and, then, only if each wins some of the time. Teasing exchanges, when worked repetitively, result in the initiator's liking the reciprocator, but the liking is not shared. The reciprocators generally come to hate the initiator. The opposite happens in an exploitive exchange unless it degenerates into an open fight, in which case, each will hate the other.

Only in a normal exchange do both parties experience predominantly pleasant reactions from the other. Only in a normal exchange do the direct learning processes facilitate both parties' learning to provide even more pleasant consequences for the other. Only in a normal exchange do all of the cues which signal reinforcement, including the individuals themselves, become conditioned reinforcers which evoke pleasant sensations. Of course this picture is slightly overdrawn. There are costs, aversive consequences—such as effort, fatigue and other opportunities for exchange foregone—which in part balance the pleasant consequences. However, these costs are self-generated, the result of the individual's own decisions and limitations. They are not born as a result of the other's behavior. Hence people will not be ambivalent about the other party to such exchanges. Thus, the normal exchange is highly stable, unless for some reason it degenerates into one of the other forms. As we have seen, degeneration can be avoided if the parties involved learn how to modify one another's behavior via positive reinforcement, through the use of reward and nonreward and, thus, avoid punishment, negative reinforcement, altogether. The essence of maintaining a normal exchange is striking a bargain, that is, amicably deciding the terms of the exchange. This can be done through negotiations or implicitly as it is done in our experimental classes. The latter is more subtle, avoiding long arguments and recriminations. The children in such instances simply hold back until they receive that which is satisfying to them and the teachers try different things until they find something that the children like and which they are willing to give in exchange for, what is to the teachers, a satisfactory work pattern. For the above theoretical advantages, the normal exchange is deserving of more exploration as a model for human relations.

INTELLIGENCE

We have put off discussing the development of intelligence and related matters until now primarily because the subject is so complex and requires extensive background. In the third chapter a series of experiments on language acquisition was presented. One of these involved six kindergarten classes and the relationship between remedial language development and IQ change. It was found that using the Bereiter-Regan Conceptual Skills Program, together with an appropriate token exchange, the inner-city children in the experiment learned standard language in which they are generally weak, language that involves symbolic reasoning and mediates learning in the classroom. The result of this training was a net increase of fifteen points in IQ. To us this change in IQ was a welcomed result, for it seemed to be hard evidence that these children had experienced a substantial increase in general intellectual ability. However, the data do run counter to the concept of fixed hereditary intelligence and to Jensen's (1969) main argument that IQ cannot be changed much by instruction. Hence, the data are seen by some as problematic, as in need of explanation. We will start by defining intelligence.

Long ago, well after intelligence tests had demonstrated their usefulness, Boring, the famous psychologist, wryly suggested that intelligence ought to be defined as that which intelligence tests measure. At this juncture, his may be a reasonable way to proceed. In the first place, intelligence has always been assumed to involve mental age, a mental ability that normally increases as people get older, as they become more and more experienced in working physical and social exchanges. Hence, it may be thought of, in part, as an acquired expertise.

The IQ score, itself, which gauges the intelligence of a particular individual, is the ratio of mental age to chronological age multiplied by 100. The metric for mental age is obtained by averaging the accumulative acquisitions of samples of individuals of the various age groupings. In other words, a mental age of four is the average score on a battery of "intelligence" items of a large and representative sample of four-year olds; a mental age of five is the average of a large and representative sample of five-year olds; and so on. This means that an IQ of 100 is an acquisition rate of the mental ability called intelligence that is about average for the population as a whole. Basically then, the assumption is that the faster one learns to work the items on an intelligence test, the more intelligent one is. In thinking about it, this is not an unreasonable way to gauge intelligence, and it has the further convenience of relating IQ to learning theory, for the acquisition rate of an ability or expertise is a prime variable in learning theory.

Therefore, the genus for our definition of intelligence is: a kind of mental ability whose magnitude is gauged by its acquisition rate. To complete the definition we need a differendum to differentiate intelligence from other kinds of mental abilities. Again, we will proceed inductively, this time relying on the work of Carl Spearman. In his long distinguished career Spearman found that practically all tests of mental ability are intercorrelated, some of them quite substantially. As he factor analyzed these correlations, he found further that all of the tests were loaded, some of them more highly than others, on a general factor which he called *g*. Spearman (cf. 1946) suggested that when the term intelligence is used, it should refer to this factor common to all tests of mental ability. Spearman then went one step further. He examined those tests of mental ability most heavily loaded with *g* to determine their content. His inference: they seemed to involve what he characterized as "the ability to educe relations and correlates." Over the years educational psychologists have come to accept Spearman's technical definition of intelligence as *g* and also the meaning he attributed to it.

Spearman chose his verb carefully; to educe is to deduce and to infer. Hence, intelligence refers to the acquisition rate of the ability to use both deductive and inductive logic in relating and correlating. It is this definition which leads to the hypothesis that intelligence should be increased by language training, for language is a conventional set of symbols which people use deductively and inductively to communicate relations and correlates to one another. This does not mean that we are suggesting, contrary to the psychogenetic data, that heredity is not a partial determinant of IQ. It plainly is. Rather, we are suggesting that heredity and environment interact in influencing acquisition rates that are ultimately measured as *g*. But at present the data suggest there are two sets of related hereditary and environmental variables.

Quality of the Cortex and IQ

It is generally assumed (cf. Hebb, 1949; Krech, 1969; Jensen, 1969) that the acquisition rates measured as IQ increase as the quality of the tissues and the biochemistry of the cortex improves. Such a theory is very straightforward since the cognitive or symbolic functions are known to occur in the cortex and it is not difficult to imagine how heredity, which is determined for the individual when the ovum and the sperm unite at the time of conception, can effect the quality of the tissue, the biochemistry and, hence, rates of acquisition of the ability to educe relations and correlates.

However, the data suggest that physiology of the cortex may also be modified by environmental experience. Data from animal experiments indicate that species' specific learning, i.e. maze learning for rats and probably language learning for children, produces changes in the quality of the tissue and the biochemistry of the cortex (cf. Krech, 1969). The effect is apparently analogous to that of physical exercise on the musculature of the body. The appropriate use of the tissue strengthens it. These physiological changes are then reflected in increased acquisition rates which show behaviorally as very substantial transfer effects.

The transfer effects of a first language acquisition series on a second is illustrated in Figure 10.4. If we did not know better we might infer that the two curves were generated by two different persons one brighter than the other—as judged by the higher initial level of performance, the faster rate of acquisition and the higher equilibrium rate after acquisition. Actually, the two curves were generated by the same individuals, four preschoolers, in first and second acquisition series. The qualitatively better acquisition rate

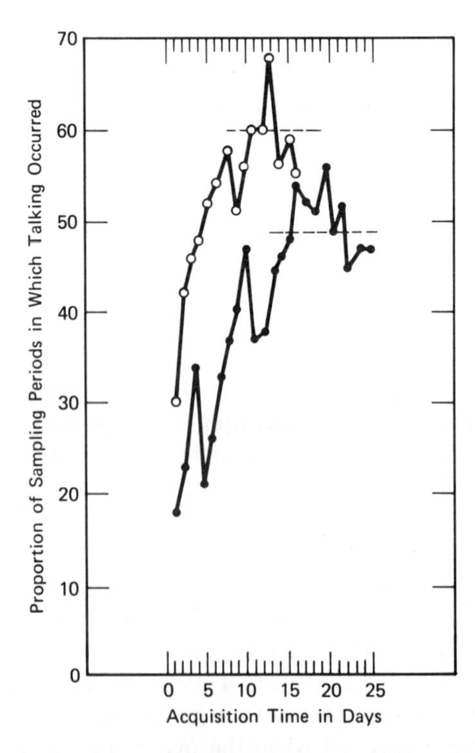

Figure 10.4. Proportion of sampling periods in which talking occurred in first (filled dots) and second (unfilled dots) acquisition series. (Original data, Figure 3.1, B1 and B2 periods.) Equilibria are indicated by dotted lines.

during the second series is evidently the result of having gone through the first.

In other words, a child's learning environment may influence the acquisition rates measured as IQ by providing or withholding certain very basic learning experiences the transfer of which would effect the rate of later learning experiences. For example, if the social environment did not reinforce the acquisition of certain classes of language, the child would consequently not benefit from the expected transfer effects which, in turn, should depress the rate of other acquisitions measured as IQ.

Quality of the Autonomic Nervous System and IQ

It is the autonomic nervous system that responds to reinforcers in ways that persons experience as pleasant or adverse feelings. Hence, the autonomic nervous system activates a person to work his environment for reinforcers and, thereby, regulates acquisition rates, including those ultimately measured as IQ. The hereditary quality of the tissue and the biochemistry of the autonomic nervous system may thus influence IQ a number of ways but: (a) some autonomic mechanisms might be more responsive to conventional reinforcers than others and (b) the ease or degree to which emotions or feelings can be conditioned may vary from one autonomic mechanism to another.

The related environmental variables have to do with the strength of the reinforcers for those behaviors related to the acquisitions measured as IQ. As we have seen, a wide variety of acquisition rates may be increased by increasing the strength of the related reinforcers. However, when the reinforcers are limited to conditioned reinforcers, as they generally are in the traditional educational system, it becomes crucial that children go through the acculturation experiences in the home or elsewhere which condition them to respond to those reinforcers. These experiences are apparently analogous to so-called imprinting which is evidently essential for the normal development of certain other species, for example, graylag geese (Lorenz, 1966) and rhesus monkeys (Harlow and Harlow, 1965).

In other words, the above theory suggests that while heredity does have an important influence on the acquisition rate, measured as IQ, certain environmental variables (E) interact with the hereditary variables (H) to change the magnitude of H and E's relationships to IQ and thus may change the relative contributions of H and E.

Actually, Jensen (1969) recognizes in the equations he cited from Sir Cyril Burt's investigations that H and E do interact in determining IQ (but perhaps not as much as we have suggested here). Also, minimal interaction is described by what Jensen refers to as the threshold hypothesis. According to Jensen the environments which almost all children encounter as they are growing up are in the normal range in that they allow the children to acquire an IQ up to their hereditary potential. The exceptions are environments involving extreme isolation, such as orphanages of the past. Such minimal, unresponsive social environments apparently have catastrophical effects on the IQ's of the inhabitants regardless of their hereditary potentials; almost all children who grow up in such environments develop IQ's in the defective range.

This threshold theory is nicely supported by a long term experiment conducted by Skeels (1966) who followed the intellectual development of two samples of children from early infancy until adulthood. At the outset, both samples of children were in an orphanage where they spent their time in a cottage with thirty to thirty-five children of the same sex under the care of a matron and three or four untrained older girls who had grown up in the orphanage. The matron and her helpers even mended the children's clothing, cleaned and maintained the cottage. Consequently the result was rather severe regimentation: the children were trained to sit down, to stand up, to walk, in fact to do most things in unison. Also, the activities were meager because of inadequate equipment. In fact, the children spent most of the time sitting around in chairs. Also they were reinforced very little for the acquisition of language or for other pro-normal behavior patterns. In particular, the situation was such that the children were probably not conditioned to respond to the reinforcers that are conventionally used in school, such as the approval of an adult and getting the right answers.

In any event, the sample of children who spent their entire childhood in the orphanage, who comprised what Skeels called his comparison group, experienced a massive IQ loss during the first few years in the orphanage—at sixteen months the median IQ was 88, at thirty-eight months it was 63 and at forty-nine months it was 61. In other words, during their first four years in the orphanage the children in the comparison group experienced a cumulative loss in their median IQ of 27 points.

Through a fortunate accident Skeels found what appeared to be a better learning environment for the thirteen children in what he called his experimental group. At an average age of seventeen months the experimental children were transferred from the orphanage to a state hospital for the mentally retarded and there placed individually in wards with older mentally defectives (most were young adults with mental ages ranging between twelve and thirteen years). Offhand one might be concerned about the prospects for these youngsters in such a situation, but the older patients apparently gave them very intensive, loving care. In fact, all but three were taken over by one individual who, in effect, became their foster parent. The others in the wards were supportive, attentive, kind but less involved, like aunts or neighbors. In addition, between the wards there developed a kind of competition to see which could teach their young charges the most.

Skeels was aware of this situation when twelve of the thirteen transfers were made. In any event as the staff psychologist at both the institutions he saw to it that Stanford-Binet IQ measures were taken on the experimental children at an average age of fifteen months, two or three months before they were transferred from the orphanage. At that time the children in the experimental group had all tested in the mentally defective range with a median IQ of 65. When they were tested a second time, at a median age of thirty-seven months, their median IQ was 93 points, an increase in the median of 28 points. At that juncture, it was possible to place eleven of the thirteen experimental children in adoptive homes. These adopted children were tested again when they were almost six years of age and at that time their median IQ was 96 points which would indicate an overall gain in the median of 31 points.

Unfortunately, Skeels' follow-up study of these children as adults did not include an IQ test. However, the data show that the experimental children made an average adaptation. All but two were married; the average income was slightly above that for Iowa where most of them still lived; on the average they and their spouses graduated from high school; their occupations were slightly better than average; all who got married became parents and their twenty-eight children had a median IQ of 105.

As adults only one person in the contrast group married, had a good occupation and otherwise made what would be called a normal adaptation. He evidently responded, beginning at age six, to a special educational program that was introduced at the orphanage. The others, however, were extremely marginal people who had completed on the average three grades by the time they were adults. Five were still institutionalized and the others worked at the most menial occupations—doing dishes, cleaning up in a cafeteria, cleaning up yards, etc.

Clearly, then, Skeels' data support Jensen's threshold hypothesis. Those children who at an early age were taken out of the extremely debilitating environment developed normal IQ's and made normal adaptations. The comparison group that stayed in the debilitating environment of the orphanage experienced a decline in IQ and, with one exception previously noted, made defective or at best marginal adaptations as adults.

However, a second study was done by Skodak and Skeels (1949) involving the long term intellectual development of adopted children. As Skodak and Skeels observed, most adopted children apparently have very intense loving relationships with their foster parents who, because they want children so badly, spend an unusual amount of time talking with and teaching them. The result, as Skodak and Skeels' data amply indicate, their IQ's as well as their academic achievement are generally much higher than might be expected had the children been reared by their natural parents. The average IQ, 115 points at age thirteen, is approximately 20 points higher than the average IQ's of their natural mothers and of those children generally reared in homes where the father's occupations equaled those of their natural fathers. Evidently these adopted children generally benefited from very substantial transfer effects, and they were evidently conditioned to respond maximally to the conventional reinforcers used in schools.

Remember, according to the threshold hypothesis once a child experiences a learning environment in the normal range, he is supposed to develop to his full potential. Certainly the environment of homes established by mothers with an IQ of 95 and fathers whose occupations are in the two lowest categories of Edward's seven-point scale[4] are in the normal range, as are the environments produced by the families of adopted children. Yet when put in the latter homes, the adopted children developed IQ's that averaged 20 points higher than expected. Hence these data are counter to the threshold hypothesis.

Also, Bereiter and Engelmann (1966) have done a series of experiments which have consistently produced rather substantial shifts in IQ's in inner-city preschoolers, shifts which also run counter to Jensen's hypothesis. They designed a curriculum to help these children develop language as a medium for learning and for reasoning, in addition to reading and simple arithmetic. Reinforcement was limited to approval and disapproval, but the teaching process was designed so feedback to the children was both immediate and consistent or relatively so. In five experiments, Bereiter and Englemann have been successful in increasing individual Stanford-Binet IQ's by 9 points in a year's time.

Bereiter (1969) did another very interesting experiment. He decided to teach one class of preschoolers the items on the Stanford-Binet to see how much IQ could be inflated. To his surprise, the increment in this class was only 7 points on the Stanford–Binet and 7 points on the WPPSI IQ test which was used as a check for non-specific effects. This experiment is important because when taken in conjunction with the other experiments, it, too, suggests that the acquisition rate measured as IQ is largely a transfer effect of prior acquisitions of verbal language, reading and arithmetic abilities.

Our IQ experiments reported in Chapter 3 also included language training and some training in reading and arithmetic. In addition, we used token reinforcers with material backups which are substantially stronger than conditioned reinforcers alone; they support a much higher acquisition rate.

[4] These are the standard status categories developed for and used by the US Census.

In any event, the seven month MA (mental age) increments were substantially larger than those obtained by Bereiter: as may be recalled from Chapter 3, the net median increase in IQ was 15 points.

In general, then, the above studies are consistent with the theory that hereditary and environmental variables interact to influence the acquisition rates measured as IQ. Specifically, they suggest the following: (1) Measured IQ may be changed substantially by changing the quality of the children's learning environments. The net changes may range from 9 to 30 points. Furthermore, it is quite possible to induce a 15 point increase in the IQ's of black children and thus erase the usual IQ difference between blacks and whites. (2) The measured increases in IQ were obtained when children were put into an environment where the frequency of reinforcement for language acquisition (verbal and graphic) was substantially increased and where the strength of the reinforcers for language acquisition was increased. (3) The strength of the reinforcers for language acquisition was increased by adding material reinforcers to the conventional conditioned reinforcers and by conditioning the children to respond more intensely to the conventional conditioned reinforcers. (4) Finally, measured changes in IQ will be permanent if the related changes in the children's learning environments are permanent, but they will be transient if the related changes are transient. In other words, like other acquisition rates, those measured as IQ will stabilize or equilibrate at a level supported by the learning environment.

Hence, based on learning theory, we are suggesting an equilibrium theory of IQ which postulates a substantial interaction between environmental and hereditary variables in the determination of IQ. (5) Learning environments vary dramatically in their effectiveness: in the content of what is reinforced, in the strength of the reinforcers, in the immediacy and the consistency of reinforcement. In general, the more effective the learning environment, the higher the acquisition rate and if what is being acquired involves educing relations and correlates, i.e. verbal and graphic language, then mental age will increase at an increasing rate until that rate stabilizes or equilibrates at the level supported by the environment. (6) If one holds the learning environment constant, then individuals will vary with respect to IQ, mostly in relation to their hereditary capacity. (7) If it were possible to equate individuals on hereditary variables which determine IQ and to assign them to learning environments of variable effectiveness, their IQ would vary almost entirely in proportion to the effectiveness of the environment. (8) However, with most people heredity and environment interact to influence the acquisition rates that are measured as IQ. This means that both H and E variables influence the relation of the other to IQ and, therefore, as the experimental data reviewed have suggested, it is quite possible to manipulate the essential dimensions of learning environments and thus produce substantial changes in IQ.

CONCLUSION

We suggest that so many past attempts to increase IQ and to accelerate academic achievement have failed because the instructional environments were not designed to capitalize on the essential operating characteristics of the biological learning mechanisms. The changes in IQ and in the rate of academic achievement reported in this book were obtained simply because those essential variables were manipulated appropriately. In other words, these successes were built on a foundation of a more or less solid theory of how the environment and the hereditary variables interact to effect acquisition rates measured as IQ. This is not the only occasion in which it has been possible to change the values of both H and E rather markedly, as is conveniently noted by Jensen in the case of tuberculosis (1969).

At one time tuberculosis had a very high hereditability; the tuberculosis bacilli were extremely widespread throughout the population so the main factor in determining whether or not an individual contracted tuberculosis was not the probability of exposure (the environmental variable) but the individual's inherited physical resistance to such bacilli (the hereditary variable). Because of public health programs tuberculosis bacilli are now relatively rare, and differences in exposure (E) rather than physical predisposition (H) is the most important determinant of who contracts tuberculosis. In an analogous way, using the H and E variables that influence IQ, we may learn how to help many of those children who now grow up as mentally disadvantaged, more or less wards of society.

Even so, the data are not complete. There is some possibility that our equilibrium theory of intelligence could ultimately be rejected in favor of Jensen's threshold hypothesis. Even so, at this juncture the equilibrium theory stands as an attractive alternative. As Burt (1969) suggests, the data thus far do not seem to suggest that it is futile to try to improve IQ, even of so-called disadvantaged inner-city children. In fact, it seems that when inner-city children are placed in an appropriate learning environment with meaningful reinforcers for learning, with an appropriate curriculum which supplements language training in their home environment, they learn at a rate at least equal to or above the national norms.

A MATTER OF TASTE?

Not infrequently we encounter people who, although they are impressed with the results our teachers obtain, express an aversion for the idea of rewarding children for talking or for studying. "It's demeaning," they say, "to give children material rewards for doing something they should do anyway."

Perhaps, but we have a different perspective. It is hardly intelligent, hardly humane to ignore the operating characteristics of children's biological learning mechanisms, to design learning environments just on the basis of superstition or taste. It is also demeaning because such environments, if not pathogenic, are almost inevitably ill-suited to acculturative learning; children who work them never do as well as they might in a more powerful learning environment. If the design of children's physiology is such that they perform and learn more easily and at a maximal rate in an environment which can be worked for material reinforcers, then why not allow them such a learning environment? Why make it more difficult for them? Why deny them their potential development? We use material rewards with college and graduate students. To those with the best high school and undergraduate records, the reinforcers, although delayed, include tuition and a living allowance, "a free ride." And the professional scholars, the professors, are advanced in rank and paid in proportion to the amount and excellence of their scholarly work. Similarly, adults in all other fields of endeavor are paid, not always in proportion to the excellence of their performance, but generally so. Why? Because mankind found centuries ago that it is much more productive, efficient and humane to pay a man for the excellence of his work than to enslave him, forcing him to work to avoid pain of punishment with just an allowance of food and clothing.

Actually the ideal of study as its own reward is a survival of a notion that originally gained currency in the old world in various contexts. One context was the aristocracy. Only the nobility, and few others, were educated, not for practical reasons, but mainly to be dilettante scholars, to pursue their studies as a form of conspicuous leisure.

The fact is that dilettante scholars have seldom made substantial contributions to knowledge; those have generally been the work of professionals, who were paid in proportion to their scholarly excellence. In the modern world education has lost most of its decorative functions. In this age of expertise it provides the training required to earn a living.

The relationship between the education of family head and family income is shown in Figure 10.5. These data illustrate perhaps what everyone knows, that income increases with educational achievement. However, if the data are translated into lifetime earning differentials and lifetime tax differentials as they are for the data on white families, then a rather surprising result emerges. If, by one means or another educational achievement of the family head is extended four years (for example to twelve instead of eight years or to sixteen instead of twelve), the lifetime family earnings increase by about $100,000 and the lifetime taxes paid to the various governments increase by about $23,000. If by one means or another, educational achievement were increased eight years (for example from eight to sixteen years), lifetime earnings would increase by about $250,000 and taxes paid, by

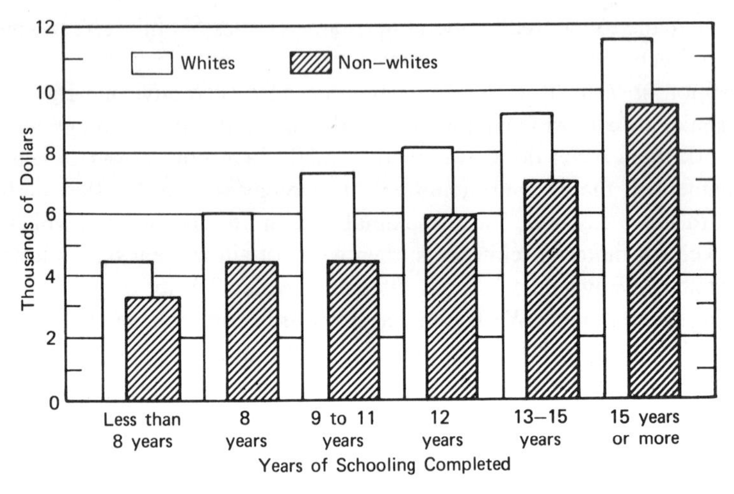

Figure 10.5. Median family income by years of school completed and color of Head. Source: Statistical Abstract of the United States, 1968, p. 327.

about $58,000. It should be noted that the above figures are conservative, as might be surmised from the assumptions used in the calculations (see footnote "a" to Table 10.5). Even so, as calculated the economic benefits

Table 10.5. Hypothetical Difference in Lifetime Income and Taxes if Higher Educational Level Had Been Achieved.[a]

	Hypothetical Education					
	8 Years		12 Years		16 Years or More	
Present Education	Income[b]	Taxes[b]	Income[b]	Taxes[b]	Income[b]	Taxes[b]
Less than 8 years	$74	$17	$169	$39	$325	$75
8 years	—	—	95	22	251	58
12 years	—	—	—	—	105	24

[a] Assumptions: 45 working and taxable years. 1966 income data for white families (Stat. Abstract of U. S., 1968, p. 327) which means figures exclude inflation and/or deflation, and productivity increases. Taxes are computed at 23 percent of income, the approximate figure found for all income classes except those with incomes in excess of $15,000 who pay 35 percent (Kolko, 1964). Economists include social security payments as taxes and lump all welfare receipts including social security benefits into one category, transfer payments. Transfer payments are constant across all family income levels, about $400 in 1960. The above figures do not include compensations for transfer payments, since that is a constant.

[b] Thousand dollar units.

of improving educational achievement are impressive. When added to the human benefits, they are convincing reasons why it is in society's interest to finance the research and development of educational achievement of the less able. A similar argument could be made for educational programs which turn psychotic or other behaviorally disabled persons into normally functioning adults. Only in that case the benefits would be substantially greater.

ONE LAST WORD

Nevertheless, the educational programs we have developed and reported here are not by any means finished products. We have reported our work, primarily so other investigators could start checking out our procedures and results in their own experimental classrooms and perhaps in the process improve upon what we have done. Even so, it is no longer necessary that inner-city children be schooled in a blackboard jungle and end up with cumulative deficits in academic achievement. It is no longer necessary that hyperaggressive boys disrupt classrooms for a few years only to be turned out on society as hostile failures. It is no longer necessary for autistic children, saddest of all, to tear up their families for a few years only to languish for the rest of their lives mutely vegetating in the back wards of mental hospitals.

Appendixes

APPENDIX A

The Mathematical Properties of Learning Curves

This appendix is included in this book for three specific reasons.[1] (1) The mathematical properties of learning curves are interesting and important in themselves. (2) In a mathematical analysis transfer and other such important effects can be understood in precise ways. (3) A mathematical analysis allows a rigorous comparison of our results with those obtained using automatic data taking devices and, thus, allows a crucial cross check on the adequacy of our measurement and other methodological procedures.

The word mathematics may scare away some readers. Even so, the writing is not difficult—although it does assume an understanding of basic algebra and basic analytic geometry, including logarithms.

ACQUISITION CURVES

Although one might never guess it from looking at the raw data, acquisition curves have precise mathematical properties. At least when the methodology of an experiment approximates, even roughly, the expected standards, acquisition data consistently approximate a power function.

These mathematical properties have been known for some time, and they apply to group as well as to individual acquisition curves. Examples of the former are given in Figures A.1 and A.2. The first of these is an organizational acquisition curve involving production rates during and after the startup of a side trimmer in a steel plant. Such acquisition curves are typical in all of the twenty industries which Baloff (1966) has studied.

Figure A.2 involves the acquisition curves of four-person groups of college students solving missing-symbol problems in communication network experiments (conducted by Robert L. Burgess, 1969, for his doctoral dissertation under the direction of the first author). Notice that the data in

[1] Hamblin took the major responsibility for writing this appendix.

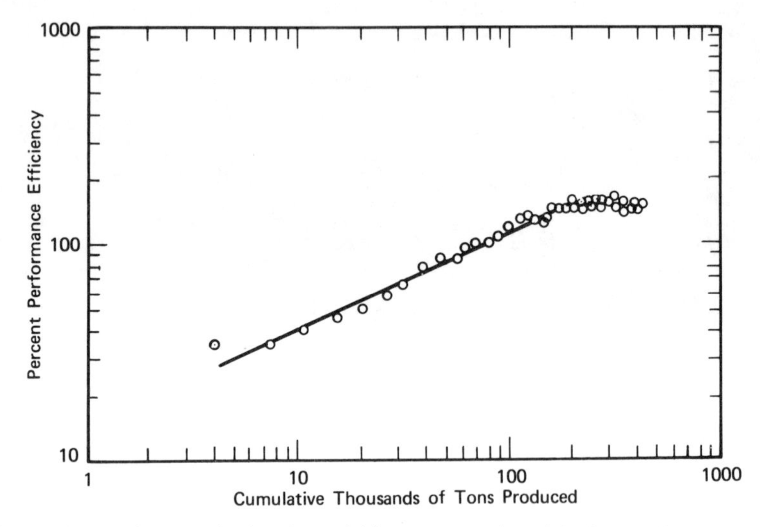

Figure A.1. An organizational acquisition curve on logarithmic coordinates generated during the startup of a side trimmer in a steel plant. The acquisition and final equilibrium phases are represented. (Adapted from Baloff, 1963.)

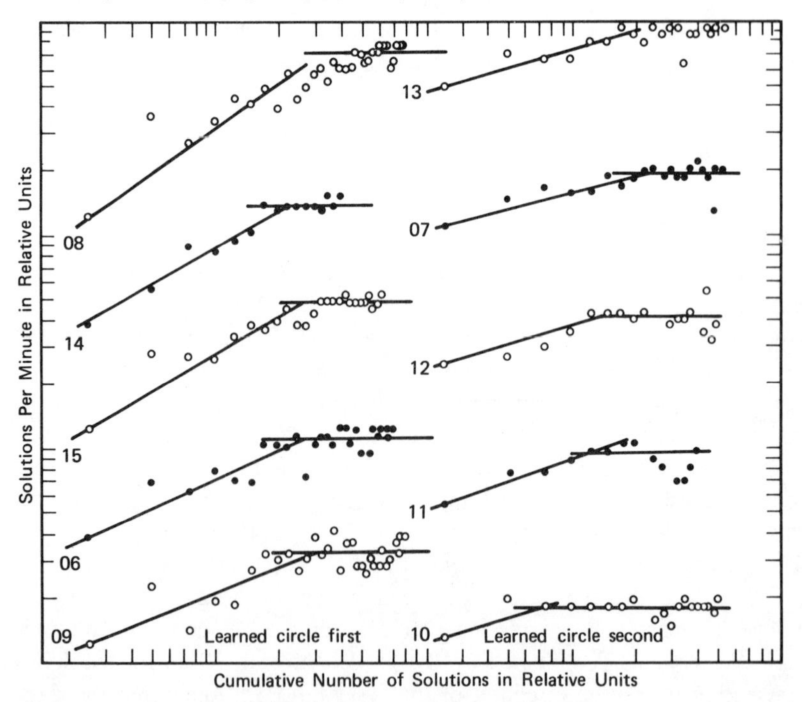

Figure A.2. Acquisition curves plotted on logarithmic coordinates using rate data generated by four-person groups in a communications network experiment by Burgess (1969). To position plots on the logarithmic coordinates, each set of data was multiplied by an appropriate constant (an allowable transformation for ratio scales). Hence the units are relative. Plot by Hamblin.

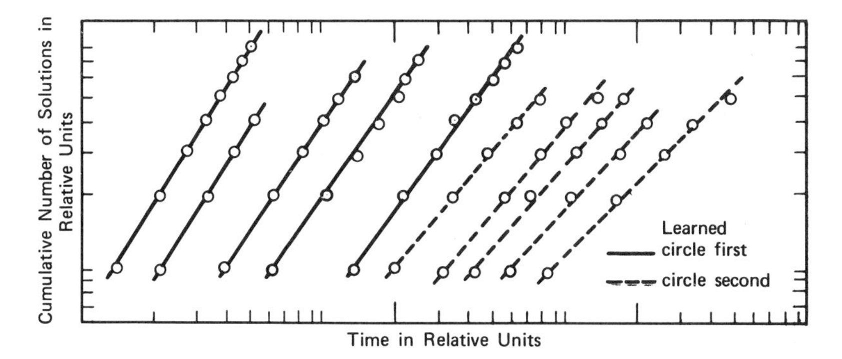

Figure A.3. Cumulative acquisition curves plotted on logarithmic coordinates using data generated by ten four-person groups in a cummunications network experiment by Burgess (1969). Data for each group was multiplied by an appropriate constant to position plots so all units are relative. Plot by Hamblin.

both of these instances are somewhat noisy. They do not fit the theoretical or expected function perfectly.

The fit is somewhat improved if the responses are measured accumulatively instead of as rates. The plots in Figure A.3 illustrate this for the same data shown in Figure A.2. The cumulative curves in this figure give a very close approximation to the theoretical or expected function. In these plots the noise is all but eliminated because cumulating data is a subtle way of averaging out random variations. Examples of individual cumulative curves plotted on logarithmic coordinates are given in Figure A.4. These were taken from a review article by J. C. Stevens and Savin (1962). A similar set of curves are plotted in Figure A.5 from data from our experiments presented in earlier chapters.

It is very interesting that acquisition curves take the same mathematical form both within and across species. The reader may have noted earlier that two of the learning curves in Figure A.4 were generated by animal subjects. Without looking at the legend, it is impossible to tell which curves are which. This invariance across species rules out the possibility that the shape of the acquisition curve in the human animal is a cultural artifact.

The invariance of the curve generated under controlled conditions, always a power function, suggests also that acquisition is a determined or automatic process not unlike the stimulus-response functions characteristic of the neuro-sensory human and animal systems. The accumulated research in neuro-physics, for example, shows that the frequency of neurons firing in sensory receptors and in the related cortical areas is determined, that is, increases automatically, as a power function of stimulus magnitude. Similarly in psychophysics, the magnitudes of sensations, as discovered by S. S. Stevens (1962), increase as a power function of the magnitude of their related stimuli. It appears that the acquisition mechanisms are similarly built to

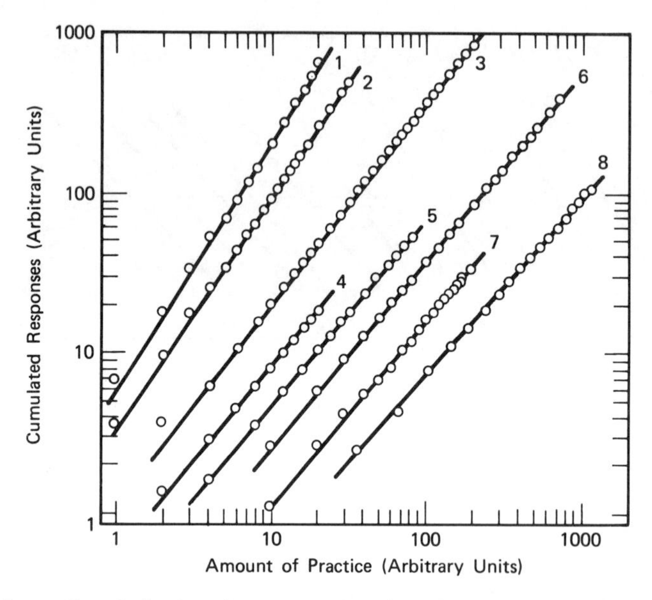

Figure A.4. Cumulative learning curves plotted on logarithmic coordinates. The table beneath the graph gives the equation of each curve, the nature of the variables measured, and the range of values plotted on the abscissa. In order to avoid crowding, a few points are omitted near the top of some of the functions. Otherwise all available data are plotted. (J. C. Stevens and H. B. Savin, 1962.)

Learning Task	Equation	Abscissa	Ordinate	No. Subjects	References
1. Nonsense syllables	$P = 5.7t^{1.56}$	Trials (1–20)	No. correct anticipations	40	Tsao (1948)
2. Pursuit Rotor	$P = 0.064t^{1.46}$	Minutes (1–31)	Minutes on target	25	Dore & Hilgard (1937)
3. Ball Tossing	$P = 0.0356t^{1.25}$	No. throws (200–20,000)	No. in target area	1	Braden (1924)
4. U-Maze	$P = 0.027t^{1.19}$	Trials (25–250)	No. correct responses	4 (rats)	Anderson (1937)
5. Coding Letters	$P = 16t^{1.18}$	Minutes (1–20)	No. letters	97	Gentry (1940)
6. Writing upside down	$P = 25t^{1.18}$	Minutes (1–70)	No. letters	45	Kientzle (1946)
7. Operant Extinction	$P = 3.47t^{1.17}$	Minutes (3–57)	Decrement in No. responses	1 (rat)	Catania (unpublished data)
8. Typesetting	$P = 46.4t^{1.10}$	Hours (12.7–1227)	No. ems set	50	Kelly & Carr (1924)

respond directly to reinforced practice so throughout acquisition the rate of the behavior being repetitively reinforced increases as a power function of cumulative practice or of acquisition time.

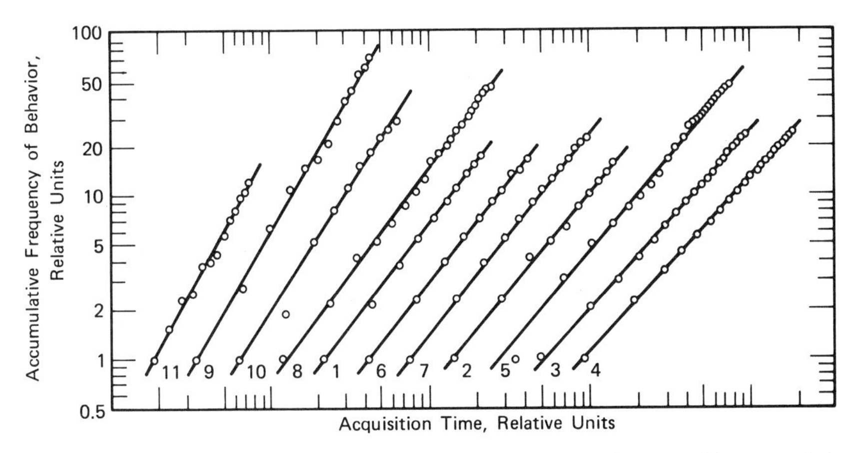

Figure A.5. Eleven acquisitions from experiments in earlier chapters with accumulative measures of behavior plotted on logarithmic coordinates by Acquisition Time. For the purposes of this presentation the curves were positioned arbitrarily using a procedure equivalent to multiplying the ratio scales of behavior and time by constants, allowable transformations which change neither the slope nor the relative fit of the data to the expected function.

Number	Source	Period	Data (B)	Equation
	Fig.			
1	2.5	C	Test items correct, tutored tasks	$B = 6.7T^{1.28}$
2	2.5	C	Time working in peer tutoring teams	$B = 16T^{1.20}$
3	5.4	B1	Studying, hyperactives, primary class	$B = 6.7T^{1.08}$
4	5.5	B1	Studying, hyperactives, intermediates	$B = 7.2T^{1.07}$
5	5.2	B1–C–B2	Cooperation, hyperaggressive preschoolers	$B = 7.7T^{1.17}$
6	5.1	A1	Aggression, hyperaggressive preschoolers	$B = 7.6T^{1.26}$
7	3.1	B1	Talking, inner city preschoolers	$B = 15T^{1.25}$
8	3.1	B2	Talking, inner city preschoolers	$B = 9T^{1.34}$
9	5.3	B2	Studying, hyperaggressive preschoolers	$B = 2.3T^{1.77}$
10	5.3	B3	Studying, hyperaggressive preschoolers	$B = 25T^{1.53}$
11	5.4	A1	Disruptions, hyperactive primary class	$B = 2.2T^{1.77}$

Not all of our experiments yielded data which when plotted resulted in the expected acquisition function. For example, the aforementioned data from the peer tutoring experiment with the "famous eight" do not, evidently because of inadequate experimental controls. The cumulative data for each of the three experimental groups are plotted on logarithmic coordinates in Figure A.6. Each of the three curves in that figure should have been straight lines, but only B's data yield the expected result. Evidently there was a basic midstream change in experimental conditions in A and C, possibly the termination of the conflicts between tutors and their pupils. However, we will never know because the tutoring was unobserved.

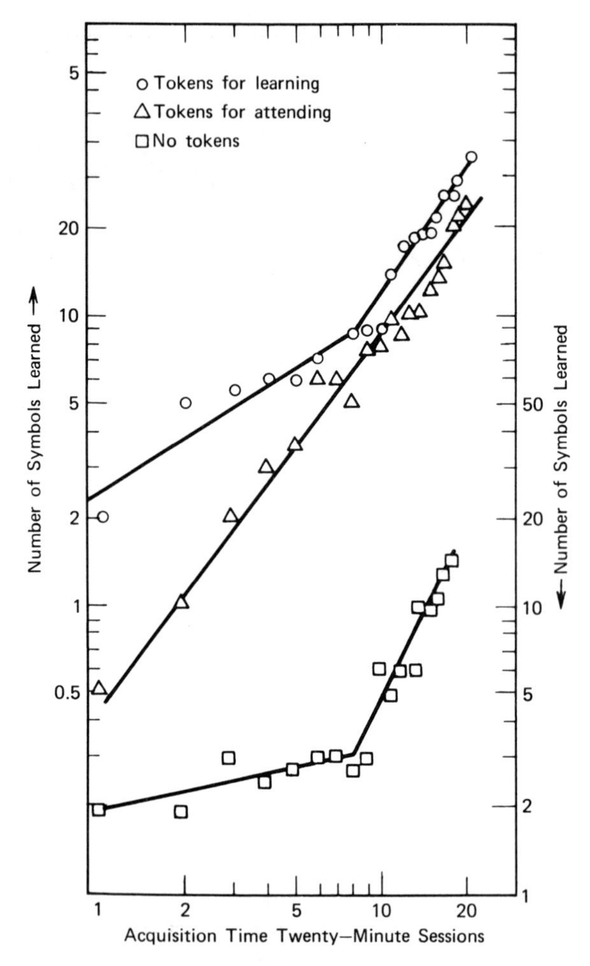

Figure A.6. Three cumulative acquisitions—number of symbols learned, "famous eight" —plotted on logarithmic coordinates. Original plot, Figure 3.6.

Also, to fit a function accurately it is necessary to have at least five and preferably seven data points. In some of our experiments, as noted in the last chapter, acquisition occurred immediately or nearly so, within one or two time periods. This seems to happen when the behavior being reinforced is already in the children's expertise repertoire so acquisition does not involve expertise learning, just contingency clarification which can occur rapidly. An example is the acquisition of studying in the B2 periods by the once hyperaggressive boys in the primary and intermediate classes, see Figures 5.4 and 5.5. They had already acquired the expertise requisite for studying during their respective B1 periods.

However, in almost all instances where acquisition did occur over several experimental sessions, the resulting plots do approximate the expected power function passably, if not well.

In Figure A.7 the studying data generated by the hyperactive boys in the primary and intermediate classes provide a good example, for introductory purposes. The data are less noisy than usual, and hence, give a rather good fit to the expected function.

The general equation which describes the acquisition lines in Figure A.7 is as follows:

$$B = c(T - T_0)^n$$

when B is a measure of the rate of the behavior being reinforced in each successive experimental session; T_0 a constant which may be thought of as the origin of acquisition time; T an accumulative measure of acquisition time usually in terms of experimental sessions; n, the exponent; and c, a multiplicative constant which will be referred to as the unity constant because of the way it is calculated.

T_0 is essential to determine before plotting the data. It is defined as the number of the session which marks the end of the initial equilibrium, just before the transition into acquisition takes place. The data in Figure A.7 were obtained from Figures 5.4 and 5.5, the B1 sessions. The transition into acquisition occurred in both instances during the 18th experimental

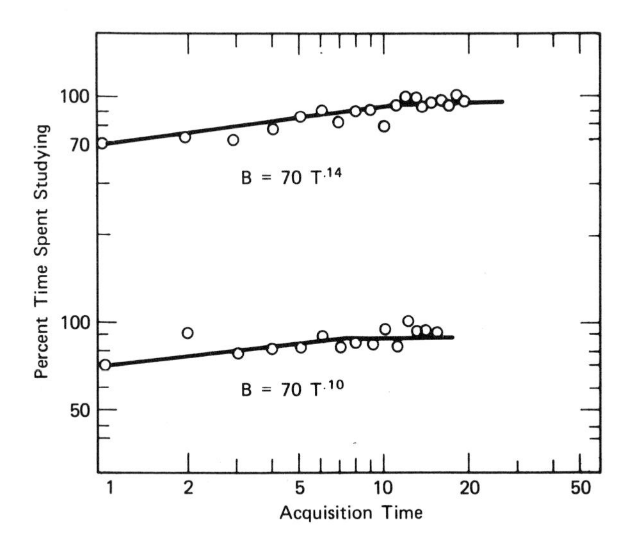

Figure A.7. Two acquisition series—percent time spent studying hyperactive primary and intermediate classes—plotted in logarithmic coordinates. Original plots, Figures 5.4 and 5.5, B1 conditions.

session, the session the contingencies were changed. Hence, T_0 is session 17 which in the corrected time measure $(T - T_0)$, makes session 18 equal to 1, in effect the first of the acquisition sessions. Thus, as suggested earlier, T_0 is an origin constant which turns a running measure of experimental time into a ratio measure of acquisition time.

The exponents, measured as the slope of the acquisition line, are in these examples .10 and .14. The unity constant c is the value of B on the acquisition line when $(T - T_0)$ equals one. In both of these examples, c happens to be .70. If the unity constant is standardized as a percentage of the final equilibrium, there turns out to be a very regular inverse curvilinear relationship between it and the acquisition exponent. In other words as the acquisition exponent increases in magnitude, the unity constant decreases in magnitude, at a decreasing rate. This is pictured in Figure A.8 for our acquisition data, some of it pictured in this appendix. A similar relationship was found by Baloff (1967) in his industrial acquisition data. There also appears to be a curvilinear relationship between the acquisition exponent and the number of sessions before final equilibrium. However, this relationship is weaker, the data being more noisy.

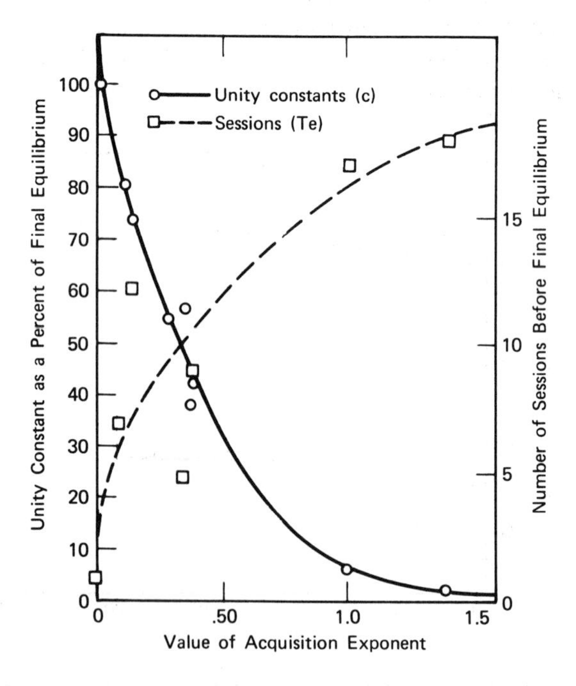

Figure A.8. Covariation of parameters in acquisition equation $B = c(T\text{-}T_0)^n$. Data are from several experiments.

The plots on logarithmic coordinates are useful for several reasons. For example, they are a convenient gauge of the adequacy of experimental methodology. It is rather surprising to find that the acquisition curves generated in our better controlled man-man learning environments are every bit as precise as those typically generated in man-machine learning environments where the measurement is mechanical, automatic and highly accurate. This is particularly true since none of the data takers, in fact, none of the experimenters had any idea that their data would be put to this kind of use.[2]

The Transfer Effect

The plots on logarithmic coordinates also highlight many of the properties of acquisition, particularly the exponents, unity constants and sessions until final equilibrium yield rather precise summary measures of acquisition rate. As an illustration, consider the logarithmic plots in Figure A.9. The exponents and the unity constants, of the two acquisition lines differ, as do the number of sessions until final equilibria. As suggested in the last chapter, if these acquisition curves were generated by two different persons, the one who generated the top one would be considered brighter. His unity constant is higher (.33 vs. .18), his exponent lower (.28 vs. .38) and his acquisition time shorter (9 vs. 13 sessions) all of which indicate superior acquisition.[3]

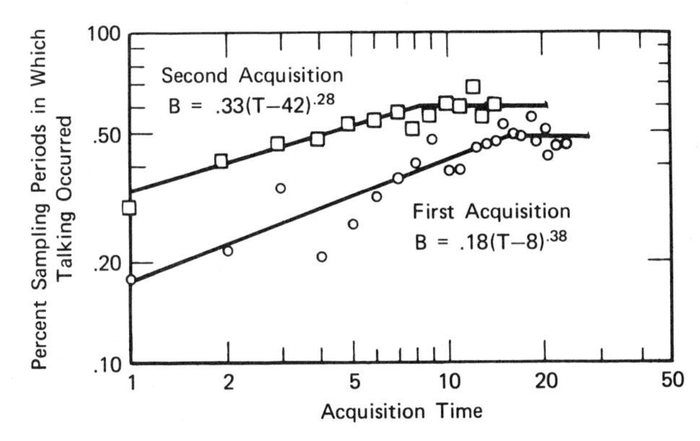

Figure A.9. First and second language acquisitions, four inner-city preschoolers, plotted on logarithmic coordinates. Original plots, Figure 3.1.

[2] These analyses were an afterthought of Hamblin as a way of bringing together in summary the results of the earlier chapters. It may be recalled Hamblin collaborated on most of the experiments. Although at the time he was certainly aware of the possibilities, he had not discussed, even considered this kind of analysis. These analyses, then, were post experimental. That the logarithmic plots fit the expected function as well as they do came as a surprise, albeit a pleasant one.

[3] The rule that smaller acquisition exponents involve faster acquisitions may seem contradictory at first but that in fact is what happens as may be noted in Figure A.10.

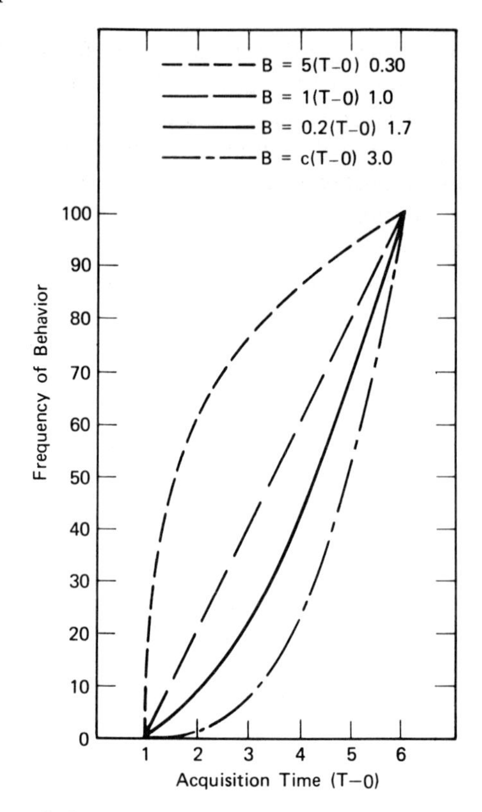

Figure A.10. Theoretical curves representing acquisition series with different exponents. Note: the smaller the exponent, the faster the acquisition of behavior.

By looking at the plots of the original data on linear coordinates in Figure 3.1 and in Figure 10.4, it is possible to see that this is in fact a correct inference—the upper plot does represent superior acquisition in every way. The rate of talking was higher at the outset, the acquisition curve was steeper, acquisition time shorter and the final equilibrium higher. However, in that figure it is quite obvious that the two acquisitions were by the same individuals, four inner-city preschoolers, in the B2 and B1 periods of our language acquisition experiment. In other words, as suggested in Chapter 10 the qualitatively better acquisition during B2 was evidently a transfer effect, the result of the prior acquisition which occurred during B1.

As may be noted in Table A.1, the second acquisition is characterized by a shorter latency to the new equilibrium (1.5 sessions vs. 9 sessions), a larger unity constant (a median behavioral rate which is 87 percent of the final equilibrium vs. 57 percent), and a smaller acquisition exponent (evidently a median near zero vs. a median of .35). These very consistent

Table A1. Transfer-of-Learning Effects: Acquisition—Hyperaggressive Boys.

	First Acquisition				Second Acquisition			
New	Experimental Period	Latency, New Equilibrium	Unity Constant %	Acquisition Exponent	Experimental Period	Latency, New Equilibrium	Unity Constant %	Acquisition Exponent
Preschoolers								
Studying	B1-C-B2	17 sessions	7%	1.0	B3	3 sessions	28%	—
Cooperation	B1-C-B2	9 sessions	43	.38	B3	2 sessions	61	—
Aggression	A1	5 sessions	57	.35	A2	1 session	100	—
Primary Class								
Studying	B1	12 sessions	74	.14	B2	1 session	100	—
Disruptions	A1	18 sessions	2	1.40	A2	1 session	100	—
Intermediate Class								
Studying	B1	7 sessions	81	.10	B2	2 sessions	82	—
Disruptions	A1	1 session	100		A2	3 sessions	87	—
Median		9 sessions	57%	.35		1.5 sessions	87%	less than .10[a]

[a] When acquisition occurs in fewer than five sessions it is inappropriate to plot the data and determine an acquisition exponent. However, in such instances the exponent approaches zero, the asymptote. Hence, the designation "less than .10."

differences combine to show how the transfer of earlier acquisitions can effect the rate of subsequent acquisitions in a substantial way.

The Strength of the Reinforcers

Although most of our experimental effort in this book has been designed to show the effect of increasing and decreasing the strength of reinforcers, we have precious little data to show the effect on rate of acquisition, *per se*. In most instances where weak reinforcers were used, a low level equilibrium rather than a slow acquisition resulted. There was one exception: the cooperation data for the hyperaggressive preschoolers (Figure 5.2). During A1, the teacher's approval was apparently enough of a reinforcer for these boys to enable them to acquire a cooperative pattern. The data, while noisy, when plotted on logarithmic coordinates (Figure A.11) suggest an acquisition exponent circa .56. During the B1-C-B2 periods, cooperation continued to be repetitively reinforced with the teacher's approval and, in addition, with tokens and material backups. Hence, the reinforcers for cooperation were stronger during B1-C-B2 than during A1. The acquisition plot of the B1-C-B2 cooperation data is also given on logarithmic coordinates in Figure A.11; these data, while again noisy, nevertheless give an exponent circa .38. Therefore, the data suggest the principle that the stronger the reinforcer, the faster the acquisition rate as indicated by the smaller acquisition exponent.

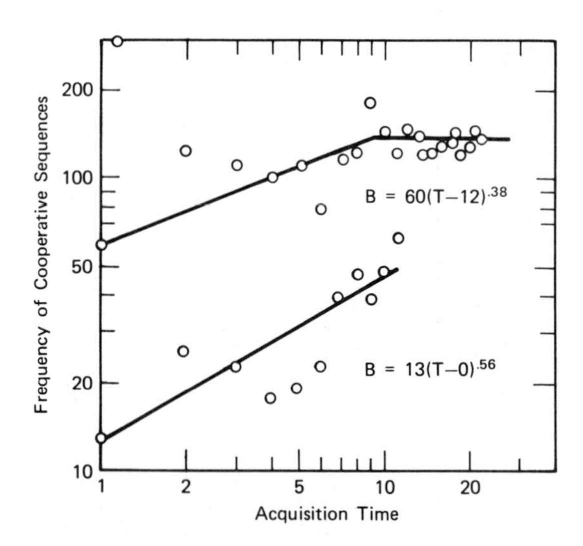

Figure A.11. Two acquisition series—frequency of cooperative sequences with approval, tokens, and material backups as reinforcers (top plot, B1-A2) and with just approval as a reinforcer (bottom plot, A1)—plotted on logarithmic coordinates. Original plots, Figure 5.2, hyperaggressive preschoolers.

The Social Nature of the Acquisition Data

As noted, all of our data were generated in social or man-man learning environments. Thus the acquisition curves generated in this research are each evidently the function of a compromise between the two parties of an instructional exchange, a child or children on the one hand and tutor or teacher on the other.

This is illustrated in the acquisition plot in Figure A.12 where the freqency of the criterion response of the child is plotted in concert with the reinforcing response of the teacher. Note that the teacher's response rate lagged at times behind that of the child, indicating perhaps that she was allowing the child to pace the exchange.

However, the picture is further elaborated by the data in Figure A.13. Here, the frequency with which the mother makes a request, i.e. signals an exchange, is plotted in concert with the child's response. In this case, the child's response pattern lags behind the mother's. These data suggest, then, that both parties to the exchange experience acquisition: the child acquires the expertise involved in his criterion response, and the mother acquires the ability to manage an exchange, if not generally, then with her particular child. Even so, most of the variance in acquisition curves, perhaps 90 percent, is generally a function of the child's behavior. At least it should be if the exchange is run well, for the better acquisition environments, mechanical or social, are apparently self-pacing.

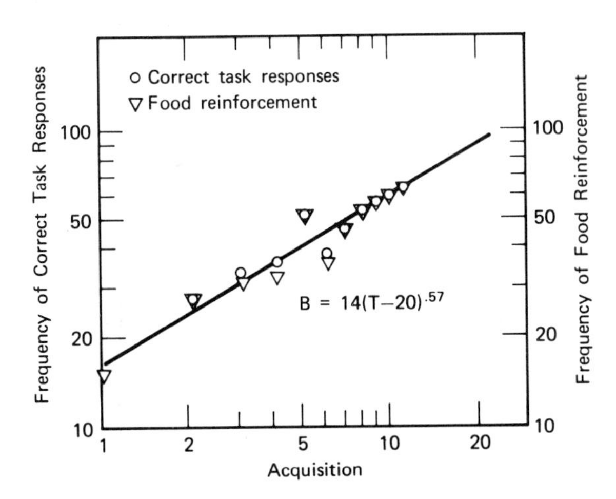

Figure A.12. Two acquisition series—frequency of correct task responses and frequency of food reinforcement, by an autistic boy and his mother—plotted on logarithmic coordinates.

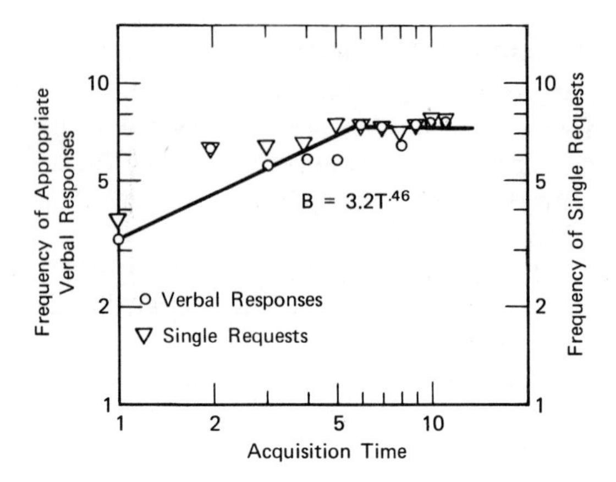

Figure A.13. Acquisition series—frequency of appropriate verbal responses and frequency of single requests, by an autistic child and his mother—plotted on logarithmic coordinates.

Contingency Learning

Contingency learning seems to take place via discovery, imitation and instruction. The contingency learning involved earlier, in Figure A.9, occurred primarily via peer imitation. The teacher, when a child did not know the answer to a query, generally called upon another child, either from within or outside the group, who did know the answer. The data in Figure A.14 also involved the learning of verbal contingencies via imitations; the data were generated by an autistic child. The symbolic contingency learning involved in Figure A.15 occurred as a result of instruction. These are the

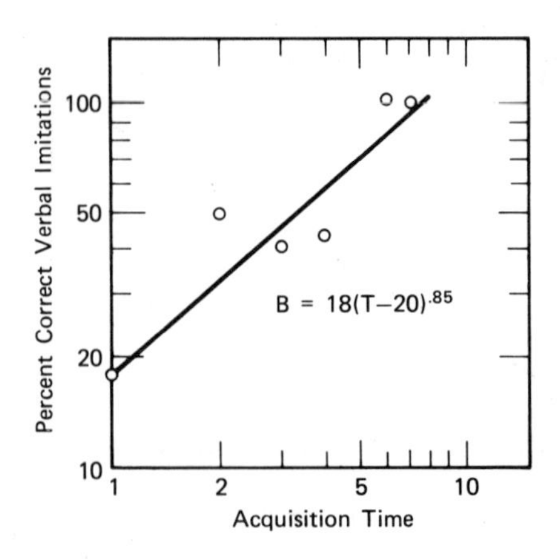

Figure A.14. Acquisition of verbal imitation by a mute autistic boy. Original data, Figure 8.7.

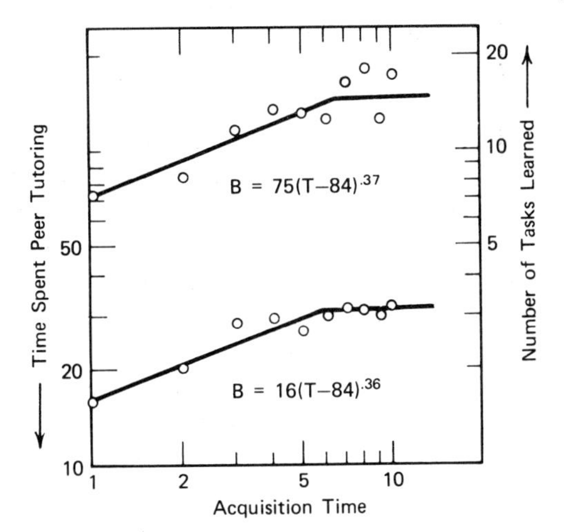

Figure A.15. Two simultaneous acquisition series, time spent peer tutoring and number of tasks learned, Webster preschoolers—plotted on logarithmic coordinates. Original plot, Figure 2.5, condition C.

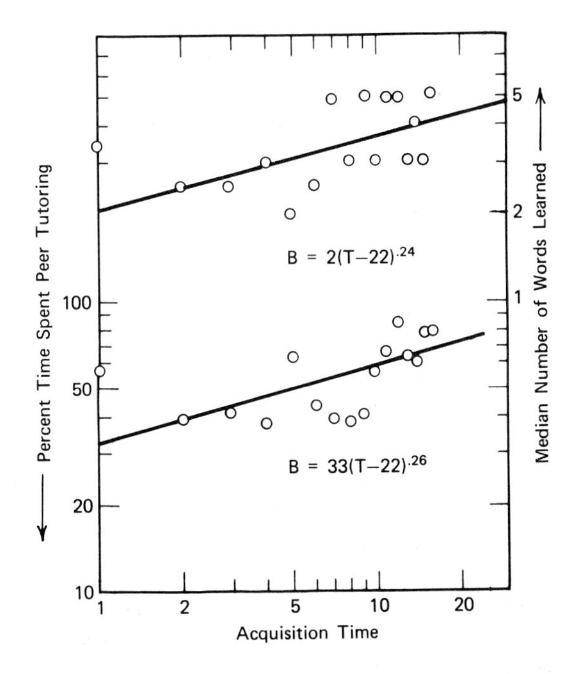

Figure A.16. Two simultaneous acquisition series—percent time spent peer tutoring and median number of words learned, Washington University preschoolers—plotted on logarithmic coordinates. Original plots, Figures 2.2 and 2.3.

data generated by the Webster preschoolers who were being tutored by their peers. In this instance they were told the contingencies and were reinforced by their peers in subsequent repetitive presentations when they demonstrated they knew, at criterion level, the contingencies involved. The tasks, it will be recalled, involved mostly reading and arithmetic contingencies. These data are from evidently well-controlled experiments; they and the other plot in the figure (A.15) incidentally illustrate the covariation of reinforced practice and learning to criterion. The acquisition exponents are nearly identical (.36 vs. .37), the unity constants are nearly identical (when standardized as a percentage of the final equilibrium both are about 50 percent); and the number of sessions to final equilibrium are the same (6 in each case). This result was obtained because in repetitively reinforcing contingency learning we indirectly reinforced the component behavior, that is working and tutoring. A similar result apparently obtains with data from the Washington University Preschool in Figure A.16. However, the experiment was evidentally so ill-controlled, the data so noisy, that the interpretation suggested in the figure is problematic.

IN SUMMARY

Galileo, the first to do mathematical experiments, observed that the secret relationships of variables in nature are decodable into the language of mathematics. We have seen in this appendix that acquisition curves may be described rather accurately as power functions; there seem to be several kinds, some involving rate data, some involving cumulative data, and the latter data give a better fit to the theoretical function. However, the rate data picture the equilibria which obtain after acquisition. For that reason they were analyzed here.

The equations which describe acquisition were then noted, and variables which are related to the parameters of the acquisition equations were then detailed with illustrative data.

Although the presentation may be technical for the average social, behavioral science reader, what really happens in transfer and other learning effects appears to be measurable only in the context of an appropriate mathematical analysis. Admittedly, it is costly to learn enough mathematics to become literate, that is to be able to read and write mathematics as a theoretical language. Yet mathematics is such a superior way to characterize relationships among variables that those who really care about understanding the operating characteristics of the biological learning mechanisms will be quite willing to pay the price.

APPENDIX B

References

Aarons, A. C., Gordon, B. Y., & Stewart, W. A. *Linguistic-cultural differences and American education.* North Miami Beach, Fla.: Florida FL Reporter, 1969.

Anderson, A. C. The effect of equalizing reward upon the breakdown of a discrimination habit, and its bearing upon reminiscence. *Journal of Comparative Psychology,* 1937, *23,* 421–437.

Ayllon, T., & Azrin, N. *Token economy: A motivational system for therapy and rehabilitation.* New York: Appleton-Century-Crofts, 1968.

Azrin, N. H., Hake, D.F., & Hutchinson, R. R. Elicitation of aggression by a physical blow. *Journal of the Experimental Analysis of Behavior,* 1965, *8*(1), 55–77.

Azrin, N. H., Hutchinson, R. R., & Hake, D. F. Pain-induced fighting in the squirrel monkey. *Journal of the Experimental Analysis of Behavior,* 1963, *6*(4), 620.

Azrin, N. H., Hutchinson, R. R., & Sallery, R. D. Pain-aggression toward inanimate objects. *Journal of the Experimental Analysis of Behavior,* 1964, *7*(3), 223–228.

Azrin, N. H., Ulrich, R. E., Hutchinson, R. R., & Norman, D. G. Effect of shock duration on shock-induced fighting. *Journal of the Experimental Analysis of Behavior,* 1964, *7*(1), 9–11.

Baloff, N. *Manufacturing startup: A model.* (Doctoral dissertation, Stanford University) Ann Arbor, Michigan: University Microfilms, 1963. No. 64–5570.

Baloff, N. Startups in machine-intensive production systems. *Journal of Industrial Engineering,* 1966, *17,* 25–31.

Baloff, N. Estimating the parameters of the startup model: An empirical approach. *Journal of Industrial Engineering,* 1967, *18,* 248–253.

Bandura, A. *Principles of behavior modification.* New York: Holt, Rinehart, & Winston, 1969.

Bandura, A., & Walters, R. H. *Social learning and personality development.* New York: Holt, Rinehart, & Winston, 1963.

Baruch, D. W. *New ways in discipline.* New York: McGraw-Hill, 1949.

Becker, W. C., Thomas, D. R., & Carnine, D. *Reducing behavior problems: An operant conditioning guide for teachers.* Urbana, Illinois: Educational Resources Information Center on Early Childhood Education, 1969.

Bereiter, C. The future of individual differences. *Harvard Educational Review,* 1969, *39,* 310–318.

Bereiter, C., & Engelmann, S. *Teaching disadvantaged children in the preschool.* New Jersey: Prentice-Hall, 1966.

Bernstein, B. Social class, linguistic codes and grammatical elements. *Language and Speech,* 1962, *5,* 221–240.

Bernstein, B. Elaborated and restricted codes: Their social origin and some consequences. *American Anthropologist,* 1964, *66,* 1–34.

Bettelheim, B. *The empty fortress: Infantile autism and the birth of the self.* New York: Free Press, 1967.

Bijou, S. W., & Baer, D. M. *Child development: A systematic and empirical theory.* New York: Appleton-Century-Crofts, 1961.

Birnbrauer, J., Bijou, S., Wolf, M., & Kidder, J. Programmed instruction in the classroom. In L. Ullmann & L. Krasner (Eds.), *Case studies in behavior modification.* New York: Holt, Rinehart, & Winston, 1965. Pp. 358–363.

Braden, S. R. An extensive experiment in motor learning and relearning. *Journal of Educational Psychology,* 1924, *15,* 313–315.

Burgess, R. L. *Communication networks, behavioral consequences and group learning.* (Doctoral dissertation, Washington University) Ann Arbor, Michigan: University Microfilms, 1969. No. 69–15, 217.

Burgess, R. L., & Akers, R. L. A differential association-reinforcement theory of criminal behavior. *Social Problems,* 1966, *14*(2), 128–147.

Burt, C. Intelligence and heredity. *The New Scientist,* 1969, *42,* 226–228.

Carlson, C. F. A neurological model of early infantile autism and its therapeutic implications. Paper presented at the APA Symposium on Early Infantile Autism, Columbia, Missouri, 1967.

Catania, A. (unpublished data). Cited in J. C. Stevens & H. B. Savin. On the form of learning curves. *Journal of the Experimental Analysis of Behavior,* 1962, *5*(1), 15–18.

Cheyney, A. B. *Teaching culturally disadvantaged in the elementary school.* Columbus, Ohio: Merrill, 1967.

Clark, K. *Youth in the ghetto. A study of the consequences of powerlessness and a blueprint for change.* New York: Harlem Youth Opportunities Unlimited, Inc., 1958.

Clark, K. *Dark ghetto: Dilemma of social power.* New York: Harper & Row, 1965.

Clark, K., & Parsons, T. (Eds.), *The Negro American.* Boston: Houghton-Mifflin, 1966.

Cohn, W. On the language of lower class children. *The School Review,* 1959, *67*(4), 435–440.

Cooley, C. H. *Social organization.* New York: Schocken Books, Inc., 1962.

Coleman, J. S. et al. *Equality of educational opportunity.* Washington, D.C.: U. S. Government Printing Office, OE38001, 1966.

Cruze, W. W. Maturation and learning in chicks. *Journal of Comparative Psychology,* 1935, *19,* 371–409.

Cruze, W. W. Maturity and learning ability. *Psychological Monographs,* 1938, *50,* 49–65.

Dehn, J. *An investigation of the development and maintenance of the negative behavior of autistic children.* (Doctoral dissertation, Washington University), 1969.

Deutsch, M. *The disadvantaged child.* New York: Basic Books, 1967.

Diederich, P. B. Pitfalls in the measurement of gains in achievement. *The School Review,* 1956, *64,* 59–63.

Dollard, J., Doob, L. W., Miller, N. E., Mowrer, O. H., & Sears, R. R. *Frustration and aggression.* New Haven: Yale University Press, 1939.

Dore, L. R., & Hilgard, E. R. Spaced practice and the maturation hypothesis. *Journal of Psychology,* 1937, *4,* 245–259.

Downing, J. A. *The initial teaching alphabet reading experiment.* Chicago: Scott, Foresman, 1965.

Dressel, P. L., & Mayhew, L. B. *Cooperative study of evaluation in general education.* Dubuque, Iowa: W. C. Brown, 1954.

Duncan, O. D. Is the intelligence of the general population declining? *American Sociological Review,* 1952, *17,* 401–407.

Duncan, O. D., Featherman, D. L., & Duncan, B. Socioeconomic background and occupational achievement: Extensions of a basic model. Final Report, Project No. 5-0074 (EO-191) U. S. Department of Health, Education, and Welfare, Office of Education, Bureau of Research, May, 1968.

Durkin, D. *Children who read early.* New York: Teachers College Press, 1966.

Eisenberg, L. The autistic child in adolescence. *American Journal of Psychiatry,* 1956, *112,* 607–612.

Erikson, E. H. *Childhood and society.* New York: Norton, 1950.

Erikson, E. H. *Identity, youth and crisis.* New York: Norton, 1968.

Eysenck, H. J. The effects of psychotherapy. *International Journal of Psychiatry,* 1965, *1,* 97–142.

Eysenck, H. J. New ways in psychotherapy. *Psychology Today*, 1967, *1*(2), 39–47.

Ferritor, D. *Modifying interaction patterns: An experimental training program for parents of autistic children.* (Doctoral dissertation, Washington University) Ann Arbor, Michigan: University Microfilms, 1969. No. 69–22, 526.

Ferster, C. B., & Skinner, B. F. *Schedules of reinforcement.* New York: Appleton-Century-Crofts, 1957.

Fox, D. J. *Expansion of the more effective schools program.* New York: Center for Urban Education, 1967.

Fox, D. J. A reply to the critics. *The Urban Review*, 1968, *2*(6), 27–34.

Freud, S. *Complete works.* New York: Macmillan, 1964. 24 vols.

Gates, A. I. The necessary mental age for beginning reading. *Elementary School Journal*, 1937, *37*, 497–508.

Gates, A. I., & Bond, G. L. Reading readiness: A study of factors determining success and failure in beginning reading. *Teachers College Record*, 1936, *37*, 679–685.

Gentry, J. R. Immediate effects of interpolated rest periods on learning performance. *Teachers College Contributions to Education*, 1940, (799).

Gesell, A. L., & Amatruda, C. S. *The embryology of behavior: The beginnings of the human mind.* New York: Harper, 1945.

Gesell, A. L. *Infant development; The embryology of early human behavior.* New York: Harper, 1952.

Gesell, A. L., Thompson, H. & Amatruda, C. S. *The psychology of early growth.* New York: Macmillan, 1938.

Goffman, E. *The presentation of self in everyday life.* Garden City, New York: Doubleday, 1959.

Goffman, E. *Asylums.* Garden City, New York: Doubleday, 1961.

Hamblin, J. A. *Peer tutoring, token exchange effect on reading.* Unpublished doctoral dissertation, Saint Louis University, 1970.

Hamblin, R. L., Bridger, D. A., Day, R. C., & Yancey, W. L. The interference-aggression law? *Sociometry*, 1963, *26*(2), 190–216.

Hamblin, R. L., Buckholdt, D., Bushell, D., Ellis, D., & Ferritor, D. Changing the game from "get the teacher" to "learn." *Trans-action*, 1969, *6*(3), 20–31.

Hanson, H. M. Effects of discrimination training on stimulus generalization. *Journal of Experimental Psychology*, 1959, *58*, 321–334.

Harlow, H. F., & Harlow, M. K. The affectional systems. In A. M. Schrier et al. (Eds.), *Behavior of nonhuman primates.* New York: Academic Press, 1965. Pp. 287–333.

Hays, W. L. *Statistics for psychologists.* New York: Holt, Rinehart, & Winston, 1963.

Hebb, D. O. *The organization of behavior: A neuropsychological theory.* New York: Wiley, 1949.

Hebb, D. O., & Williams, K. A method of rating animal intelligence. *Journal of General Psychology*, 1946, *34*, 59–65.

Henry, J. The natural history of the education of the deprived Negro child. Second Quarterly Report, Washington University, Contract No. OE6-2771, Department of Health, Education, and Welfare, 1967.

Holland, J. G., & Skinner, B. F. *The analysis of behavior.* New York: McGraw-Hill, 1961.

Homans, G. C. *Social behavior: Its elementary forms.* New York: Harcourt, Brace, & World, 1961.

Hunt, J. McV. *Intelligence and experience.* New York: Ronald Press, 1961.

Hunt, J. McV. The psychological basis for using preschool enrichment as an antidote for cultural deprivation. *Merrill-Palmer Quarterly*, 1964, *10*, 209–248.

Hurlock, E. B. *Child development.* (4th ed.) New York: McGraw-Hill, 1964.

I. R. C. D. Bulletin. *A Bi-Monthly Publication from the Information Retrieval Center on the Disadvantaged*, 1965, *1*, 5.

Jaquith, J. R. *Alphabet and speech: A study of the relations between graphic and phonological symbolism.* (Doctoral dissertation, Indiana University) Ann Arbor, Michigan: University Microfilms, 1968. No. 69–18, 695.

Jensen, A. R. Learning abilities of Mexican-American and Anglo-American children. *California Journal of Educational Research*, 1961, *12*, 147–159.

Jensen, A. R. Learning ability in retarded, average, and gifted children. *Merrill Palmer Quarterly*, 1963, *9*(2), 123–140.

Jensen, A. R. The culturally disadvantaged: Psychological and educational aspects. *Educational Research Bulletin*, 1967, *10*(1), 4–20.

Jensen, A. R. How to boost IQ and scholastic achievement. *Harvard Educational Review*, 1969, *39*, 1–12.

John, V. P. The intellectual development of slum children: Some preliminary findings. *American Journal of Orthopsychiatry*, 1963, *33*, 813–822.

Kallmann, F. J. The genetic theory of schizophrenia; an analysis of 691 schizophrenic twin-index families. *American Journal of Psychiatry*, 1946, *103*, 309–322.

Kanner, L. Autistic disturbances of affective contact. *Nervous Child*, 1943, *2*, 217–250.

Kanner, L. Early infantile autism. *Journal of Pediatrics*, 1944, *25*, 211–217.

Kelley, C. M., & Carr, H. A. The curve of learning in typesetting. *Journal of Experimental Psychology*, 1924, *7*, 447–456.

Kety, S. S. Biochemical theories of schizophrenia. *Science*, 1959, *129*, 1528–1532, 1590–1596.

Kientzle, M. J. Properties of learning curves under varied distributions of practice. *Journal of Experimental Psychology*, 1946, *36*, 187–211.

Kolko, G. *Wealth and power in America.* New York: Praeger, 1962.

Kozloff, M. Parents' introduction to behavior therapy. Unpublished internal document, CEMREL, St. Louis, 1968.

Kozloff, M. *Social and behavioral change in families of autistic children.* (Doctoral dissertation, Washington University) Ann Arbor, Michigan: University Microfilms, 1969. No. 70–10, 961.

Krech, D. Psychoneurobiochemeducation. *Phi Delta Kappan*, 1969, *50*(7), 370–375.

Kuo, Z. Y. The influence of embryonic movements upon the behavior after hatching. *Journal of Comparative Psychology*, 1932, *14*, 109–122.

Levitt, E. E. Psychotherapy with children: A further evaluation. *Behavior Research and Therapy*, 1963, *1*(1), 45–51.

Lewis, W. W. Continuity and intervention in emotional disturbance: A review. *Exceptional Children*, 1965, *31*(9), 465–475.

Lorenz, K. *On aggression.* New York: Harcourt, Brace, & World, 1966.

Lovaas, O. I. A behavior therapy approach to treatment of childhood schizophrenia. *Minnesota Symposia on Childhood Psychosis*, 1967.

Lovaas, O. I. A program for the establishment of speech in psychotic children. In H. N. Sloane, Jr. & B. D. MacAulay, *Operant procedures in remedial speech and language training*. Boston: Houghton-Mifflin, 1968. Pp. 125–154.

Lovaas, O. I., Berberich, J., Perloff, B., & Schaeffer, B. Acquisition of imitative speech in schizophrenic children. *Science*, 1966, *151*, 705–707.

Lovaas, O. I., Freitag, G., Gold, V. J., & Kassorla, I. C. Experimental studies in childhood schizophrenia: Analysis of self-destructive behavior. *Journal of Experimental Child Psychology*, 1965, *2*(1), 67–84, *2*(2), 108–120.

Lovaas, O. I., Freitag, G., Kinder, M., Rubenstein, B., Schaeffer, B., & Simmons, J. Establishment of social reinforcers in two schizophrenic children on the basis of food. *Journal of Experimental Child Psychology*, 1966, *4*(2), 109–125.

Lovaas, O. I., Schaeffer, B., & Simmons, J. Q. Building social behavior in autistic children by use of electric shock. *Journal of Experimental Research and Personality*, 1965, *1*(2), 99–109.

Madsen, C. H., Jr., Becker, W. C., Thomas, D. R., Koser, L., & Plager, E. An analysis of the reinforcing function of "sitdown" commands. In R. K. Parker (Ed.), *Readings in educational psychology*. Boston: Allyn and Bacon, 1968. Pp. 265–278.

Maier, N. R. F. *Frustration: The study of behavior without a goal.* Ann Arbor: University of Michigan Press, 1961.

Maltzman, I. On the training of originality. *Psychological Review*, 1960, *67*(4), 229–242.

Maltzman, I., Simon, S., Raskin, D., & Licht, L. Experimental studies in the training of originality. *Psychological Monographs; General and Applied*, 1960, *74*(6), whole #493.

Mead, G. H. *Mind, self, and society: From the standpoint of a social behavorist.* Chicago: University of Chicago Press, 1934.

Mead, G. H. *On social psychology: Selected papers.* Chicago: University of Chicago Press, 1964.

Moore, O. K., & Anderson, A. R. The responsive environments project. In R. D. Hess & R. M. Baer (Eds.), *Early education.* Chicago: Aldine, 1968. Pp. 171–190.

Morphett, M. V., & Washburne, C. W. When should children begin to read? *Elementary School Journal*, 1931, *31*, 496–503.

Neill, A. S. *Summerhill.* New York: Hart, 1960.

Newton, E. S. Verbal destitution: The pivotal barrier to learning. *Journal of Negro Education*, 1960, *24*, 497–499.

Patterson, G. R., & Gullion, M. E. *Living with children: New methods for parents and teachers.* Champaign, Ill.: Research Press, 1968.

Pavlov, I. P. *Conditioned reflexes.* New York: Dover Publications, 1960.

Pfeiffer, C. A. *Teaching preschoolers complex skills using a programmed exchange.* (Doctoral dissertation, Washington University) 1969.

Piaget, J. *The language and thought of the child.* New York: Harcourt Brace, 1926.

Piaget, J. & others. *Judgment and reasoning in the child.* New York: Harcourt Brace, 1928.

Piaget, J. *The child's conception of physical causality.* New York: Harcourt Brace, 1930.

Piaget, J. *The moral judgment of the child.* Glencoe, Ill.: Free Press, 1948.

Piaget, J. *The origins of intelligence in children.* New York: International Universities Press, 1952.

Pitman, I. J. Learning to read: An experiment. *Journal of Royal Society of Arts*, 1961, *109*, 149–180.

Pryor, K. Behavior modification: The porpoise caper. *Psychology Today*, 1969, *3*(7), 259.

Redl, F., & Wineman, D. *The aggressive child.* New York: Free Press, 1957.

Reese, E. P. *Analysis of human operant behavior*, Dubuque, Iowa: W. C. Brown, 1966.

Riesen, A. H. Plasticity of behavior: Psychological aspects. In H. F. Harlow & C. S. Woolsey (Eds.), *Biological and biochemical bases of behavior.* Madison: University of Wisconsin Press, 1959. Pp. 425–450.

Rimland, B. *Infantile autism: The syndrome and its implications for a neural theory of behavior.* New York: Appleton-Century-Crofts, 1964.

Risley, T. R. The effects and side effects of punishing the autistic behaviors of a deviant child. *Journal of Applied Behavior Analysis*, 1968, *1*, 21–35.

Risley, T. R., & Wolf, M. M. Experimental manipulation of autistic behavior and generalization into the home. In R. Ulrich, T. Stachnik, & J. Mabry (Eds.), *Control of human behavior.* Glenview: Scott, Foresman, 1966. Pp. 193–199.

Risley, T. R., & Wolf, M. M. Establishing functional speech in echolalic children. *Behavior Research and Therapy*, 1967, *5*(2), 73–88.

Risley, T., Wolf, M., & Mees, H. Application of operant conditioning procedures to the behavior problems of an autistic child. In R. Ulrich, T. Stachnik, & J. Mabry (Eds.), *Control of human behavior.* Glenview: Scott, Foresman, 1966. Pp. 187–193.

Rosenthal, R., & Jacobson, L. *Pygmalion in the classroom.* New York: Holt, Rinehart, & Winston, 1968.

Rutter, M. Concept of autism: A preview of research. *Journal of Child Psychology and Psychiatry*, 1968, *9*, 1–25.

Signor, R. Hyperactive children. *Washington University Magazine*, 1967, *37*(2), 19–25.

Skeels, H. M. *Adult status of children with contrasting early life experiences.* Chicago: University of Chicago Press, 1966.

Skinner, B. F. *The behavior of organisms: An experimental analysis.* New York: Appleton-Century, 1938.

Skinner, B. F. *Science and human behavior.* New York: Macmillan, 1953.

Skodak, M., & Skeels, H. M. A final follow-up study of one hundred adopted children. *Journal of Genetic Psychology*, 1949, *75*, 85–125.

Smith, J. M., & Smith, D. E. P. *Child management: A program for parents.* Ann Arbor: Ann Arbor Publishers, 1966.

Spearman, C. Theory of general factor. *British Journal of Psychology*, 1946, *36*, 117–131.

Spearman, C., & Jones, L. W. *Human ability.* New York: Macmillan, 1950.

Stephens, J. M. *The process of schooling.* New York: Holt, Rinehart, & Winston, 1967.

Stevens, J. C., & Savin, H. B. On the form of learning curves. *Journal of the Experimental Analysis of Behavior*, 1962, *5*(1), 15–18.

Stevens, S. S. The surprising simplicity of sensory metrics. *American Psychologist*, 1962, *17*, 29–39.

Stewart, M. A., Pitts, F. N. Jr., Craig, A. G., & Dieruf, W. The hyperactive child syndrome. *American Journal of Orthopsychiatry*, 1966, *36*(5), 861–867.

Stoddard, D. *Comparative analysis of training programs in behavior modification.* Unpublished doctoral dissertation, Washington University, 1970.

Sutherland, E. H., & Cressey, D. R. *Principles of criminology.* Chicago: Lippincott, 1960.

Terrace, H. S. Discrimination learning with and without errors. *Journal of Experimental Analysis of Behavior*, 1963, *6*, 1–27.

Terrace, H. S. Wavelength generalization after discrimination learning with and without errors. *Science*, 1964, *140*, 318–319.

Thomas, D. R., Becker, W. C., & Armstrong, M. Production and elimination of disruptive classroom behavior by systematically varying teacher's behavior. *Journal of Applied Behavioral Analysis*, 1968, *1*, 35–45.

Thompson, W. R., & Heron, W. The effects of restricting early experience on the problem-solving capacity of dogs. *Canadian Journal of Psychology*, 1954, *8*, 17–31.

Tsao, J. C. Studies in spaced and massed learning: I. Time period and amount of practice. *Quarterly Journal of Experimental Psychology*, 1948, *1*, 29–36.

Ullmann, L. P., & Krasner, L. (Eds.), *Case studies in behavior modification.* New York: Holt, Rinehart, & Winston, 1965.

Ulrich, R. E., & Azrin, N. H. Reflexive fighting in response to aversive stimulation. *Journal of the Experimental Analysis of Behavior*, 1962, *5*(4), 511–520.

Veblen, T. *Theory of the leisure class.* New York: Viking Press, 1968.

Vetter, H. J. *Language behavior and psychopathology.* Chicago: Rand McNally, 1969.

Weikart, D. P. Perry preschool project progress report, Ypsilanti, Michigan Public Schools. Unpublished mimeographed paper, June 1964. Cited by C. Bereiter & S. Engelmann, *Teaching disadvantaged children in the preschool.* New Jersey: Prentice-Hall, 1966.

Williams, C. D. The elimination of tantrum behavior by extinction procedures. In L. P. Ullmann & L. Krasner (Eds.), *Case studies in behavior modification.* New York: Holt, Rinehart, & Winston. Pp. 295–297.

Wittick, M. Language arts for the disadvantaged. In J. M. Beck & R. W. Saxe (Eds.), *Teaching the culturally disadvantaged pupil.* Springfield, Ill.: Charles C. Thomas, 1965. Pp. 109–149.

Woodcock, R. W., & Davies, C. O. *The Peabody rebus reading program.* Circle Pines, Minn.: American Guidance Service Inc., 1969.

Author Index

Subject Index